PEDIATRIC COLLECTIONS
Food Insecurity

EDITED BY:

Kimberly Montez, MD, MPH, FAAP
Associate Editor, Diversity, Equity, Inclusion and Justice, *Pediatrics* Executive Editorial Board
Past Vice Chair of the Executive Committee, Council on Community Pediatrics

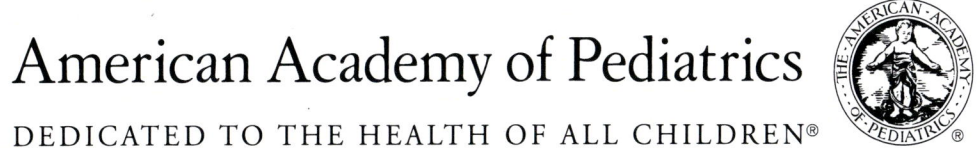

American Academy of Pediatrics
DEDICATED TO THE HEALTH OF ALL CHILDREN®

Published by the American Academy of Pediatrics
345 Park Blvd.
Itasca, IL 60143

The American Academy of Pediatrics is not responsible for the content of the resources mentioned in this publication. Web site addresses are as current as possible but may change at any time. Products are mentioned for information purposes only. Inclusion in this publication does not imply endorsement by the American Academy of Pediatrics.

APC046

Print ISBN: 978-1-61002-811-0
eBook ISBN: 978-1-61002-812-7

PEDIATRIC COLLECTIONS
Food Insecurity

Table of Contents

Food Insecurity

ix **Collection Introduction**
Kimberly Montez, MD, MPH, FAAP

1 **Community-Led Interventions to Address Food Inequity**
Advocacy Case Study | *Original Publication* | January 18, 2024

8 **Farm to Families: Clinic-based Produce Provision to Address Food Insecurity During the Pandemic**
Advocacy Case Study | *Original Publication* | September 22, 2022

16 **Accuracy of a Single Financial Security Question to Screen for Social Needs**
Article | *Original Publication* | December 1, 2023

24 **Food Insecurity Screening and Intervention in United States Children's Hospitals**
Research Article | *Original Publication* | September 19, 2022

32 **Food Insecurity Screening of Hospitalized Patients: A Descriptive Analysis**
Brief Report | *Original Publication* | May 12, 2022

37 **Evaluating Screening to Assess Endorsement of Food Insecurity in the Inpatient Setting**
Brief Report | *Original Publication* | March 8, 2024

42 **Quality Improvement to Identify and Address Food Insecurity During Pediatric Hospitalizations**
Research Article | *Original Publication* | November 4, 2024

52 **Progress and Potential: Addressing Food Insecurity in Caregivers of Hospitalized Children**
Commentary | *Original Publication* | November 4, 2024

55 **Disparities and Biases in Food Insecurity Screening Among Admitted Children**
Brief Report | *Original Publication* | June 20, 2024

59 **Food Insecurity and Experiences of Discrimination Among Caregivers of Hospitalized Children**
Article | *Original Publication* | November 21, 2023

69 **Reducing Caregiver Hunger During Pediatric Hospitalization**
Quality Report | *Original Publication* | April 20, 2023

78 **Food Insecurity and Community-Based Food Resources Among Caregivers of Hospitalized Children**
Research Article | *Original Publication* | June 17, 2024

90 **Addressing Food Insecurity Among Hospitalized Children: Upstream and Downstream Approaches**
Commentary | *Original Publication* | June 17, 2024

93 **Identifying Food Insecurity in Cardiology Clinic and Connecting Families to Resources**
Quality Report | *Original Publication* | April 28, 2022

103 **Establishing a Permanent Food Pantry in a Pediatric Emergency Department**
Advocacy Case Study | *Original Publication* | September 12, 2023

108 **SNAP Participation and Emergency Department Use**
Article | *Original Publication* | January 30, 2023

117 **Perspectives From Urban WIC–Eligible Caregivers to Improve Produce Access**
Article | *Original Publication* | January 5, 2023

127 **Caregiver Perspectives on Improving Government Nutrition Benefit Programs**
Article | *Original Publication* | October 8, 2024

137 **Caregiver Perspectives on Underutilization of WIC: A Qualitative Study**
Article | *Original Publication* | January 18, 2022

149 **Assessing and Improving WIC Enrollment in the Primary Care Setting: A Quality Initiative**
Quality Report | *Original Publication* | July 13, 2023

158 **Health Care as a Partner in Federal Nutrition Programs: Call for Advocacy**
Pediatric Perspectives | *Original Publication* | November 10, 2022

161 **Cost-effectiveness of Improved WIC Food Package for Preventing Childhood Obesity**
Article | *Original Publication* | January 23, 2024

169 **Trends in Severe Obesity Among Children Aged 2 to 4 Years in WIC: 2010 to 2020**
Article | *Original Publication* | December 18, 2023

179 **Universal Free School Meals Policy and Childhood Obesity**
Article | *Original Publication* | March 18, 2024

188 **Food Insecurity and Childhood Obesity: A Systematic Review**
Review Article | *Original Publication* | June 13, 2022

203 **Food Insecurity and Cardiometabolic Markers: Results From the Study of Latino Youth**
Article | *Original Publication* | March 16, 2022

213 **Pediatric Formulas: An Update**
Article | *Original Publication* | July 1, 2024

About AAP Pediatric Collections

Pediatric Collections is a series of selected pediatric articles that highlight different facets of information across various AAP publications, including AAP Journals, AAP News, Blog Articles, and eBooks. Each series of collections focuses on specific topics in the field of pediatrics so that you can keep up with best practices, and make an informed response to public health matters, trending news, and current events. Each collection includes previously published content focusing on specific topics and articles selected by AAP editors.

Visit http://collections.aap.org to view the latest Pediatric Collections.

Food Insecurity

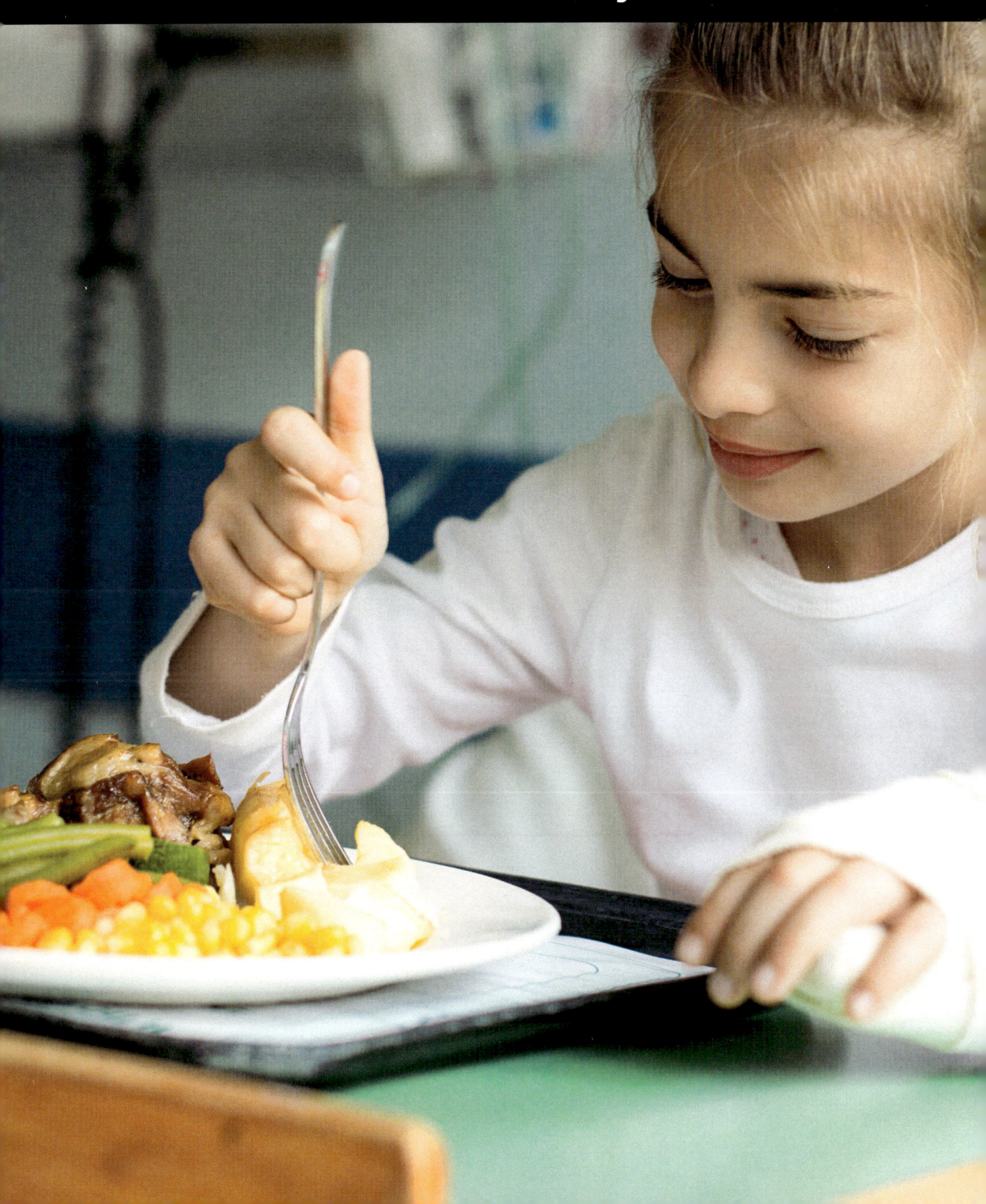

Food Insecurity
Collection Introduction

Kimberly Montez, MD, MPH, FAAP
Associate Editor, Diversity, Equity, Inclusion and Justice, *Pediatrics* Executive Editorial Board
Past Vice Chair of the Executive Committee, Council on Community Pediatrics

Food insecurity, which refers to the inadequate access to sufficient food for an active and healthy life, has been on the rise in recent years, following its historic low during the COVID-19 pandemic and the implementation of momentous economic relief measures. In 2023, the prevalence of food insecurity among households with children was 18%, up from 13% in 2021.[1] Food insecurity disproportionately affects single parents, members of racial and ethnic minorities, low-income individuals, and households with young children. Food insecurity negatively affects health throughout the life course, leading to poor psychosocial and physical health outcomes, as well as academic achievement. It also accounts for $52.9 billion in health care costs.[2]

Healthcare systems, regulatory bodies, and quality- and standard-setting organizations are increasingly recognizing the harm that health-related social needs, including food insecurity, have on health outcomes as well as their associated costs. In 2024, the Centers for Medicare & Medicaid Services instituted a requirement that at least one question be included in health risk assessments from a list of specified screening tools on 3 domains: housing stability, transportation access, and food security. The Joint Commission, the hospital accreditation body, issued new standards requiring that hospitals screen for health-related social needs and provide community resource information to those who screen positive.

Since the publication of the American Academy of Pediatrics (AAP) policy statement on food insecurity in 2015, "Promoting Food Security for All Children," screening for and addressing food insecurity in pediatric clinical settings has transformed from being innovative to becoming a standard of care.[3] Research on effective screening and intervention practices has continued to grow. Although the AAP and Food Research & Action Center published "A Toolkit for Pediatricians to Address Food Insecurity," little guidance from regulatory bodies exists on evidence-based clinical screening and intervention practices for food insecurity.[4] *Pediatric Collections: Food Insecurity* is the latest AAP endeavor to help pediatricians and clinicians who care for children through cutting-edge research, current knowledge, and advocacy practices for addressing food insecurity in clinical settings.

This collection covers a variety of food insecurity and nutrition-related topics. For example, screening and intervention practices for food insecurity in the hospital and subspecialty settings are growing areas of research. Similarly, while the federal nutrition programs, such as the Supplemental Nutrition Assistance Program and the Special Supplemental Nutrition Program for Women, Infants, and Children, are evidence-based at mitigating food insecurity, providing direct connections to those programs in clinical settings is relatively novel; caregiver perspectives on how to increase engagement with these programs are unique. Several quality reports and advocacy case studies highlight potential interventions that are both scalable and adoptable.

Although the field of pediatrics has come a long way in screening for, intervening on, and researching food insecurity, future efforts should focus on how healthcare systems can meaningfully contribute to improving health outcomes in this space. As screening and intervention become more widely adopted, new initiatives should be rigorously evaluated to inform best practices. Research should focus on exploring both the potential negative and positive consequences on workflows and experiences of care by staff and families; health information technology is another ripe area for investigation; value-based care, cost-effectiveness of programs, and reimbursement by payors are other areas of needed evaluation. As pediatricians and clinicians who care for children, we have a unique opportunity to mold the future of the field and promote food security for all children. I hope this collection will add to your toolbox for how to mitigate food insecurity in clinical settings.

References

1. Rabbitt MP, Reed-Jones M, Hales LJ, Burke MP. Household Food Security in the United States in 2003 (Report No. ERR-337). United States Department of Agriculture, Economic research Service. 2024. https://doi.org/10.32747/2024.8583175.ers
2. The Healthcare Costs of Food Insecurity. Feeding America. Accessed October 29, 2024. https://public.tableau.com/app/profile/feeding.america.research/viz/TheHealthcareCostsofFoodInsecurity/HealthcareCosts
3. Council on Community Pediatrics, Committee on Nutrition, et al. Promoting Food Security for All Children. *Pediatrics*. 2015;136(5):e1431-1438.
4. Ashbrook A, Essel K, Montez K, Bennett-Tejes D. Screen and Intervene: A Toolkit for Pediatricians to Address Food Insecurity. American Academy of Pediatrics and Food Research & Action Center. Accessed October 29, 2024. https://frac.org/wp-content/uploads/FRAC_AAP_Toolkit_2021.pdf

Community-Led Interventions to Address Food Inequity

Michelle C. Gorecki, MD, MPH,[a] Vivian Sevilla, MBA, LSSGB,[b] Kristen Gasperetti, MPA,[b] Lauren Bartoszek, PhD,[c] Madeline Chera, PhD,[d] Kimberly Cutler, BS,[b] Chika Okano, BS,[b] Binny M. Samuel, PhD, MBA,[e] Constance Stewart, MBA,[b] Carley L. Riley, MD, MPP, MHS,[f,g] on behalf of the System to Achieve Food Equity Learning Network*

Approximately 1 in 6 children in the United States, and 1 in 5 children in our local county (Hamilton County, Ohio), are food insecure. Here, we describe a novel community–academic partnership to address food inequity through distributed leadership and shared power with local neighborhood leaders. Using neighborhood-level data and community voice, 3 Cincinnati neighborhoods with high rates of poverty and food insecurity were selected as the primary intervention targets. Neighborhood leadership councils with community members representing each neighborhood were created. These councils requested intervention proposals and then decided which community designed interventions would receive grant funding. The academic partner provided grant funding distribution, quality improvement support, and data guidance and support for all partners, as well as community engagement support if desired by the community-led intervention leaders. In its first year (2021–2022), 9 interventions were funded, moving more than $250 000 into community-designed and community-led interventions to promote food security in 3 disadvantaged neighborhoods. Through leveraging community partnerships, these initiatives supplied 89 039 equivalent meals, including 56 244 pounds of produce, serving at least 3106 families in 3 neighborhoods in Cincinnati. Critical to the success of the initiatives were distributed leadership, shared power, word of mouth, and community engagement. The success of this type of community–academic partnership shows promise to address a wide variety of social and health challenges.

[a]Division of General and Community Pediatrics, [b]James M. Anderson Center for Health Systems Excellence, and [f]Division of Critical Care, Cincinnati Children's Hospital Medical Center, Cincinnati, Ohio; [c]The Health Collaborative, Cincinnati, Ohio; [d]Green Umbrella, Cincinnati, Ohio; [e]Carl H. Lindner College of Business, University of Cincinnati, Cincinnati, Ohio; and [g]Department of Pediatrics, University of Cincinnati College of Medicine, Cincinnati, Ohio

Dr Gorecki analyzed the data and drafted the initial manuscript; Ms Sevilla provided quality improvement expertise and support, conceptualized the intervention, designed the data collection instrument, and critically reviewed and revised the manuscript; Ms Gasperetti coordinated the advocacy work, collected the data, and critically reviewed and revised the manuscript; Dr Bartoszek participated in the stewardship team and critically reviewed and revised the manuscript; Dr Chera participated in the stewardship team, contributed to project assessment, and critically reviewed and revised the manuscript; Ms Cutler collected and analyzed the data and critically reviewed and revised the manuscript; Ms Okano provided quality improvement expertise and support, collected the data, and critically reviewed and revised the manuscript; Dr Samuel provided data management and analytics expertise, influenced the stewardship team process design and participated in the stewardship team, and critically reviewed and revised the manuscript; Ms Stewart coordinated the advocacy work, collected the data, and critically reviewed and revised the manuscript; Dr Riley conceptualized and designed the initiative, supervised data collection, analyzed the data, critically reviewed, and revised the manuscript; and all authors approved of the final manuscript and agree to be accountable to all aspects of this work and have participated in this advocacy work.

*A list of network affiliates appears in the Acknowledgments.

DOI: https://doi.org/10.1542/peds.2023-063116

Accepted for publication Aug 9, 2023

Address correspondence to Carley Riley, MD, MPP, MHS, Cincinnati Children's Hospital Medical Center, 3333 Burnet Ave, MLC 2005, Cincinnati, OH 45229. E-mail: carley.riley@cchmc.org

PEDIATRICS (ISSN Numbers: Print, 0031-4005; Online, 1098-4275).

The System to Achieve Food Equity Learning Network (SAFE) began as a response to the COVID-19 pandemic surge in food insecurity. Nationally, rates of food insecurity rose dramatically during the pandemic, with an estimated increase of an additional 7 million children from 2018, to a total of 18 million children.[1] This increase was experienced locally in Cincinnati, Ohio. The experience of food insecurity during childhood is associated with a myriad of negative health, socioemotional, and developmental effects.[2,3] Pediatricians are called on to address childhood food insecurity.[4] The primary goal of SAFE's collective effort in response was to increase food security and improve nutrition quality for all 66 000 children living in Cincinnati, with a focus on children who live in households and neighborhoods experiencing a disproportionate burden of food insecurity. The network brought together key partners to address food insecurity, including the local hospital system, local government, the regional food policy council, nonprofit organizations including food pantries, the school system, and the library system. By initiating open lines of communication between these critical stakeholders, SAFE was beginning to build a learning network.[5]

As a first step, SAFE mapped childhood poverty and emergency free-food distribution sites across Cincinnati as a means of identifying geographic areas likely

To cite: Gorecki MC, Sevilla V, Gasperetti K, et al. Community-Led Interventions to Address Food Inequity. *Pediatrics.* 2024;153(2):e2023063116

ADVOCACY CASE STUDY

experiencing a gap between anticipated need and current supply. To focus our learning, guided by neighborhood-level data and community voice, SAFE chose 3 neighborhoods to target its initial collective response: Avondale, East Price Hill, and Lower Price Hill. These 3 neighborhoods have faced decades of underinvestment, in no small part because of the redlining practices of the 1930s through which the Home Owners Loan Corporation likely labeled them as "hazardous,"[6] thus making it nearly impossible to obtain a mortgage and driving away investment. In 2020, residents in Avondale, East Price Hill, and Lower Price Hill self-identified their race as 81%, 36%, and 48% Black, respectively, and households self-reported incomes of 33%, 27%, and 66% below the federal poverty level, respectively.[7] These rates of poverty are significantly higher than the United States average of approximately 12%.[8] East Price Hill also has a significant Latino population, with 20% of residents self-identifying as Hispanic/Latino.[7] By selecting these neighborhoods, SAFE also aimed to address inequities driven and sustained by systemic racism.[9]

In November 2021, with a desire to grow and address food insecurity beyond emergency food distribution, SAFE launched its community-led intervention initiative. The goal of this initiative was to facilitate innovative, family-centered, and community-led interventions to catalyze transformational change to improve food security. The SAFE learning network invited individuals and organizations to submit project proposals to improve food security in any of the selected neighborhoods. Embedded in the mission of the initiative was coproduction.[5] Neighborhood leadership councils informed, assessed, and selected the community-created interventions that would receive funding to support their neighborhood. The stewardship team reviewed the input from the neighborhood leadership councils, considered the social impact of the interventions, and determined the financial award that would be distributed to the recipients (aiming to prevent inequitable disbursement of funds). In addition, the stewardship team strived to support new or emerging community leaders who would receive funding, looking for ways to support their development, success, and ensure sustained future growth. In the pursuit of equity, shared power and a collaborative culture were essential.

METHODS AND PROCESS

The SAFE Learning Network was awarded $475 000 of grant funding from a foundation, with more than $250 000 to be stewarded through the academic partner to fund community-designed, community-chosen, and community-led initiatives to promote food equity. The remaining budget was used for a community connector position at a nonprofit, a community engagement specialist, and funding for additional research and infrastructure. The idea to finance community-led food equity interventions was first presented and discussed at regularly scheduled SAFE meetings. SAFE sought community-led interventions that were based in improvement science and would include measurable tests of change.

In pursuit of codesign and distributed leadership, SAFE created neighborhood leadership councils of 5 to 7 community members from the 3 neighborhoods of focus (Avondale, East Price Hill, and Lower Price Hill; Fig 1). Existing relationships between the academic partner and many families and community members allowed SAFE to quickly create the neighborhood leadership councils. Our hospital system has previously created neighborhood leadership councils for disease-specific conditions such as asthma. Additionally, our Center for Clinical & Translational Science & Training has strong community connections with a long history of

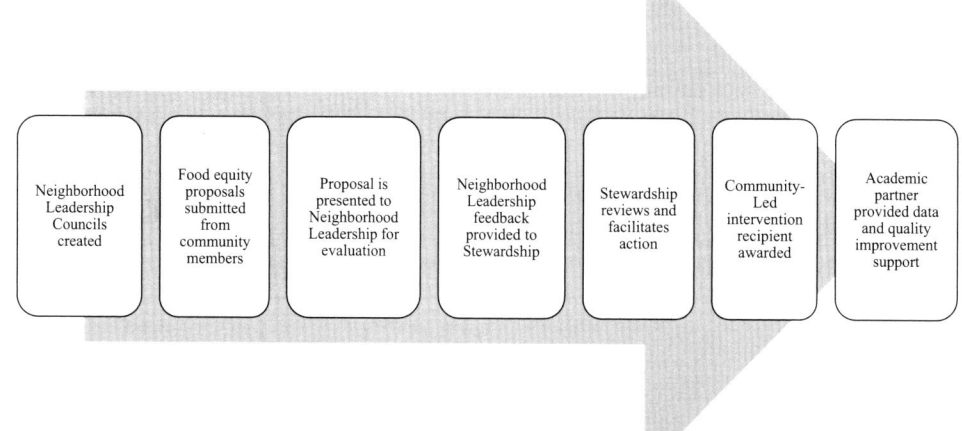

FIGURE 1
Timeline of community-led intervention process.

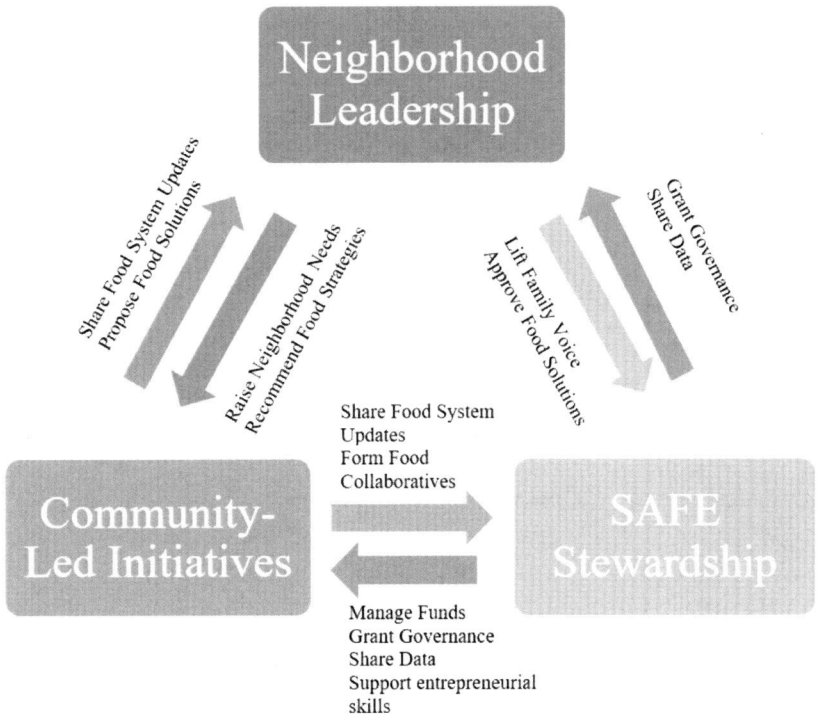

Neighborhood Leadership

Share Food System Updates
Propose Food Solutions

Raise Neighborhood Needs
Recommend Food Strategies

Lift Family Voice
Approve Food Solutions

Grant Governance
Share Data

Community-Led Initiatives

SAFE Stewardship

Share Food System
Updates
Form Food
Collaboratives

Manage Funds
Grant Governance
Share Data
Support entrepreneurial
skills

FIGURE 2
Model of approach used to ensure distributed leadership and shared power through checks and balances during this work.

community-engaged work. Proposals to address food equity in the 3 neighborhoods of focus were solicited from community members via flyers and social media. Proposals were then presented to the neighborhood leadership councils for codesign and evaluation. Neighborhood leadership evaluated the proposal using a rubric (Supplemental Table 2). The stewardship team had 10 members, including 5 representatives of the academic partner, and 5 members of nonprofit organizations. Based on assessments made by the neighborhood leadership team, the stewardship team evaluated the impact of the proposed initiatives and determined the financial award. One way coproduction was woven into the fabric of this initiative was through a model of shared governance to ensure equitable evaluation and selection of the interventions (Fig 2). The model consisted of a neighborhood leadership council in each of the neighborhoods and a stewardship team.

Data to be collected/tracked were determined by the intervention leader with support from the academic partner. Once funding was distributed, the academic partner provided data management, quality improvement, and community engagement support as wanted or as needed by the community-led intervention leaders. For example, during biweekly meetings with quality improvement specialists, intervention leaders' learnings and data were captured using the A3 method template.[10] Built into the

design of this advocacy work was a series of checks and balances to ensure distributed leadership and shared power (Fig 2).

Outcomes

The community-led intervention process brought together key stakeholders and allocated decision-making to the community by having the neighborhood leadership councils codesign and determine which community designed and led interventions to fund. More than $250 000 funded 9 different interventions (Table 1). Funded interventions ranged from supporting the expansion of existing programs, to investing in new programming of existing organizations, to supporting the startup of first-time interventions. Given the rolling nature of application acceptance, most intervention learnings and results were captured within the first 6 months of intervention initiation. The chosen interventions included a community garden, a mobile food pantry, shelf-stable food delivery, produce delivery, and a resident-designed, launched, and operated nonprofit grocery and deli enterprise offering a range of needs-based free-food programming. Collectively, the community-led initiatives were able to supply more than 89 039 meals, including 56 244 pounds of produce, serving at least 3106 families, and they provided nutrition and cooking education to 3 neighborhoods in Cincinnati. The amount of meals and produce distributed by partners per dollar

TABLE 1 Overview of Community-Led Initiatives to Address Food Inequity

Community-Led Initiative and Target Neighborhood	Description	Neighborhood Leadership Comments	Award Amount	Use of Funding	Outcome Measure
HyperFarm Avondale	Use hydroponic indoor farming to provide fresh, local produce delivered weekly to local families.	"The neighborhood is in need of accessing fresh local food." "Great and innovative way to provide fresh food to the community."	$90 100	Purchased an indoor hydroponic farming system ($80 000). Because of delays with zoning and electricity, pivoted. Partnered with food delivery company to deliver produce from community gardens (some vegetables not available from gardens were purchased in bulk).	62 families were registered and received biweekly deliveries of 15-20 lb of fresh produce. This totaled 3152 lb of fresh produce over 3 mo.
Queen Mother's Market: Avondale Community Garden	Establish a community garden, provide hands-on experience in gardening; offer education related to nutrition, healthy meal planning and food choices	"Includes education of fruits and vegetables to relatable health issues in the community of Avondale. Shifting the mind set of why fruits and vegetables are important will be key."	$20 000	Garden beds, gardening equipment	30 families received boxes of produce from the garden weekly for 3 mo.
Last Mile Mobile Market Avondale	Use a refrigerated van to use as a mobile food pantry to take rescued food from grocers and food establishments to provides local access to boxes of free, fresh food including meat, dairy, produce, and bread.	"Yes, without a grocery store being in Avondale residents are limited to what they have available. I like that this mobile van offers a variety of food options. Many times families do not feel that they have options, so this will like more of a choice." "Spreading the word is important."	$50 000	Staffing and volunteer recruitment. Also funded refrigerated van maintenance, insurance, and fueling. Shelving units to outfit the refrigerated van and materials needed for food distribution events (folding tables, tent, whiteboard, gloves, bags)	Total of 34 972 lb of food distributed. Average of 45 shoppers per distribution day.
Childhood Food Solutions Avondale	Deliver shelf-stable basic groceries to local families. Provide extra boxes as requested with aim of getting families through days when they have no other option for food.	"Assisting in filling the meal gap, but the food may not be sustainable. They are giving people food, but the food is very unhealthy." "Not a long-term solution."	$20 000	Groceries, boxes, and delivery.	163 families received a total of 448 food boxes on a monthly or biweekly basis. Conducted survey of recipients to see how boxes helped families: With 97 responses in the past 4 mo, families reported: Less stress - 59% More money for groceries - 58% Not going to bed hungry - 51% More energy - 40%
Meiser's Fresh Grocery & Deli Lower Price Hill	Support opening and pilot of new community-designed, driven, and operated grocery store. Supply and manage inventory of free food and affordable food (WIC, SNAP, and Produce Perks). Establish system to track inventories, customer activity and sales. Advertise Meiser's Green Giveaways.	N/A (test applicant, did not present to neighborhood leadership group. Leaders remarked that the relationship with the SAFE Learning Network led to their first use of improvement science methodology, and allowed for cross-neighborhood and interorganizational collaborations).	$12 000	Additional 10 h/wk for 3 mo for an associate ($15/h). Associate training and community outreach. Transaction processing costs and service subscription. Purchasing inventory to become a WIC-qualified location ($10 000).	10 307 meals worth of food sold. 515 households registered for Green Giveaways over first year from opening. Store hours were expanded from 30 to 60 h/wk. Median sales increased from about $1300 per week to >$4000 in transactions each week. Cooking tools and household items were distributed so that families had the necessary items to prepare desired meals and recipes.

TABLE 1 Continued

Community-Led Initiative and Target Neighborhood	Description	Neighborhood Leadership Comments	Award Amount	Use of Funding	Outcome Measure
Isaiah 55 Inc The Kanggy Garden Project Lower Price Hill	Provide a mobile delivery service to provide healthy, prepared meals and meal kits.	"Yes, we need healthy foods and also have the food delivered to people with instructions and a meal they can cook themselves."	$10 000	Coolers, insulated delivery bags, food	122 families received hot meal/meal kits weekly for up to 6 wk.
Feeding the Future- Lord Gym's Ministries East Price Hill	Sponsor 65–80 children to learn how to make 5 easy meals in a crockpot, after which the children keep the crockpot.	"This intervention could generate excellent output/ good impact at the community." "This neighborhood is very much depending on the SAFE program. I would like to thank you all for contributing your time and concerns to my community. One team one mission."	$25 000	Crockpots, food, and commercial kitchen equipment	2804 meals served, 67 households where children learned how to cook meals in a crockpot/kept crockpot after.
MyWhy East and Lower Price Hill	Provide a pay-as-you-go farmer's market.	"I think they have a well-developed plan. I also like that they partner with other organizations. There is strength in collaboration."	$15 050 (SNAP, WIC, Produce Perks cover 2/3 of market, this is remaining 1/3)	Marketing materials, fruit distribution, farmer's markets.	37 567 lb of fresh produce distributed.
Eat 2 Live Food Equity Lower Price Hill	Sponsor 10 local families to learn how to make healthy and nutritious meals	"The community needs to learn about cooking, budgeting and having a Black man teach these classes is a bonus."	$10 000	Cookware, recipe ingredients, space rental. Participants who regularly attended also received grocery gift cards.	234 meals served over 6 wk (September and October 2022)

invested varied in part because some interventions, such as the grocery store, sold produce in addition to free giveaways. Other community-led interventions have additional sources of funding that allowed them to have larger reach than would be expected based on the SAFE funding alone. A summary of the first year of the SAFE Learning Network's work is available online.[11]

Lessons Learned

Key learnings emerged from the community-led initiatives that are highly relevant for those planning to conduct similar work. The use of distributed leadership (all interventions were community-designed, -chosen, and -led) neutralized power dynamics and was essential to the production of relevant, meaningful, and effective interventions. The positive outcomes from this approach demonstrate how it is far superior to the "savior" approach in which external organizations intervene in communities autonomously without engaging with communities.[12] The shared power model of the community-led initiatives allowed for high levels of community support before the start of any interventions. Because the intervention leaders live and work in the communities they were serving, the leaders also noted better and more timely feedback from the community. Furthermore, the approach saw enhanced

success of the individual interventions from increased word of mouth in part because a trusted messenger (the community member leading the intervention) was the one spreading the word about the community-led interventions. Some interventions far surpassed their initial goals. Another key learning was the value of the role of the academic partner as an anchor institution.[13] The academic partner was able to convene and support major stakeholders through a combination of its positive reputation in the community and had significant resources available to support interventions. Also, the stewardship team strived to provide additional entrepreneurial development of intervention leaders. They were searching for ways to support the continued growth of intervention leaders as innovators.

A few challenges emerged at the learning network level. One was restrictions regarding the funding timeline. The academic partner had only 1 year from when the funding was initially distributed to report back to the funder. Fortunately, the funder's reporting requirements were less intensive compared with other funders. An additional challenge was that the academic partner had key staff turnover during the first year of this work. Furthermore, leaders of the community interventions had worries about the funding and experienced some stress surrounding the use of funds (ie, worries they would have to pay back to the academic partner if the interventions were not as successful as proposed). Building trust through clearly described expectations of the academic–community partnership in advance, as well as maintaining open lines of communication, will continue to be crucial for this work. Intervention leaders have noted that open lines of communication helped shift the dynamic from grantee/grantor toward peer to peer.

Additional learnings were gained from qualitative feedback from families about different approaches among the interventions themselves. For example, families praised interventions that gave them choice and at times they expressed disappointment when healthy options were limited, or when there were limited options overall. Families experienced dignity when they felt they had options similar to a grocery store and when there was more intention in giving them options. We would encourage those considering interventions to support food equity in the future to prioritize offering choices to families to increase participation and support dignity. Many interventions addressed common barriers reported by families (Table 1), such as transportation. Families reported food acquisition cost as a significant driver of their food insecurity, and cost was addressed through most interventions by making food free to families. However, some families reported experiencing increased dignity when the intervention used a "pay what you can" or "specials, sales and rewards" model, instead of receiving free food perceived as a "hand out" to prevent feelings of stigma or negative connotations around the word "free." The enormous degree to which families in our community are experiencing food insecurity underscores the need to advocate for an improved food system and policies that will address underlying drivers of food insecurity.

The community-led intervention leaders faced many barriers, primarily because of current local and federal policies. Many food-insecure families experience cyclical monthly needs, typically with less need during the first few calendar days of the month after public benefits have been distributed.[14] This pattern quickly became notable to many leaders of the community-led initiatives, and they adjusted their processes to better meet this cycle. In addition to advocating for changes to public benefits, it is important to consider weekly variation in food needs when planning food equity interventions. Other leaders faced zoning issues, requiring adjustments in plans because of local regulations. Multiple initiative leaders have mentioned frustration with broader food policies preventing them from optimal execution of projects and discussed the need for a more centralized citywide food distribution process to support the development of justice-oriented enterprises. This again underscores the ongoing need to advocate for changes to our food systems and policies to better address hunger and food insecurity in the United States. Through partnership with learning network member, the Greater Cincinnati Regional Food Policy Council, SAFE continues to connect community leaders with systems and policy change advocacy opportunities.

Many interventions faced barriers from other social determinants of health negatively affecting their local community. For example, the community garden experienced less involvement after there was a nearby gun violence incident. Leaders also commented that families' stress and experience of trauma affected their ability to engage in some interventions. Home delivery programs were limited in reach because of housing insecurity, leading some families to stop participating in the intervention. Intervention leaders also faced unanticipated expenses. For example, the cost to maintain an inventory of food was greater than expected for some. As with all advocacy work striving to address social determinants of health, it is important to consider the broader social–political context families live in and acknowledge the role of structural racism's toxic influence at all levels.[9]

CONCLUSIONS

In its first year (2021–2022), the SAFE Learning Network funded 9 community-designed, chosen, and led interventions to promote food equity. The community-led initiatives supplied more than 89 000 meals, including more than 56 000 pounds of produce, and served more than 3100 families in 3 neighborhoods in Cincinnati over the course of 4 to 6 months. Keys to success of the initiatives included shared power, distributed leadership, word of mouth, and community engagement. Common challenges faced by intervention leaders included policy barriers (both local food regulatory policies and national public benefits policies) and interrelated social determinants of health affecting their neighborhoods. Kroger's Zero Hunger Zero Waste foundation has granted SAFE an additional year of funding for continued support of the community-led interventions. We are working with the intervention leaders to determine how best to use these funds to continue to support successful interventions and ensure sustainability. The SAFE Learning Network has continued to learn alongside our local community, striving to achieve empowering distributed leadership. Overall, we found the model of a neighborhood leadership council informing a stewardship team to be an excellent way to put decision-making power in the community. We are planning to move toward a networkwide collaborative model of stewardship, to continue to pursue shared power and distributed leadership. The success of this advocacy work demonstrates a potential model of collaboration that could be used to address a wide variety of social and health challenges.

ACKNOWLEDGMENTS

The authors thank Shannon Carr, Anthony J. Fairhead, Matt M. Hawkins, Rebecca M. Hennessey, Mary Beth Knight, and Kai Stoudemire for critically reviewing and revising the manuscript. Thank you to the leaders, team members, and volunteers of the initiatives to address food inequity and the members of the Neighborhood Leadership Councils of Avondale, East Price Hill and Lower Price Hill. Thank you to all members of the System to Achieve Food Equity: All Children Thrive Learning Network, 84.51°, Childhood Food Solutions, Cincinnati and Hamilton County Public Library, Cincinnati Children's Hospital Medical Center, Cincinnati Public School, City of Cincinnati Office of Environment and Sustainability, Cincinnati City Council, Chef Mike's Burning with Style Culinary Services, Freestore Foodbank, Greater Cincinnati Regional Food Policy Council, Green Umbrella, Hamilton County Recycling and Solid Waste, Hyperfarm, Isaiah 55, Inc, Kroger's Zero Hunger Zero Waste Foundation, La Soupe, Last Mile Food Rescue, Lehigh University, Lord's Gym, MyWhy, Queen Mothers Market, The Health Collaborative, Walnut Hills Redevelopment Foundation, UMC Food Ministry, University of Cincinnati, University of Louisville, and Your Store of the Queen City.

ABBREVIATION
SAFE: System to Achieve Food Equity

FUNDING: The community-led initiatives were funded by a grant from The Zero Hunger Zero Waste Foundation. Dr Gorecki's effort on this project was supported by the National Research Service Award in Primary Medical Care, T32HP10027, through the Health Resources and Services Administration. The other authors received no additional funding.

CONFLICT OF INTEREST DISCLOSURES: The authors have indicated they have no potential conflicts of interest to disclose. The Health Resources and Services Administration had no role in the design and conduct of the study. Sunny Parr, the executive director of Zero Hunger Zero Waste Foundation, was a member of the System to Achieve Food Equity Learning Network Stewardship Team.

REFERENCES

1. Gundersen C, Hake M, Dewey A, Engelhard E. Food insecurity during COVID-19. *Appl Econ Perspect Policy.* 2021;43(1):153–161

2. Thomas MMC, Miller DP, Morrissey TW. Food insecurity and child health. *Pediatrics.* 2019;144(4):e20190397

3. Johnson AD, Markowitz AJ. Associations between household food insecurity in early childhood and children's kindergarten skills. *Child Dev.* 2018;89(2):e1–e17

4. COUNCIL ON COMMUNITY PEDIATRICS; COMMITTEE ON NUTRITION. Promoting food security for all children. *Pediatrics.* 2015;136(5): e1431–e1438

5. Parsons A, Unaka NI, Stewart C, et al. Seven practices for pursuing equity through learning health systems: notes from the field. *Learn Health Syst.* 2021;5(3):e10279

6. Overbey S. Redlining in Cincinnati: effects on Black well being. Available at: https://storymaps.arcgis.com/stories/d76e295c27bc45deba 50273ac9fc06fd. Accessed November 15, 2022

7. Department of City Planning and Engagement. *2020 Census Data: 2020 Cincinnati Statistical Neighborhood Approximations.* City of Cincinnati; 2021

8. US Census Bureau. Poverty status in the past 12 months. Available at: https://data.census.gov/table?q=poverty+status+in+the+past+12+months &tid=ACSST1Y2021.S1701. Accessed September 6, 2023

9. Yearby R. Structural racism and health disparities: reconfiguring the social determinants of health framework to include the root cause. *J Law Med Ethics.* 2020;48(3):518–526

10. Flinchbaugh J. *A3 problem solving: applying lean thinking.* Lean Learning Center; 2012:533–538

11. The System to Achieve Food Equity (SAFE) Learning Network. The System to Achieve Food Equity (SAFE) Year One Report 2021–2022. Available at: https://static1.squarespace.com/static/60d494b4d5d35b54 59cb43a8/t/63849f9e8671157ecfe88dfc/1669636008538/SAFE+Year+ One+Report.pdf. Accessed June 14, 2023

12. Key KD, Furr-Holden D, Lewis EY, et al. The continuum of community engagement in research: a roadmap for understanding and assessing progress. *Prog Community Health Partnersh.* 2019;13(4):427–434

13. Ubhayakar S, Capeless M, Owens R, Snorrason K, Zuckerman D. *Anchor Mission Playbook.* Rush University Medical Center and The Democracy Collaborative; 2017

14. Laraia BA. Food insecurity and chronic disease. *Adv Nutr.* 2013;4(2): 203–212

Farm to Families: Clinic-based Produce Provision to Address Food Insecurity During the Pandemic

Rachel Brown, MPH,[a] Georgia Reilly, MPH,[b] Falguni Patel, MPH,[c] Carly Freedman, BS,[c] Senbagam Virudachalam, MD, MSHP,[a,d,e,f,g,h] Danielle Cullen, MD, MPH, MSHP[a,g,h,i]

With rising rates of food insecurity (FI) during the pandemic, we implemented a clinic-based, community-supported agriculture program at 2 outpatient centers in low-income areas associated with an urban children's hospital and evaluated (1) the program's ability to reach FI families without preceding eligibility criteria, and (2) caregiver experiences and preferences for programming. Free boxes of produce were distributed weekly to caregivers of pediatric patients during a 12 week pilot period. Ability to reach the target population was measured by number of participating families and caregiver demographic information. We purposively sampled 31 caregivers for semistructured interviews on a rolling basis to understand program preferences. Content analysis with constant comparison was employed to code interviews inductively and identify emerging themes. Of 1472 caregivers who participated in the program, nearly half (48.3%) screened positive for FI, and 45% were receiving federal food assistance. Although many caregivers were initially "surprised" by the clinic-based program, they ultimately felt that it reinforced the hospital's commitment to "whole health" and perceived it to be safer than other food program settings during the pandemic. Several programmatic features emerged as particularly important: ease and efficiency of use, kindness of staff, and confidentiality. This advocacy case study demonstrates that a community-supported agriculture program in the clinical setting is an acceptable approach to supporting food access during the pandemic, and highlights caregiver preferences for a sustainable model. Furthermore, our data suggest that allowing families to self-select into programming may streamline operations and potentially facilitate programmatic reach to families who desire assistance.

[a]PolicyLab, [e]Center for Pediatric Clinical Effectiveness, [d]Department of Pediatrics, Divisions of General Pediatrics and [i]Emergency Medicine, [c]Children's Hospital of Philadelphia, Philadelphia, Pennsylvania; [b]University of Pennsylvania Center for Public Health Initiatives, Philadelphia, Pennsylvania; [f]Community Health and Literacy Center, Philadelphia, Pennsylvania; [g]Leonard Davis Institute of Health Economics, Philadelphia, Pennsylvania; and [h]University of Pennsylvania Perelman School of Medicine, Philadelphia, Pennsylvania

Ms Reilly, Ms Patel, Ms Freedman, and Dr Cullen conceptualized and designed this advocacy study, and participated in all stages of program implementation and evaluation, manuscript drafting, and review; Ms Brown contributed to the conceptualization and design of the study, participated in all stages of program implementation and evaluation, designed the data collection tools, supervised data collection, conducted the initial analyses, drafted the initial manuscript, and reviewed and revised the manuscript; Dr Virudachalam contributed to study design and data evaluation, and reviewed and revised the manuscript; and all authors approved the final manuscript as submitted and agree to be accountable for all aspects of the work.

DOI: https://doi.org/10.1542/peds.2022-057118

Accepted for publication Jun 27, 2022

Address correspondence to Rachel Brown, MPH, PolicyLab, Children's Hospital of Philadelphia, 2716 South St, Philadelphia, PA 19146. E-mail: brownr19@chop.edu

PEDIATRICS (ISSN Numbers: Print, 0031-4005; Online, 1098-4275).

FUNDING: Supported by a CHOP Children's Fund Community Impact Award, Hardon Family. The funder had no role in the design and conduct of the study.

CONFLICT OF INTEREST DISCLAIMER: The authors have indicated they have no conflicts of interest relevant to this article to disclose.

To cite: Brown R, Reilly G, Patel F, et al. Farm to Families: Clinic-based Produce Provision to Address Food Insecurity During the Pandemic. *Pediatrics.* 2022;150(4):e2022057118

The coronavirus disease 2019 (COVID-19) pandemic deepened challenges for the nearly 1 in 4 children who were already food insecure (FI) in Philadelphia and created new barriers to food access for families who never previously struggled.[1,2] This sustained period of FI has been driven by the convergence of numerous structural- and individual-level factors including: pandemic-related unemployment that disproportionately affected low-income families; school closures that curtailed regular access to federal lunch programs for >1 million children in Pennsylvania; and unprecedented demand for charitable food system resources compounded by social distancing measures that limited capacity to meet community need.[3–5] Furthermore, although the severity of barriers to food access has fluctuated over time, their effect on FI has endured. In Philadelphia, the

ADVOCACY CASE STUDY

childhood FI rate is projected to reach 28.6% in 2022, from a prepandemic rate of 21%.[1]

Produce access during the pandemic has proved particularly difficult for low-income families, a population with historically low rates of fruit and vegetable consumption.[6-8] Both FI and poor diet quality have associations with children's health, including increased rates of hospitalization and anemia, as well as increased risk of coronary heart disease, hypertension, and stroke in adulthood.[9-13] Cost-subsidized, community-supported agriculture (CSA) programs, also known as seasonal farm shares, have been identified as a feasible and acceptable approach to addressing these disparities.[14-16] Recent research also supports the effectiveness of subsidized CSA programs situated in clinical settings in improving diet quality.[17,18]

Many social program models condition eligibility on disclosure of need through social risk screening tools.[19] Emerging evidence suggests that prerequisite screening may exclude many who want support because of discordance between screening results and desire for resources.[20-24] In pediatric settings, documentation of need in the child's medical record may increase stigma and fear of negative repercussions that may deter program participation among families who would benefit.[25,26]

This advocacy case study describes the implementation and evaluation of Farm to Families, a clinically-based, free CSA launched in response to intensified FI during the COVID-19 pandemic. In addition to meeting immediate need by providing free boxes of fruits and vegetables, we assessed whether a CSA situated in a pediatric clinical care setting is feasible and acceptable to pediatric caregivers, and the program's ability to reach the intended population of FI families without preceding eligibility criteria.

METHODS AND PROCESS

Setting

Farm to Families was initiated at 2 Children's Hospital of Philadelphia (CHOP) clinical care sites in West Philadelphia: 1 primary care site and 1 outpatient subspecialty care site. Poverty levels in the neighborhoods surrounding both CSA sites exceed 45%.[27] In 2020, these outpatient centers saw a combined 374 635 patients; 31% were Black or African American, 11% Hispanic or Latino, and 44% had Medicaid.

Stakeholders

The CHOP Office of Community Relations facilitated an expedited partnership with a local nonprofit, St. Christopher's Foundation for Children (SCFC), that included delivery of produce boxes from a local cooperative of >100 organic family farmers. SCFC has collaborated with health care institutions in Philadelphia since 2010, operating a subsidized CSA to increase access to fresh produce in low-income neighborhoods.[28]

The time and expertise of hospitalwide partners, including physicians, researchers, community relations experts, and child and family life specialists, informed program development and operations. Each location was operated primarily by a site manager, a designated hospital employee responsible for on-site logistics and produce box distribution, as well as volunteer hospital employees.

Program Design and Operation

Farm to Families was implemented as a pilot program to provide a free box of organic fruits and vegetables to any family that visited the outpatient care sites. There were no eligibility, exclusion, or application criteria. Farm to Families operated once per week from July 7 to October 1, 2020, aligned with the sites' hours of highest patient volume to maximize reach. Produce was ordered weekly from SCFC, and packaged and delivered to each site the morning of program operation, without a need for on-site refrigeration. Box contents varied weekly according to the farm cooperative's produce availability. For the first 6 weeks of programming, boxes distributed at the outpatient subspecialty care site were supplied without cost by the United States Department of Agriculture's Farmers to Families Food Box grant program, a federal initiative to purchase and distribute produce during the COVID-19 pandemic.[29] Produce boxes were otherwise paid for by a combination of institutional funding and individual donations at the price of $14 per box.

Site managers and volunteers staffed tables in high-traffic areas of each clinic and invited caregivers to participate. The program was not advertised before initiation; thus, the initial participant population comprised families visiting the sites for appointments. A scheduled appointment was not a prerequisite for participation, and families were encouraged to return weekly. Boxes included a recipe card that identified the fruits and vegetables being provided and offered preparation suggestions. Tote bags to assist with transportation of the produce were printed with the web address of a searchable regional resource map (www.CommunityResource Connects.org).

Challenges

Most challenges to program implementation were related to the COVID-19 pandemic. Infection prevention measures limited the availability of on-site personnel for program staffing. The pandemic also increased the difficulty of predicting patient flow and volume, introducing challenges related to estimating the number of produce boxes each site had the capacity to distribute. To address this, each site received 50 produce boxes at program launch and increased distribution incrementally until capacity was reached. Weekly meetings were held with program staff to adjust the quantity of boxes per site and to troubleshoot operational difficulties.

Data Collection

One adult caregiver of each participating family completed a brief registration survey before receiving their first produce box. The survey was offered in English and Spanish, with an integrated text-to-voice option to address literacy barriers. Staff were available to read the survey questions aloud upon request; supplemental translation services were also available. Given heightened infection prevention measures, families were encouraged to complete the survey on their smartphone with use of a quick response code. If a caregiver did not have a smartphone or encountered technological challenges, a designated study tablet (iPad) was available for survey completion. Survey responses were recorded directly into Research Electronic Data Capture database software.[30]

Caregivers were additionally offered participation in a semistructured telephone interview within 2 weeks of initial participation to explore their perceptions and preferences related to the CSA. Caregivers who opted-in for an interview were purposively sampled on a rolling basis to achieve representation across demographic characteristics, FI status, program site, and frequency of participation to contextualize qualitative findings. Interviews were conducted until thematic saturation was reached. At the conclusion of each interview, participants were again offered a text message providing food and other social resources. Interview participants received a $25 eGifter Choice gift card.

All study procedures were deemed exempt from review by the CHOP Committee for the Protection of Human Subjects.

Reach

Tracking the proportion of clinic visitors who received CSA boxes was not a goal of the program in its pilot phase. However, we measured reach in terms of patterns of box distribution that could inform full implementation of the program, including the number of produce boxes distributed weekly by site and participant demographic information. The registration survey included demographic questions, the Hunger Vital Sign 2-item FI screen, and questions about the caregiver's participation in the Supplemental Nutrition Assistance Program (SNAP) and the Special Supplemental Nutrition Program for Women, Infants, and Children (WIC).[31-33] All caregivers were offered a text message with food and other social resources.

Acceptability

Acceptability was measured by frequency of repeat program use, interest in future use, and qualitative findings. Repeat participation was tracked weekly, by participant name, at each Farm to Families site. Caregivers were offered the option to be notified if low-cost produce boxes were made available once the free pilot ended. A semi-structured interview guide was developed to explore program acceptability and elicit perceptions of specific program features, including operational structure, setting, and box contents (Supplemental Information).

Impact on Produce Preferences and Perceptions

The semistructured interview additionally assessed the impact of Farm to Families on participants' produce preferences and perceptions. Questions explored how the produce box affected caregivers' dietary and shopping patterns, attitudes toward produce consumption, and food preparation.

Data Analysis

Frequencies and descriptive statistics are reported for all program participants. We conducted Fisher's exact test, χ^2 test, and 2 sample t tests to detect significant differences in demographic characteristics between all program participants and interview participants. Statistical analyses were performed using R version 4.1.1 (2021) and RStudio version 1.4 (2021) software packages.[34,35]

Qualitative data were coded and analyzed using QSR NVivo 12 software.[36] Dominant themes in the interview guide informed the development of a codebook. The constant comparison method was employed to guide an integrated approach in which inductive coding was used to expand upon the initial start list of codes and iteratively refine the codebook. A team of 3 researchers with qualitative research training coded the first 3 transcripts independently and then reconvened to update the codebook to reflect emerging themes. This team met weekly to assess interrater reliability and

TABLE 1 Participant Demographics

	Total Participants: 1472 N (%)	Interview Participants: 31 N (%)	P
Age, y			.12
18 or under	32 (2.2)	2 (6.5)	
19–30	280 (19.0)	4 (12.9)	
31–40	613 (41.7)	14 (45.2)	
41–50	353 (24.0)	4 (12.9)	
51 or over	189 (12.8)	7 (22.6)	
Sex			.26
Female	1228 (83.4)	29 (93.0)	
Male	235 (16.0)	2 (7.0)	
Nonbinary	3 (0.2)	0 (0.0)	
Ethnicity			.99
Not Hispanic or Latino	1113 (75.6)	24 (77.4)	
Hispanic or Latino	158 (10.7)	3 (9.7)	
Unknown/not reported	201 (13.6)	4 (12.9)	
Race			.52
Black or African American	699 (47.5)	17 (54.8)	
White	433 (29.5)	7 (22.6)	
Asian American	92 (6.2)	2 (6.5)	
American Indian/Alaska Native	28 (1.9)	1 (3.2)	
>1 race	52 (3.5)	2 (6.5)	
Native Hawaiian or other Pacific Islander	4 (0.3)	0 (0.0)	
Other/not listed	73 (5.0)	0 (0.0)	
Household size, mean (SD)			
Adults	2.2 (0.9)	2.3 (0.9)	.54
Children	2.2 (1.2)	2.5 (1.4)	.25
FI			
Yes	711 (48.3)	18 (58)	.37
SNAP benefits recipient			
Yes	552 (37.5)	16 (51.6)	.16
WIC benefits recipient			
Yes	348 (23.6)	11 (35.5)	.19
Repeat program use			
Yes	214 (14.5)	16 (51.6)	<.001***
Total program visits, mean (SD)	2.8 (2.4)	4.0 (3.3)	.003***

*** Indicates statistical significance ($P < .05$).

resolve coding disagreements through consensus.

Outcomes

Reach

During the pilot period, 2010 boxes of produce were distributed across the 2 program sites. Each site began by distributing 50 boxes per week, increasing incrementally to a maximum of 70 and 100 boxes at the primary care and subspecialty care sites, per week, respectively.

A total of 1472 unique caregivers participated in Farm to Families during the pilot period. Caregivers reported an average of 2.2 adults and 2.2 children in their household.

Among program participants, 47.5% identified as Black or African American, 83.4% were female, and 41.7% were between the ages of 31 and 40 years. Nearly half (48.3%) screened positive for FI. Forty-five percent of participants were receiving WIC or SNAP benefits, with 37.5% receiving SNAP benefits and 23.6% receiving WIC benefits. The majority (56.3%) of caregivers opted in to receive a text message with information about food and other social resources (Table 1).

Acceptability

The majority of program participants (77%) indicated interest in receiving information about Farm to Families if the program transitioned to a fee-for-service model. Among FI participants, 85.3% reported interest in future programming. A total of 215 (14.6%) families participated in the program more than once during the pilot period; of these, 62.8% returned once, 15.8% returned twice, and 21.4% returned 3 or more times. Among return participants, 49.3% screened positive for FI.

The majority (79.7%) of program participants consented to be contacted for a phone interview. After providing informed consent, 31 caregivers participated in a semistructured interview lasting ~30 minutes, conducted by 2 research team members trained in qualitative interview methodologies. The caregivers interviewed were proportionally representative of all program participants on the basis of demographic characteristics (Table 1). Ten (32.3%) of the interviewees had repeat CSA participation at the time of interview; rates of repeat CSA participation were significantly higher among interviewed caregivers (51.6%) as compared with overall program participants (14.5%) by the end of the 12 week program pilot. Twelve of the 31 transcripts were double-coded to confirm interrater reliability over time, producing an average κ statistic of 0.84.

Five major features of Farm to Families emerged in the semistructured interviews as particularly important to programmatic acceptability: the trustworthiness of the clinical setting as a food provider during a pandemic; ease and efficiency of program use with the grab-and-go model located near an exit; quality of the produce provided; kindness of staff; and confidentiality and respect

TABLE 2 Factors Related to Programmatic Acceptability

Factors Related to Programmatic Acceptability	Representative Quotation
Clinical setting	"Well, it was strange at first to be honest … But I think, because … the fact that they were allowed to be within the hospital and everything, gave us kind of that level of trust like, 'Okay, like the foods clearly going to be fine and everything.'"[10]
	"I like that the doctor's office is kind of trying to cater to the whole family and not just, like, pushing medicine as a solution to sickness… I think it is a nice indicator that they're looking at the whole picture."[11]
Ease and efficiency of program use	"It was perfect because it was actually, it was at the entrance and exit. So, we did it as we were leaving. So, we just literally got our box and went right down to the parking garage."[18]
Quality of produce	"Everything was fresh. It wasn't like, you know, I didn't feel like it was just, like, leftover food."[7]
Kindness of staff	"I still love interacting with them. I walk in there, they know who my daughter and I are, and every week, they're like, 'Hey, it's good to see you.'"[25]
Confidentiality and respect	"Like, around our neighborhood, you can go and get free boxes and stuff. But it's everybody from the neighborhood. It's people that you know that are, like, helping out. I would say, with the doctor's office, it's more, like, private. It's more privacy. It's more discreet. Nobody knows anything. Nobody judges you because everybody's in line."[26]
	"It was an opportunity that was helping the parents that came into the hospital with their children with any needs with no discrimination. Everybody felt equal."[22]

Brackets indicate interview participant number.

while participating so that there was " … no discrimination. Everybody felt equal." [participant 22] (Table 2).

Impact on Produce Preferences and Perceptions

Qualitative interviews elucidated 4 major areas of impact of the Farm to Families program: reallocation of finances, household attitudes toward produce, children's exposure to and acceptance of produce, and self-efficacy to purchase and prepare produce (Table 3).

Many caregivers explained that receiving weekly produce boxes enabled the reallocation of finances and alleviated some stress related to food access. Several caregivers experiencing FI described how this supplemental food made it easier to "stretch" their federal benefits through the month.

Another common theme reported by caregivers was that the CSA boxes cultivated favorable attitudes toward produce and healthy eating among members of their household.

Furthermore, many caregivers suggested that the CSA altered their family's beliefs about foods that were previously viewed unfavorably. As 1 caregiver explained: "It's a different way, it is a healthier way of eating. And it's a good way of introducing your kids, and not only just your kids, yourself and your family, to different things I've never tried." [participant 3]

Most caregivers also reported that the CSA improved children's exposure to and acceptance of produce and described improvements to their children's overall diets as a result of participation. Several caregivers also emphasized their children's curiosity about unfamiliar fruits and vegetables included in the box. One caregiver described how the program affected her family's diet: "They eat more fruits and vegetables … because we had it, because it was ready. It was here. So, now, I'll be buying more of it when it runs out, because they get accustomed to eating it." [participant 8]

Finally, participation in the CSA fostered caregivers' desire and comfort level to purchase and prepare fruits and vegetables. Caregivers valued the opportunity to sample new produce items before spending limited funds to purchase them and indicated that the boxes expanded opportunities for healthy meal planning.

Lessons Learned

This advocacy case study demonstrates the feasibility and acceptability of a clinic-based, free CSA during the COVID-19 pandemic, offered without prerequisite screening in clinics serving low-income families. It also highlights this model's potential to improve produce access among participating families and positively impact their exposure to and interactions with produce, even during an unprecedented time of stress and financial strain. Furthermore, the disproportionate rate of FI among program participants (48.3%) as compared with the general population of Philadelphia (21%), in

TABLE 3 Impact of Program on Produce Preferences and Perceptions

Factors Related to Programmatic Impact	Representative Quotation
Reallocation of finances	"Because then, that money could go toward something else for, like, meat or bread or anything else that we would need... But I always like to get the box first now because I don't want to buy double produce of what I got in the box."[26]
	"...I'm trying to make the food I have last a month because I can only get food at the beginning of the month, and then the fruits in between every week has been a Godsend because I've been able to extend my food that long now."[25]
Household attitudes toward produce	"It's a different way, it is a healthier way of eating. And it's a good way of introducing your kids, and not only just your kids, yourself and your family, to different things I've never tried."[3]
	"We never used to buy kale and, now, I love it. Because I never knew what to do with it ... I don't like it raw, but it's really good cooked. So, I would have never knew that because I would have never bought it at the store."[26]
Children's exposure to and acceptance of produce	"I felt happy about it because I went home and I was able to go through the box with my children ... some things we buy, some things we don't. So, they got to explore a little, as well. I think it was just a nice surprise."[4]
	"They eat more fruits and vegetables. So, it's really because we had it, because it was ready. It was here. So, now, I'll be buying more of it when it runs out, because they get accustomed to eating it."[8]
Attitudes regarding purchase and preparation of produce	"I never really went through the produce section like that, because, like I said, my children didn't really expand or eat much. Now, I go in there and I have my normals that I always picked up ... I've now picked up some more and, as I go through the produce, I look at things differently and I'm like, 'Hm, what can I explore with this or that?' So, it's opened my horizon to a lot of different things."[25]

Brackets indicate interview participant number.

conjunction with recent literature documenting discordance between social risk screening results and desire for social resources, suggests the promise of a model that allows families to self-select into programming.[1,22,23] This strategy has the added benefit of eliminating the administrative burden of implementing screening while reaching families who desire assistance, not only those who screen positive for FI.

The qualitative data highlight key programmatic features of a free, clinic-based CSA that is acceptable to caregivers, including ease and efficiency of program use, produce quality, kindness of staff, and confidentiality and respect while participating. These findings suggest areas of emphasis for program replication because caregivers reported that these factors were among the most important in their decision to participate.

Caregivers reported that program participation mitigated some barriers to obtaining food by reducing the frequency of shopping trips and enabling reallocation of finances to needs other than food. These findings are particularly significant during a time when federal nutrition programs and the emergency food system struggle to meet increased demand, and high-need families are harder to reach through traditional channels.[5,37,38] Furthermore, this advocacy case study corroborates existing evidence that clinically based, social-risk programming can successfully reach and serve FI families.[14,21,39,40] Because most caregivers were interested in receiving text message-based information about community resources, our findings also highlight an opportunity for health care institutions to leverage existing programs to connect families with social support services.

Interview participants also indicate that the CSA cultivated favorable attitudes toward produce, increased interest in purchasing produce, and built confidence in preparing produce through exploration of recipes and exposure to new ingredients. The impact of the program on families' consumption of fruits and vegetables corroborates previous evidence that a cost-subsidized CSA can address the dual health risks of FI and poor diet quality by increasing the household availability and acceptability of produce.[14-18] This finding holds particular importance during a pandemic when access to healthy foods is further reduced.[6]

This advocacy case study also demonstrates the immense value of community–clinical partnerships, particularly during a pandemic when a rapid approach is essential to meet families' urgent FI needs. Operationalizing SCFC's Farm to

Families model at CHOP and leveraging their established relationship with local farmers facilitated access to produce boxes on an accelerated timeline.

Although the Farm to Families pilot program demonstrates successful implementation of a clinic-based, free CSA during the pandemic, our study has several limitations. The program may not have consistently reached families experiencing the deepest levels of FI because these families may lack the financial, child care, or transportation resources to visit the doctor's office and participate in the program with the same regularity as families who do not face these challenges. To address this, future study will evaluate the feasibility of a home delivery option. Additionally, surveys and interviews were completed by 1 member of each household, therefore responses may not reflect the experience of every person in the home. Although we took steps to ensure representative sampling for interviews, participants who agreed to be interviewed may have viewed the program more favorably than those who did not. Additionally, it is possible that participants with higher levels of repeat participation may have had preexisting positive perceptions of produce unrelated to the program that influenced their decision to return. Because this was a pilot program serving families on a first-come, first-served basis with a predetermined number of CSA boxes, we cannot accurately predict participation patterns over time, or the proportion of clinic visitors who would participate if program capacity were increased. Further study is needed to understand the optimal frequency and duration of the program.

CONCLUSIONS

This advocacy case study demonstrates the feasibility, acceptability, and impact of a free CSA based in a pediatric health care setting during a time of increased FI. Furthermore, the program's implementation without preceding eligibility criteria suggests that allowing families to self-select into programming may streamline operations and potentially facilitate programmatic reach to families who desire assistance. Future work will optimize pricing structures as we transition to a low-cost produce box model, and evaluate the impact of home-delivery.

ACKNOWLEDGMENTS

We thank St. Christopher's Foundation for Children, as well as Children's Hospital of Philadelphia (CHOP) Department of Family Relations, CHOP Advanced Practice Nurses Manager Andrea Bailer, MSN, CRNP, the Garden at CHOP Karabots Pediatric Care Center, and CHOP Office of Community Relations for their partnership in implementing the Farm to Families program sites at CHOP. We also thank the clinical teams who contributed to program operations at each site.

ABBREVIATIONS

CHOP: Children's Hospital of Philadelphia
COVID-19: coronavirus disease 2019
CSA: community-supported agriculture
FI: food insecurity/food insecure
SCFC: St. Christopher's Foundation for Children
SNAP: Supplemental Nutrition Assistance Program
WIC: Special Supplemental Nutrition Program for Women, Infants, and Children

---

REFERENCES

1. Feeding America. Map the meal gap. Accessed: https://map.feedingamerica.org. Accessed August 9, 2021

2. Coleman-Jensen A, Rabbitt MP, Gregory CA, Singh A. *Household Food Security in the United States in 2020*. US: Department of Agriculture Economic Research Service; 2021:55

3. Parker K, Horowitz JM, Brown A. Pew Research Center. About half of lower-income Americans report household job or wage loss due to COVID-19. Available at: https://www.pewresearch.org/social-trends/2020/04/21/about-half-of-lower-income-americans-report-household-job-or-wage-loss-due-to-covid-19/. Accessed August 9, 2021

4. Food Research & Action Center. National School Lunch Program. Available at: https://frac.org/programs/national-school-lunch-program. Accessed August 10, 2021

5. Zack RM, Weil R, Babbin M, et al. An overburdened charitable food system: making the case for increased government support during the COVID-19 crisis. *Am J Public Health*. 2021; 111(5):804–807

6. Litton MM, Beavers AW. The relationship between food security status and fruit and vegetable intake during the COVID-19 pandemic. *Nutrients*. 2021;13(3):712

7. Leung CW, Epel ES, Ritchie LD, Crawford PB, Laraia BA. Food insecurity is inversely associated with diet quality of lower-income adults. *J Acad Nutr Diet*. 2014; 114(12):1943–53.e2

8. Hanson KL, Connor LM. Food insecurity and dietary quality in US adults and children: a systematic review. *Am J Clin Nutr*. 2014;100(2):684–692

9. Cook JT, Frank DA, Levenson SM, et al. Child food insecurity increases risks posed by household food insecurity to young children's health. *J Nutr*. 2006; 136(4):1073–1076

10. Cook JT, Frank DA, Berkowitz C, et al. Food insecurity is associated with adverse health outcomes among human infants and toddlers. *J Nutr*. 2004; 134(6):1432–1438

11. Casey PH, Simpson PM, Gossett JM, et al. The association of child and household

food insecurity with childhood overweight status. *Pediatrics.* 2006;118 (5):e1406–e1413

12. Skalicky A, Meyers AF, Adams WG, Yang Z, Cook JT, Frank DA. Child food insecurity and iron deficiency anemia in low-income infants and toddlers in the United States. *Matern Child Health J.* 2006;10(2): 177–185

13. Boeing H, Bechthold A, Bub A, et al. Critical review: vegetables and fruit in the prevention of chronic diseases. *Eur J Nutr.* 2012;51(6):637–663

14. Quandt SA, Dupuis J, Fish C, D'Agostino RB Jr. Feasibility of using a community-supported agriculture program to improve fruit and vegetable inventories and consumption in an underresourced vurban community. *Prev Chronic Dis.* 2013;10:E136

15. Hoffman JA, Agrawal T, Wirth C, et al. Farm to Family: increasing access to affordable fruits and vegetables among urban Head Start families. *J Hunger Environ Nutr.* 2012;7 (2-3):165–177

16. Hanson KL, Kolodinsky J, Wang W, et al. Adults and children in low-income households that participate in cost-offset community supported agriculture have high fruit and vegetable consumption. *Nutrients.* 2017;9(7):726

17. Berkowitz SA, O'Neill J, Sayer E, et al. Health center-based community-supported agriculture: an RCT. *Am J Prev Med.* 2019; 57(6 Suppl 1):S55–S64

18. Izumi BT, Higgins CE, Baron A, et al. Feasibility of using a community-supported agriculture program to increase access to and intake of vegetables among federally qualified health center patients. *J Nutr Educ Behav.* 2018;50(3):289–296.e1

19. Garg A, Brochier A, Messmer E, Fiori KP. Clinical approaches to reducing material hardship due to poverty: social risks/needs identification and interventions. *Acad Pediatr.* 2021;21(8S): S154–S160

20. Gold R, Bunce A, Cowburn S, et al. Adoption of social determinants of health EHR tools

by community health centers. *Ann Fam Med.* 2018;16(5):399–407

21. Buitron de la Vega P, Losi S, Sprague Martinez L, et al. Implementing an EHR-based screening and referral system to address social determinants of health in primary care. *Med Care.* 2019;57(Suppl 6 Suppl 2):S133–S139

22. Bottino CJ, Rhodes ET, Kreatsoulas C, Cox JE, Fleegler EW. Food insecurity screening in pediatric primary care: can offering referrals help identify families in need? *Acad Pediatr.* 2017;17(5):497–503

23. Ray KN, Gitz KM, Hu A, Davis AA, Miller E. Nonresponse to health-related social needs screening questions. *Pediatrics.* 2020;146(3):e20200174

24. Cullen D, Wilson-Hall L, McPeak K, Fein J. Pediatric social risk screening: leveraging research to ensure equity. *Acad Pediatr.* 2022;22(2):190–192

25. Cullen D, Attridge M, Fein JA. Food for thought: a qualitative evaluation of caregiver preferences for food insecurity screening and resource referral. *Acad Pediatr.* 2020;20(8):1157–1162

26. Barnidge E, LaBarge G, Krupsky K, Arthur J. Screening for food insecurity in pediatric clinical settings: opportunities and barriers. *J Community Health.* 2017; 42(1):51–57

27. Le-Scherban F, Carroll-Scott A. Drexel University Urban Health Collaborative. COVID-19 vulnerability indicators. Available at: https://drexel.edu/uhc/resources/coronavirus/vulnerability-indicators/. Accessed August 9, 2021

28. St. Christopher's Foundation for Children. Farm to Families initiative. Available at: https://scfchildren.org/farm-to-families-initiative/. Accessed August 9, 2021

29. United States Department of Agriculture. USDA Farmers to Families food box. Available at: https://www.ams.usda.gov/selling-food-to-usda/farmers-to-families-food-box. Accessed August 9, 2021

30. Harris PA, Taylor R, Thielke R, Payne J, Gonzalez N, Conde JG. Research electronic data capture (REDCap)—a metadata-driven methodology and workflow process for providing translational research

informatics support. *J Biomed Inform.* 2009;42(2):377–381

31. Hager ER, Quigg AM, Black MM, et al. Development and validity of a 2-item screen to identify families at risk for food insecurity. *Pediatrics.* 2010; 126(1):e26–e32

32. United States Department of Agriculture Food and Nutrition Service. Supplemental Nutrition Assistance Program (SNAP). Available at: https://www.fns.usda.gov/snap/supplemental-nutrition-assistance-program. Accessed August 9, 2021

33. United States Department of Agriculture Food and Nutrition Service. Special Supplemental Nutrition Program for Women, Infants, and Children (WIC). Available at: https://www.fns.usda.gov/wic. Accessed October 27, 2021

34. The R Foundation. R: A language and environment for statistical computing. Available at: https://www.R-project.org/. Accessed September 14, 2021

35. RStudio. Integrated Develpoment for R. Available at: www.rstudio.com/. Accessed September 14, 2021

36. QSR International Pty Ltd. Nvivo 12. Available at: https://www.qsrinternational.com/nvivo-qualitative-data-analysis-software/home. Accessed August 9, 2021

37. Leddy AM, Weiser SD, Palar K, Seligman H. A conceptual model for understanding the rapid COVID-19-related increase in food insecurity and its impact on health and healthcare. *Am J Clin Nutr.* 2020; 112(5):1162–1169

38. Dunn CG, Kenney E, Fleischhacker SE, Bleich SN. Feeding low-income children during the COVID-19 pandemic. *N Engl J Med.* 2020;382(18):e40

39. Cullen D, Blauch A, Mirth M, Fein J. Complete eats: summer meals offered by the emergency department for food insecurity. *Pediatrics.* 2019;144(4): e20190201

40. Cullen D, Woodford A, Fein J. Food for thought: a randomized trial of food insecurity screening in the emergency department. *Acad Pediatr.* 2019;19(6): 646–651

Accuracy of a Single Financial Security Question to Screen for Social Needs

Janel Hanmer, MD, PhD,[a] Kristin N. Ray, MD, MS,[b] Kelsey Schweiberger, MD,[b] Seth A. Berkowitz, MD,[c] Deepak Palakshappa, MD[d]

OBJECTIVES: Screening for social needs is recommended during clinical encounters but multi-item questionnaires can be burdensome. We evaluate if a single question about financial stress can be used to prescreen for food insecurity, housing instability, or transportation needs.

METHODS: We use retrospective medical record data from children (<11 years) seen at 45 primary pediatric care offices in 2022. Social needs screening was automated at well child visits and could be completed by the parent/guardian via the patient portal, tablet in the waiting room, or verbally with staff. We report the area under the receiver operating curve for the 5 response options of the financial stress question as well as sensitivity and specificity of the financial stress question ("not hard at all" vs any other response) to detect other reported social needs.

RESULTS: Of 137 261 eligible children, 130 414 (95.0%) had social needs data collected. Seventeen percent of respondents reported a housing, food, or transportation need. The sensitivity of the financial stress question was 0.788 for any one or more of the 3 other needs, 0.763 for food insecurity, 0.743 for housing instability, and 0.712 for transportation needs. Using the financial stress question as the first-step of a screening process would miss 9.7% of the families who reported food insecurity, 22.6% who reported housing instability, and 33.0% who reported transportation needs.

CONCLUSIONS: A single question screener about financial stress does not function well as a prescreen because of low sensitivity to reports of food insecurity, housing instability, and transportation needs.

[a]Department of General Internal Medicine, University of Pittsburgh, Pittsburgh, Pennsylvania, [b]Children's Hospital of Pittsburgh, University of Pittsburgh, Pittsburgh, Pennsylvania, [c]University of North Carolina at Chapel Hill School of Medicine, Chapel Hill, North Carolina; and [d]Department of Internal Medicine, Wake Forest University, Winston-Salem, North Carolina

Dr Hanmer conceptualized and designed the study, conducted the project analyses, and drafted the initial manuscript; Drs Ray, Schweiberger, Berkowitz, and Palakshappa conceptualized and designed the study; and all authors critically reviewed and revised the manuscript, approved the final manuscript as submitted, and agree to be accountable for all aspects of the work.

DOI: https://doi.org/10.1542/peds.2023-062555

Accepted for publication Oct 17, 2023

Address correspondence to Janel Hanmer, MD, PhD, Department of General Internal Medicine, University of Pittsburgh, 230 McKee Place, Suite 600, Pittsburgh, PA 15213. E-mail: hanmerjz@upmc.edu

PEDIATRICS (ISSN Numbers: Print, 0031-4005; Online, 1098-4275).

FUNDING: All phases of this study were supported by the Office of the CMIO at UPMC. Dr Palakshappa was supported by K23 HL146902. The funders had no role in the design or conduct of this study.

WHAT'S KNOWN ON THE SUBJECT: Screening for social needs is recommended by the American Academy of Pediatrics, but long screening questionnaires can be burdensome for patients and their families.

WHAT THIS STUDY ADDS: We test a single question about overall financial stress for its use as a prescreener for further questions about food insecurity, housing instability, or transportation needs. We found it does not perform adequately for this purpose.

To cite: Hanmer J, Ray KN, Schweiberger K, et al. Accuracy of a Single Financial Security Question to Screen for Social Needs. *Pediatrics*. 2024;153(1):e2023062555

ARTICLE

There is a strong relationship between unmet social needs and poor health outcomes.[1] With 1 in 5 US children living in poverty, the American Academy of Pediatrics recommends screening for health-related social needs during clinical encounters to mitigate the negative effects of poverty on child health.[1] Screening for social needs in clinical practice is generally acceptable to parents/guardians and can increase receipt of community resources.[2,3] However, screening for social needs requires time and resources, and few pediatricians report routinely screening despite supporting social needs screening.[4–6]

One possibility to reduce the burden of screening on clinics, parents/guardians, patients, and families is to use 2-step screening. With 2-step screening, an initial brief screen is used to determine the need for more comprehensive screening. A common example of this approach is the use of the Patient Health Questionnaire-2 as an initial brief screen for depression. If positive, a full Patient Health Questionnaire-9 is administered.[7] When working well, this approach can reduce respondent burden and increase screening uptake.[8] However, it could also miss families with needs if the brief screen is not sensitive and has a low negative predictive value. Financial stress is a construct related to having enough money to meet overall needs.[9] Among commonly used health-related social needs screening items, financial stress is often considered a broader assessment of needs, relative to items about more specific material needs such as food insecurity or housing instability. Therefore, it is an appealing candidate for use as an initial screening item. Here, we evaluate the ability of a single question about overall financial stress to differentiate between parents/guardians of children <11 years of age who do and do not report food insecurity, housing instability, and transportation needs.

METHODS

Population

Children's Community Pediatrics has 45 community pediatric primary care offices that span 6 urban counties and 10 rural counties and shares an electronic health record with 1 academic pediatric primary care practice. Practice size ranges from 2 to 40 clinicians and 1200 to 11 000 patients.

Routine electronic health record (EpicCare Verona, Wisconsin)-based screening for social needs began in August 2021 for all children <11 years of age who were presenting for a well-child visit. Screening could be completed in English by a parent/guardian on the patient portal, by tablet in the waiting room, or verbally with staff. Parents/guardians who preferred a language other than English were asked questions verbally with the use of an interpreter. Responses were immediately available in the medical record. We used data from children <11 years of age

assigned the questionnaire between January 1 and December 31, 2022.

Social Needs Screening Questions

The questions used in the social needs screener are the standardized questions within EpicCare and they are always administered in the same order, with the financial needs question occurring first. The questions included in the Epic Care module were validated items, derived from a 2014 Institute of Medicine (now National Academy of Medicine) report, "Capturing Social and Behavioral Domains and Measures in Electronic Health Records."[10] The overall financial stress question, "How hard is it for you to pay for the very basics like food, housing, medical care, and heating?" has 5 response options (not hard at all, not very hard, somewhat hard, hard, very hard).[11] The item on financial stress used was recommended in the Institute of Medicine report, for inclusion in electronic health record screening modules, and subsequently incorporated into EpicCare after this recommendation.[10] Screening also included questions about food,[12] housing,[13] and transportation.[14] We created binary categorizations of food insecurity, housing instability, and transportation needs (Supplemental Information).

Demographic Variables

Demographic variables were extracted from the electronic health record including the child's age, sex, race, ethnicity, and insurance provider. Race and ethnicity were collected from 2 demographic fields within the child's electronic health record, self-identified by the parent/guardian. Race and ethnicity are collected through clinical and administrative personnel at the time of the patient's first encounter and updated at parent/guardian's request. Race and ethnicity, both social constructs, are included because of the potential for experiences of racism to affect both the risk for experiencing health-related social needs and acceptability of disclosing social needs to the health care system.[15,16] Race and ethnicity are reported separately (eg, "white" includes both "non-Hispanic white" and "Hispanic white"). Race and ethnicity categories are reported if they have a frequency of 2% or more in the overall sample; categories with frequencies <2% are combined into "another race or multiple races." Insurance providers were categorized as commercial, Medicaid, other governmental, or self-pay/missing.

Analyses

We report the frequency of demographic variables and reported social needs in the entire sample and by age group (0–1, 2–5, and 6–10 years old). We also report these variables stratified by financial stress. We report the area under the receiver operating curve (AUROC) for the 5 response options of the financial stress question, as well as sensitivity, specificity, positive predictive value, and negative predictive value of the financial stress question (not hard at all versus

TABLE 1 Children's Demographics and Frequency of Parent- and Guardian-Reported Needs

	Age <2 y (n = 33321 of 34284 Eligible)	Age 2–5 y (n = 33771 of 35641 Eligible)	Age 6–10 y (n = 63322 of 67336 Eligible)	Overall (n = 130414 of 137261 Eligible)
Sex reported as female	48.8%	48.6%	48.7%	48.7%
Hispanic ethnicity	2.2%	2.2%	1.8%	2.0%
Race				
White	75.3%	78.5%	82.8%	79.8%
Black	12.5%	12.9%	11.0%	11.8%
Another race or multiple races	12.2%	9.6%	6.2%	8.4%
Insurance				
Commercial	54.3%	59.1%	65.3%	61.0%
Medicaid	36.0%	38.2%	32.0%	34.6%
Other governmental	0.8%	1.0%	1.0%	1.0%
Self-pay or missing	8.9%	1.7%	1.7%	3.5%
Financial stress				
Not hard at all	71.7%	67.9%	68.6%	69.2%
Not very hard	18.8%	21.3%	20.2%	20.2%
Somewhat hard	7.9%	9.0%	9.4%	8.9%
Hard	1.1%	1.1%	1.1%	1.1%
Very hard	0.5%	0.6%	0.6%	0.5%
Food insecurity	8.2%	9.8%	10.7%	9.8%
Housing instability	9.1%	9.4%	9.3%	9.3%
Transportation needs	4.9%	4.5%	3.8%	4.2%
Any food, housing, or transportation insecurity or need	16.2%	17.0%	17.0%	16.8%

any other response; not hard at all and not very hard versus any other response) to detect other reported social needs. These analyses are performed for the entire sample and stratified by age group. We chose to use age groups for subgroup analyses because the costs of raising children vary as they age,[17] and thus the relationships with the outcomes of interest may also vary by age. Also, some community and governmental resources, such as the Special Supplemental Nutrition Program for Women, Infants, and Children, are only available to families with children in certain age groups (<5 years of age).[18] The age groups correspond roughly to infancy, preschool age, and elementary school age in our sample.

Ethical Approval

The analysis was performed under the Univeristy of Pittsburgh Medical Center's Quality Improvement Committee Project 3373. The Quality Improvement Committee approves projects that do not meet the definition of human subjects research and therefore are reviewed by this committee instead of an institutional review board. Survey responses were collected during usual clinical care; participant consent was not required for our retrospective analyses of these deidentified clinical data.

RESULTS

Of 137261 eligible children, 127753 (93.1%) had social needs data collected at their first eligible visit and 130414 (95.0%) had data collected within at least 1 visit during 2022. Overall and by age group, demographic data and reported social needs are included in Table 1. In the entire sample, the reported racial categories were 79.8% white, 11.8% Black, and 8.4% another racial identity (including Alaska Native, American Indian, Chinese, Filipino, Guam/Chamorro, Hawaiian, Indian [Asian], Japanese, Korean, other Asian, other Pacific Islander, Samoan, and Vietnamese). In the overall sample, 48.7% of the children were female, 2.0% identified as Hispanic, and the primary insurance category was commercial (61.0%). As shown in Table 2, within each age group, reporting financial stress was associated with higher rates of other social needs (eg, in the entire sample, 1.4% of those without financial stress report food insecurity compared with 29.2% of those with financial stress [$P \leq .001$]). Children of parents reporting financial stress were more likely to identify as Hispanic ethnicity ($P \leq .001$), nonwhite race ($P \leq .001$), and be insured through Medicaid ($P \leq .001$). Likewise, children with missing social needs data were more likely to identify as Hispanic ethnicity ($P \leq .001$), nonwhite race ($P \leq .001$), and be insured through Medicaid ($P \leq .001$) (Table 3).

Reports of social needs were common (Table 1). In the overall sample, 9.8% of families reported food insecurity, 9.3% reported housing instability, 4.2% reported transportation needs, and 16.8% reported any of these needs. Overall, 30.8% of families answered the financial stress question with a response other than not hard at all and 10.6% of families answered the financial stress question

TABLE 2 Children's Demographics and Frequency of Caregiver-Reported Needs by Age Group and Report of Financial Strain

	Age <2 y (n = 33 321)			Age 2–5 y (n = 33 771)			Age 6–10 y (n = 63 322)			Overall (n = 130 414)		
	No Financial Strain (n = 23 370)	Financial Strain (n = 9220)	P	No Financial Strain (n = 22 290)	Financial Strain (n = 10 524)	P	No Financial Strain (n = 41 840)	Financial Strain (n = 19 125)	P	No Financial Strain (n = 87 500)	Financial Strain (n = 38 875)	P
Sex reported as female	48.9%	48.8%	.43	48.9%	48.4%	.40	49.1%	48.4%	.11	49.0%	48.5%	.24
Hispanic ethnicity	1.5%	2.9%	<.001	1.5%	2.6%	<.001	1.3%	2.1%	<.001	1.4%	2.4%	<.001
Race												
White	79.0%	69.7%	<.001	82.8%	72.3%	<.001	86.4%	77.5%	<.001	83.5%	74.3%	<.001
Black	9.1%	18.7%		8.9%	19.2%		7.4%	16.6%		8.2%	17.8%	
Another race or multiple races	11.9%	11.6%		8.2%	8.5%		6.2%	5.9%		8.3%	7.9%	
Insurance												
Commercial	64.1%	34.3%	<.001	70.4%	39.2%	<.001	75.3%	47.4%	<.001	71.1%	42.1%	<.001
Medicaid	26.4%	55.8%		26.8%	58.5%		21.8%	50.5%		24.3%	53.9%	
Other governmental	1.0%	0.6%		1.7%	0.7%		1.2%	0.7%		1.1%	1.0%	
Self-pay or missing	8.6%	9.3%		1.7%	1.7%		1.7%	1.4%		3.6%	3.5%	
Food insecurity	1.4%	25.7%	<.001	1.2%	28.1%	<.001	1.4%	31.4%	<.001	1.4%	29.2%	<.001
Housing instability	4.0%	22.1%	<.001	3.4%	22.0%	<.001	3.0%	23.2%	<.001	3.4%	22.6%	<.001
Transportation needs	2.7%	10.3%	<.001	2.0%	9.6%	<.001	1.6%	8.5%	<.001	2.0%	9.2%	<.001
Any food, housing, or transportation insecurity or need	6.9%	39.6%	<.001	5.7%	40.7%	<.001	5.2%	42.7%	<.001	5.8%	41.4%	<.001

TABLE 3 Children's Demographics by Age Group and Completion Status

	Age <2 y (n = 34 284)			Age 2–5 y (n = 35 641)			Age 6–10 y (n = 67 336)			Overall (n = 137 261)		
	Complete (n = 33 321)	Incomplete (n = 963)	P	Complete (n = 33 771)	Incomplete (n = 1870)	P	Complete (n = 63 322)	Incomplete (n = 4014)	P	Complete (n = 130 414)	Incomplete (n = 6847)	P
Sex reported as female	48.8%	48.5%	.97	48.6%	46.2%	.35	48.7%	47.9%	.56	48.7%	47.5%	.13
Hispanic ethnicity	2.2%	12.6%	<.001	2.2%	7.4%	<.001	1.8%	6.0%	<.001	2.0%	7.2%	<.001
Race												
White	75.3%	43.2%	<.001	78.5%	65.8%	<.001	82.8%	72.6%	<.001	79.8%	66.9%	<.001
Black	12.5%	30.1%		12.9%	21.4%		11.0%	18.9%		11.8%	21.0%	
Another race or multiple races	12.2%	26.7%		9.6%	12.8%		6.2%	8.5%		8.4%	12.1%	
Insurance												
Commercial	54.3%	23.9%	<.001	59.1%	46.7%	<.001	65.3%	54.3%	<.001	61.0%	47.9%	<.001
Medicaid	36.0%	64.2%		38.2%	50.0%		32.0%	41.8%		34.6%	47.2%	
Other governmental	0.8%	0.6%		1.0%	0.8%		1.0%	0.9%		1.0%	0.8%	
Self-pay or missing	8.9%	11.3%		1.7%	2.6%		1.7%	3.1%		3.5%	4.1%	

TABLE 4 Area Under the Receiver Operator Characteristic (AUROC), Sensitivity, and Specificity of the Single Financial Stress Question to Detect Other Needs

Insecurity or Need	5 Response Options AUROC	Not Hard at All versus Any Other Response				Not Hard at All and Not Very Hard Versus Any Other Response			
		Sensitivity	Specificity	Positive Predictive Value	Negative Predictive Value	Sensitivity	Specificity	Positive Predictive Value	Negative Predictive Value
Food insecurity	0.89	0.763	0.903	0.986	0.292	0.953	0.623	0.959	0.589
Housing instability	0.79	0.743	0.743	0.966	0.226	0.938	0.499	0.949	0.447
Transportation needs	0.73	0.712	0.671	0.980	0.092	0.911	0.447	0.974	0.180
Any food, housing, or transportation insecurity or need	0.81	0.788	0.755	0.942	0.414	0.969	0.473	0.902	0.751

with responses other than not hard at all or not very hard.

The AUROC, sensitivity, specificity, positive predictive value, and negative predictive value of the financial stress question's ability to detect other social needs are presented in Table 4 and the AUROC are illustrated in Fig 1. The AUROCs ranged from 0.73 to 0.89. When using not hard at all versus all other responses to the financial stress question, sensitivity ranged from 0.712 to 0.788, specificity ranged from 0.671 to 0.903, positive predictive values ranged from 0.942 to 0.986, and negative predictive values ranged from 0.092 to 0.414. In this sample, using the financial stress question as the first step of a 2-step screening process with not hard at all versus all other responses would have stopped screening for 69% of respondents. This would have missed 9.7% of the families who reported food insecurity, 22.6% who reported housing instability, and 33.0% who reported transportation needs.

When using not hard at all or not very hard versus all other responses to the financial stress question, sensitivity improved with a range from 0.911 to 0.969, specificity worsened with a range from 0.447 to 0.623, positive predictive values ranged from 0.902 to 0.974, and negative predictive values ranged from 0.180 to 0.751. In this sample, using the financial stress question as the first step of a 2-step screening process with not hard at all or not very hard would have stopped screening for 90% of respondents. This would have missed 37.7% of the families who reported food insecurity, 50.1% who reported housing instability, and 55.3% who reported transportation needs. The age-stratified AUROC found similar results as the overall AUROC (Supplemental Figs 2–4).

DISCUSSION

In a large sample of outpatient pediatric practices, we found that a single question about financial stress had inadequate sensitivity to be used as an initial screening question for food insecurity, housing instability, or transportation needs. Ideally, 2-step screening would employ a highly sensitive test, followed by a highly specific test,[8] to minimize respondent burden without missing families in need. We found that the financial stress question used in our electronic health record, and standardized in a widely used electronic health record, does not function well as a first-step item.

The American Academy of Pediatrics was the first national medical society to endorse health-related social needs screening.[1] Other national health care organizations have similarly recommended that clinicians screen for and assist patients with unmet social needs to improve patient care and reduce health disparities.[19–21] Additionally, national organizations, such as the Centers for Medicare and Medicaid and the Joint Commission, are in the process of setting new quality measures requiring health-related social needs screening.[22–24] Despite the growing interest and investment in integrating social needs screening in clinical care settings,[25] barriers (eg, time, family burden) exist, and it is still unclear how to most effectively implement social needs screening in busy pediatric health care settings.[26] The results of this study are consistent with and expand previous work related to health-related social needs screening in pediatric care settings. Although this is the first study to evaluate using a question regarding financial stress as a prescreen, 1 study evaluated using the 2-item Hunger Vital Sign as prescreen for other social needs.[27] Similar to our results, the authors found that utilizing the Hunger Vital Sign as a prescreen would potentially miss a large portion of families (>20%) who endorsed other health-related social needs. Further research is needed to identify alternative strategies to optimize the balance efficiency and effectiveness of social needs screening in busy clinical settings in a family-centered approach.

The findings of this study have important implications and suggest directions for future study. Perhaps the most important implication is that using a single-item financial strain prescreen would miss many families experiencing health-related social needs. This does not mean, however,

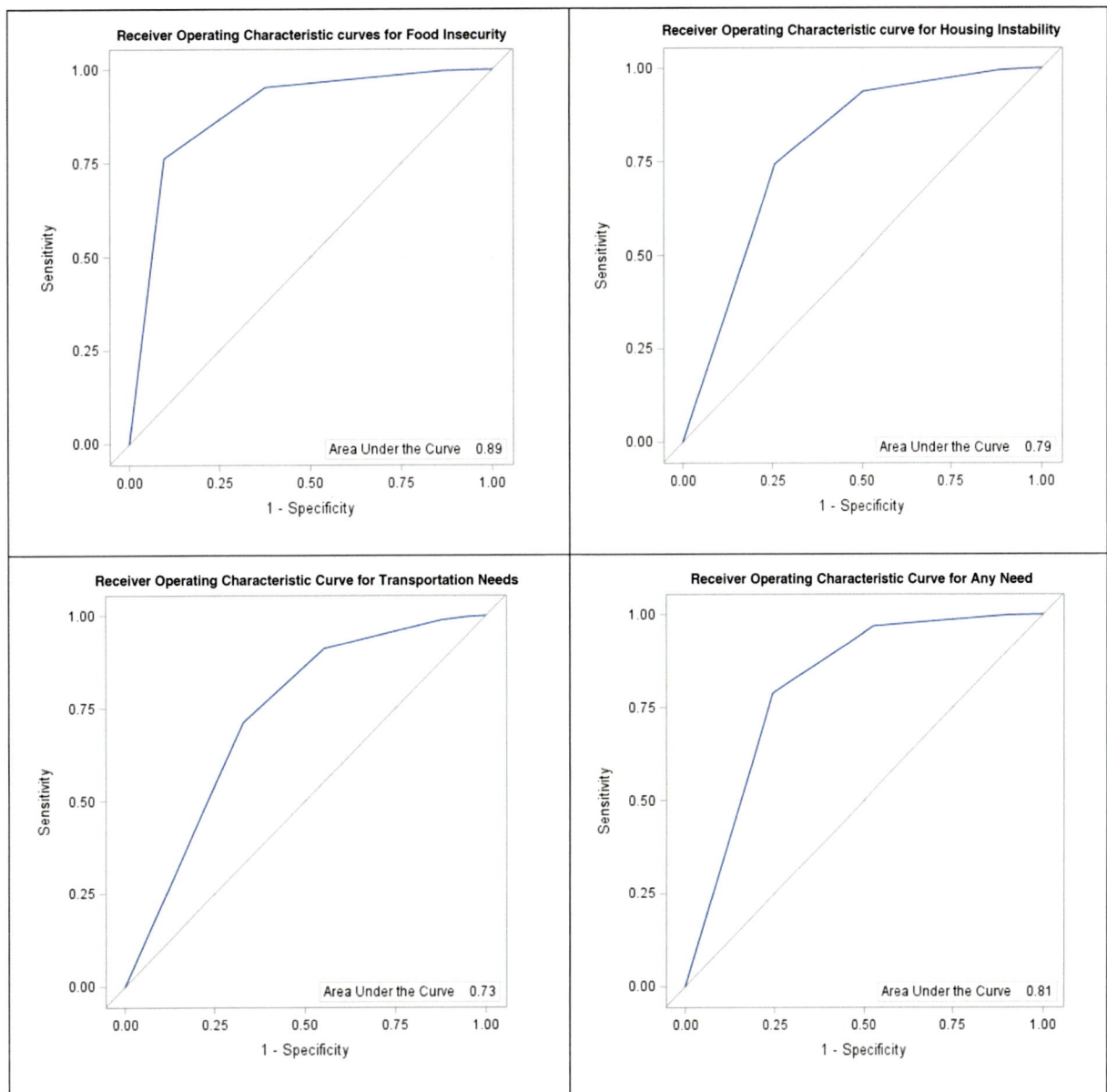

FIGURE 1
Receiver operating characteristic curves for the 5-response financial stress question's association with food insecurity, housing instability, transportation needs, and any need.

that a 2-step workflow is infeasible. Instead, future studies should investigate whether other items might have acceptable sensitivity to be used in a 2-step work flow. This work could be important for reducing the burden of screening in clinics and on families. Another interesting research question we were not able to evaluate in this study (because of the way the data are presented and stored within the electronic health record) is whether the order of questions or the mode of question administration (through the patient portal, on tablets, or verbally by clinicians or staff) affects the sensitivity of the financial strain item. Previous work on this topic has suggested that patients and caregivers often have preferences about mode of administration and may be less likely to disclose unmet social needs if asked verbally,[28–30] but it is unclear whether different modes lead to a meaningfully different relationship between responses.[2,31–33] We think this would be an important area for future investigation, because it is ideal to support modes that are concordant with patient and caregiver preferences, and elicit the most accurate information. It is important to note that, although the children with missing social needs data were relatively small, they were more likely to identify as Hispanic ethnicity, nonwhite race, and be insured through Medicaid. Insuring that social needs screening is acceptable to all patients should be a priority.

The findings of this study should be interpreted in light of several limitations. This study was conducted in a single health system in a single state and single language of administration. However, despite this, the needs identified in this sample are similar to nationally reported rates.[34] Second, the data used in this analysis were from 2022, toward the end of the coronavirus disease 2019 pandemic, a time when access to support for social needs was changing rapidly. Despite this volatility, we see no reason why these changes in the circumstances that create needs or the services available to address needs would affect the interrelationship between needs, which was the focus of this study. Thus, we would expect that the associations seen here would be generalizable to other contexts, although that could be confirmed empirically. Third, on the basis of how the data are stored in the electronic health record, we are unable to assess how the social needs questions were presented to parents/guardians or what parents/guardians perceived the intent of these questions to be. Parents/guardians may have been less likely to report social needs if they had concerns about who would have access to the results and whether reporting social needs could be used in a punitive way (eg, notifying child protective services).[35,36]

These limitations were balanced by several strengths. This study used a large sample of parents and guardians who presented to a set of outpatient pediatric clinics that span a variety of built environments (eg, urban, rural, suburban) and economic environments (eg, area deprivation index scores in the catchment area range from the fourth to 100th national percentile).[37] Further, completion of screening was high (95% of children presenting for a well-child visit during the year), suggesting that the results are representative of the patients seen in these clinics.

Developing efficient and effective evidence-based, health-related social needs screening strategies could improve implementation in clinical practice. Although 2-step screening for health-related social needs may offer benefits, we found that this specific 2-step screening strategy had inadequate performance. At this time, we recommend clinicians use multidomain screening tools to ensure they are able to detect social needs within their clinical population, ideally selected by the institution's ability to address any identified needs.

ABBREVIATION

AUROC: area under the receiver operating curve

CONFLICT OF INTEREST DISCLOSURES: The authors have indicated they have no conflicts of interest relevant to this article to disclose.

REFERENCES

1. Council on Community Pediatrics. Poverty and child health in the United States. *Pediatrics.* 2016;137(4):e20160339

2. De Marchis EH, Hessler D, Fichtenberg C, et al. Part I: a quantitative study of social risk screening acceptability in patients and caregivers. *Am J Prev Med.* 2019;57(6 Suppl 1):S25–S37

3. Garg A, Toy S, Tripodis Y, Silverstein M, Freeman E. Addressing social determinants of health at well child care visits: a cluster RCT. *Pediatrics.* 2015;135(2):e296–e304

4. Garg A, Cull W, Olson L, et al. Screening and referral for low-income families' social determinants of health by US pediatricians. *Acad Pediatr.* 2019;19(8):875–883

5. Schickedanz A, Hamity C, Rogers A, Sharp AL, Jackson A. Clinician experiences and attitudes regarding screening for social determinants of health in a large integrated health system. *Med Care.* 2019;57(Suppl 6 2):S197–S201

6. Sokol RL, Ammer J, Stein SF, Trout P, Mohammed L, Miller AL. Provider perspectives on screening for social determinants of health in pediatric settings: a qualitative study. *J Pediatr Health Care.* 2021;35(6):577–586

7. Mitchell AJ, Yadegarfar M, Gill J, Stubbs B. Case finding and screening clinical utility of the Patient Health Questionnaire (PHQ-9 and PHQ-2) for depression in primary care: a diagnostic meta-analysis of 40 studies. *BJPsych Open.* 2016;2(2):127–138

8. Fletcher RH. *Fletcher SW Fletcher GS. Clinical Epidemiology: The Essentials,* 5th ed. Philadelphia: Wolters Kluwer Health/Lippincott Williams & Wilkins; 2014

9. University of California, San Francisco, Stress Measurement Network. Financial strain. Available at: https://www.stressmeasurement.org/financial-strain. Accessed September 1, 2023

10. Committee on the Recommended Social and Behavioral Domains and Measures for Electronic Health Records; Board on Population Health and Public Health Practice; Institute of Medicine. *Capturing Social and Behavioral Domains and Measures in Electronic Health Records: Phase 2.* Washington, DC: National Academies Press; 2015

11. Puterman E, Haritatos J, Adler NE, Sidney S, Schwartz JE, Epel ES. Indirect effect of financial strain on daily cortisol output through daily negative to positive affect index in the Coronary Artery Risk Development in Young Adults Study. *Psychoneuroendocrinology.* 2013;38(12):2883–2889

12. Hager ER, Quigg AM, Black MM, et al. Development and validity of a 2-item screen to identify families at risk for food insecurity. *Pediatrics.* 2010;126(1):e26–e32

13. Children's HealthWatch. Housing instability: a new screen for adverse health issues for caregivers and children. Available at: https://childrenshealthwatch.org/housing-instability-a-new-screen-for-adverse-health-issues-for-caregivers-and-children/. Accessed September 5, 2023

14. National Association of Community Health Centers; Association of Asian Pacific Community Health Organizations; Oregon Primary Care Association; Institute for Alternative Futures. The protocol for responding to and assessing patients' assets, risks, and experiences (PRAPARE). Available at: www.nachc.org/prapare. Accessed September 5, 2023

15. Barnidge E, LaBarge G, Krupsky K, Arthur J. Screening for food insecurity in pediatric clinical settings: opportunities and barriers. *J Community Health.* 2017;42(1):51–57

16. Trent M, Dooley DG, Dougé J. Section on Adolescent Health; Council on Community Pediatrics; Committee on Adolescence. The impact of racism on child and adolescent health. *Pediatrics.* 2019; 144(2):e20191765

17. US Department of Agriculture Food and Nutrition Service. 2015 expenditures on children by families. Available at: https://www.fns.usda.gov/cnpp/2015-expenditures-children-families. Accessed September 5, 2023

18. Children First (formerly Public Citizens For Children and Youth). Insurance. Available at: https://www.childrenfirstpa.org/issues/child-health/insurance/. Accessed September 5, 2023

19. Daniel H, Bornstein SS, Kane GC, et al. Health and Public Policy Committee of the American College of Physicians. Addressing social determinants to improve patient care and promote health equity: an American College of Physicians position paper. *Ann Intern Med.* 2018;168(8):577–578

20. American Academy of Family Physicians. Assessment and action. Available at: https://www.aafp.org/family-physician/patient-care/the-everyone-project/toolkit/assessment.html. Accessed September 5, 2023

21. Byhoff E, Kangovi S, Berkowitz SA, et al. Society of General Internal Medicine. A Society of General Internal Medicine position statement on the internists' role in social determinants of health. *J Gen Intern Med.* 2020;35(9):2721–2727

22. Jacobs DB, Schreiber M, Seshamani M, Tsai D, Fowler E, Fleisher LA. Aligning quality measures across CMS—the Universal Foundation. *N Engl J Med.* 2023;388(9):776–779

23. Reynolds A. National Committee for Quality Assurance. Social need: new HEDIS measure uses electronic data to look at screening, intervention. Available at: https://www.ncqa.org/blog/social-need-new-hedis-measure-uses-electronic-data-to-look-at-screening-intervention. Accessed September 5, 2023

24. The Joint Commission. R3 report: requirement, rationale, reference. Available at: https://www.jointcommission.org/-/media/tjc/documents/standards/r3-reports/r3_disparities_july2022-6-20-2022.pdf. Accessed September 5, 2023

25. Garg A, Homer CJ, Dworkin PH. Addressing social determinants of health: challenges and opportunities in a value-based model. *Pediatrics.* 2019;143(4):e20182355

26. Dolce M, Keedy H, Chavez L, et al. Implementing an EMR-based health-related social needs screen in a pediatric hospital system. *Pediatr Qual Saf.* 2022;7(1):e512

27. Sheward R, Bruce C, Frank D, et al. Can the Hunger Vital Sign act as a prescreen for other social needs? *J Appl Res Child.* 2020;11(1):13

28. Cullen D, Woodford A, Fein J. Food for thought: a randomized trial of food insecurity screening in the emergency department. *Acad Pediatr.* 2019;19(6):646–651

29. Palakshappa D, Goodpasture M, Albertini L, Brown CL, Montez K, Skelton JA. Written versus verbal food insecurity screening in one primary care clinic. *Acad Pediatr.* 2020;20(2):203–207

30. Ray KN, Gitz KM, Hu A, Davis AA, Miller E. Nonresponse to health-related social needs screening questions. *Pediatrics.* 2020;146(3): e20200174

31. Cullen D, Attridge M, Fein JA. Food for thought: a qualitative evaluation of caregiver preferences for food insecurity screening and resource referral. *Acad Pediatr.* 2020;20(8):1157–1162

32. De Marchis EH, Hessler D, Fichtenberg C, et al. Assessment of social risk factors and interest in receiving health care-based social assistance among adult patients and adult caregivers of pediatric patients. *JAMA Netw Open.* 2020;3(10):e2021201

33. Byhoff E, De Marchis EH, Hessler D, et al. Part II: a qualitative study of social risk screening acceptability in patients and caregivers. *Am J Prev Med.* 2019;57(6 Suppl 1):S38–S46

34. Kreuter MW, Thompson T, McQueen A, Garg R. Addressing social needs in health care settings: evidence, challenges, and opportunities for public health. *Annu Rev Public Health.* 2021;42(1):329–344

35. Garg A, LeBlanc A, Raphael JL. Inadequacy of current screening measures for health-related social needs. *JAMA.* 2023;330(10):915–916

36. Cullen D, Wilson-Hall L, McPeak K, Fein J. Pediatric social risk screening: leveraging research to ensure equity. *Acad Pediatr.* 2022;22(2):190–192

37. Neighborhood Atlas. Neighborhood Atlas—mapping. Available at: https://www.neighborhoodatlas.medicine.wisc.edu/mapping. Accessed September 5, 2023

Food Insecurity Screening and Intervention in United States Children's Hospitals

Molly A. Markowitz, MD[a] Gunjan Tiyyagura, MD, MHS[a] Kaitlin Quallen, MD[a] Julia Rosenberg, MD, MHS[a]

ABSTRACT

OBJECTIVES: Food insecurity (FI) affects many United States families and negatively impacts the health of children. We assessed patterns of FI screening for United States children's hospitals, characterized screening protocols, and assessed how hospitals addressed general and inpatient-specific caregiver FI, including provision of food or meals for caregivers of admitted children.

METHODS: We conducted a cross-sectional, confidential survey of clinical team members at United States children's hospitals. We evaluated FI screening practices and responses, including which team members conduct FI screening, the types of screeners used, and interventions including social work consultations, referrals to community resources, and provision of food or meals.

RESULTS: Of the 76 children's hospital representatives (40% response rate) who participated in the survey, 67.1% reported at least some screening, and 34.2% performed universal screening for FI. Screening was conducted most frequently on the inpatient units (58.8%), with social workers (35.5%) and nurses (34.2%) administering screeners most frequently. Responses to positive screens included social work consultation (51.3%), referral to community resources (47.4%), and offering food or meals (43.4%). Eighty-four percent of hospitals provided food or meals to at least some caregivers for admitted pediatric patients. Conditional qualifications for food/meals included need-based (31.6%) and presence of breastfeeding mothers (30.3%).

CONCLUSIONS: Many United States children's hospitals screen for FI, but most survey respondents reported that their hospital did not conduct universal screening. Screening protocols and interventions varied among institutions. Children's hospitals could consider improving screening protocols and interventions to ensure that needs are identified and addressed.

www.hospitalpediatrics.org

DOI:https://doi.org/10.1542/hpeds.2022-006755

Copyright © 2022 by the American Academy of Pediatrics

Address correspondence to Molly Markowitz, MD, Department of Pediatrics, PO Box 208064, New Haven, CT 06520-8064. E-mail: molly.markowitz@yale.edu

HOSPITAL PEDIATRICS (ISSN Numbers: Print, 2154-1663; Online, 2154-1671).

FUNDING: No external funding.

CONFLICT OF INTEREST DISCLOSURES: The authors have no conflicts of interest relevant to this article to disclose.

COMPANION PAPER: A companion to this article can be found online at https://doi.org/10.1542/hpeds.2022-006871.

[a]*Department of Pediatrics, Yale School of Medicine, New Haven, Connecticut*

Drs Markowitz, Rosenberg, and Tiyyagura conceptualized and designed the study, designed the data collection instruments, coordinated and supervised data collection, collected data, carried out analyses, drafted the initial manuscript, and reviewed and revised the manuscript; Dr Quallen collected data and reviewed and revised the manuscript; and all authors approved the final manuscript as submitted and agree to be accountable for all aspects of the work.

Before the coronavirus disease 2019 (COVID-19) pandemic, 6.5% (2.4 million households) of United States households with children experienced food insecurity (FI).[1] Food insecurity is defined by the US Department of Agriculture as either[1] low food security: reduced quality, variety, or desirability of food, or[2] very low food security: disruption or reduced intake of food.[2] During the beginning of the COVID-19 pandemic, reported FI among households with children increased to 7.6% (2.9 million households).[3]

Compared to those who are food secure, children who face FI have increased risk of chronic diseases, hospitalizations, nutritional deficiencies, educational issues, and emotional and behavioral challenges.[4–9] Mothers in food insecure homes are at increased risk of anxiety and depression.[10] When a child is hospitalized, caregivers may experience multiple stressors that affect health. Not only can they experience exacerbated household FI, but they can also have isolated inpatient FI (no household FI at baseline) as a result of the admission.[11–12] Caregivers may face financial hardship from lost wages and costs associated with food, lodging, child care, and transportation.[13–17] Despite these known stressors, a 2004 study found that only 14% of US and Canadian children's hospitals routinely administered food to all caregivers and that 39% provided food to select caregivers on the basis of criteria such as demonstrated financial need or the presence of a breastfeeding mother.[18]

The American Academy of Pediatrics and other experts recommend that pediatric clinical teams screen for FI and link families to needed resources.[4,19–21] There are multiple screeners such as the Hunger Vital Sign, Well Child Care, Evaluation, Community Resources, Advocacy, Referral, Education Survey Instrument (WE CARE), and Safe Environment for Every Kid (SEEK) which include questions solely regarding access to food or as a part of a more comprehensive assessment of social needs.[22–25] There are also screening programs with integrated community referral processes such as CommunityRX

and NowPow that help health care teams identify and address FI via personalized resources lists and/or navigation programs.[26–29]

To our knowledge, the proportion of United States children's hospitals which screen for FI in the inpatient setting has not been determined. In this study, we examined the patterns of United States children's hospitals that screened for FI, characterized screening protocols, and described interventions to address

positive screens, including hospital practices to address isolated inpatient caregiver FI.

METHODS
Hospital Database

We used the Children's Hospital Association directory to compile a database of 190 United States children's hospitals, excluding specialty hospitals and institutions which exclusively provided newborn care.[28] We determined hospital

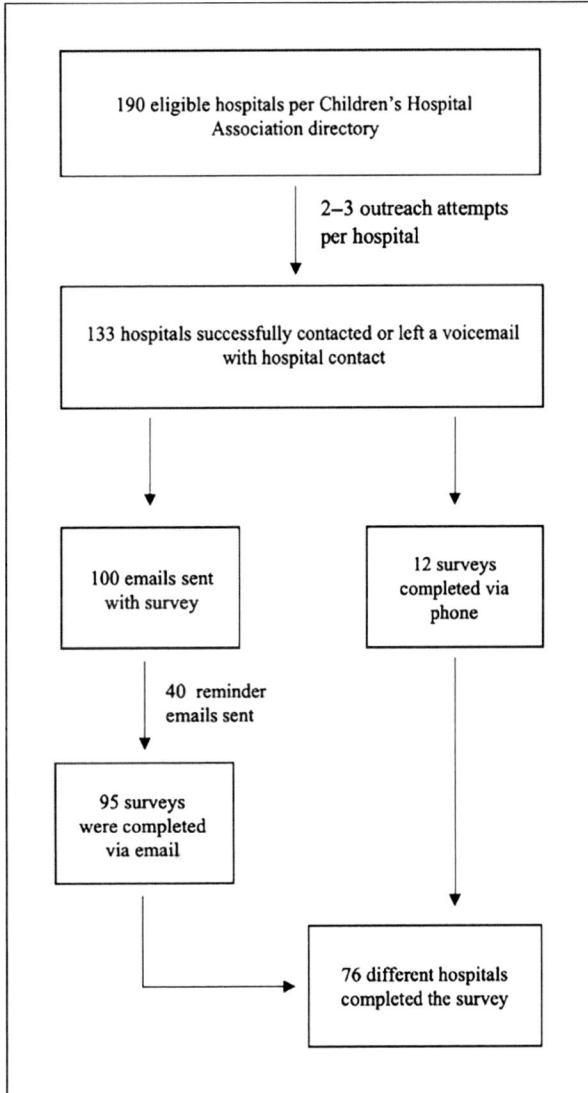

FIGURE 1 Survey assessing food provision and food insecurity screening for caregivers of admitted pediatric patients: workflow for connecting with a hospital contact and survey administration.

size (bed number) by first assessing the Children's Hospital Association directory. In cases where the bed number was not listed in the directory, it was determined via an internet search. We characterized hospital region based on United States census data and determined county-specific poverty rates using the County Health Rankings and Roadmaps.[30–31]

Survey Development

The survey was developed and refined by our research team and piloted with content experts with knowledge in survey methodology, epidemiology, and health services research who provided feedback. From the expert feedback, we modified the survey to include mostly multiple-choice (rather than free text) questions and to include specific items regarding FI screening procedures such as type of screener, when or where it is administered, and assessments of the types or qualifications for food provisions provided (Supplemental Table 4).

Survey Administration

Before the COVID-19 pandemic, in February 2020, we initially distributed the survey to 10 individuals from different children's hospitals in the United States from multiple departments including social work, nutrition, patient relations, and nursing. We specifically spoke to these care team members, rather than physicians, nurse practitioners, and physician assistants, because of known inpatient clinical workflows. After the 10 surveys were administered, we found that social work team members demonstrated the most consistent expertise in answering survey questions and willingness to participate in the study. Additionally, other groups outside of social work would often defer to the social work team at their institution when asked to complete survey questions.

Because of the COVID-19 pandemic and clinical responsibilities, research activities were paused until February 2021. We then redistributed the survey, informed by the prepandemic responses, between February 2021 through July 2021

using the following workflow[1]: We completed a Web site search for either a social work department phone number or the general phone number for the hospital.[2] We then called and asked to connect with the inpatient social work department and to speak with either a social work manager or social worker. If neither was available, we left a message requesting a call-back. At least 2 attempts were made to reach each hospital.[3] If we connected with someone from the social work department, we asked to speak with someone who had a global perspective of institutional FI screening and interventions such as a social work manager. If the social work team member shared that someone else at their institution could better answer questions regarding FI screening practices, we would attempt to connect with that individual even if they were from a different department.[4] Once a person was

identified and they agreed to participate in the study, respondents chose either E-mail or phone administration by member of the research team. E-mail respondents received 1 reminder E-mail if needed. We also redistributed the survey to the 10 institutions which completed survey before the survey modifications. There was no incentive for survey participation.

Data Analysis

After contacting all institutions, 40.0% (76 of 190) submitted at least 1 response and 9.2% (7 of 76) of those institutions submitted multiple responses (Fig 1). We consolidated multiple responses, and when there were discrepancies from the same institution, we included the affirmative responses (example: answered yes to screening for FI), recognizing that an individual may not always have a global

TABLE 1 Survey Assessing Food Provision and Food Insecurity Screening for Caregivers of Admitted Pediatric Patients: Hospital and Respondent Characteristics

	Responding Hospitals (N = 76)		Nonresponding Hospitals (N = 114)		
	n	(%)	n	(%)	P^b
Number of staffed beds					.41
< 100	13	(17.1)	27	(23.7)	
101–200	35	(46.1)	44	(38.6)	
201–300	13	(17.1)	21	(18.4)	
>300	10	(13.2)	9	(7.9)	
Could not determine	5	(6.6)	13	(11.4)	
Region					.17
Northeast	14	(18.4)	27	(22.8)	
South	26	(34.2)	40	(35.1)	
Midwest	27	(35.5)	24	(21.1)	
West	8	(10.5)	22	(19.3)	
Pacific	1	(1.3)	1	(0.90)	
Child poverty rate by county, %					.17
<10	12	(15.8)	20	(17.5)	
11–20	52	(68.4)	64	(56.1)	
>20	12	(15.8)	30	(26.3)	
Participant department					—
Social work	60	(79.0)	—	—	
Nursing	6	(7.9)	—	—	
Other	10	(13.2)	—	—	

—, not applicable.
[a] Other included: nutrition and administration.
[b] P values were calculated using χ^2.

perspective of protocols and services. Descriptive statistics were performed by using Stata 15 (StataCorp, College Station, Texas), and between-group differences were assessed by using χ^2 test. This study was deemed exempt by the university institutional review board.

RESULTS
Respondent Characteristics

There was no significant difference in the hospital demographic characteristics for hospitals which had an individual complete the survey. Social work team members constituted the majority of participants in this study (79.0%). Most hospitals had between 100 to 300 staffed beds and were located in the Midwest or Southern regions of the United States. Most (68.4%) hospitals were located in a county with a child poverty rate between 10% to 20% (Table 1).

Food Insecurity Screening

The majority (67.1%) of hospitals screened at least some individuals for FI. About one-third of institutions universally screened for FI on admission. The most frequently reported locations where FI screeners where administered included the inpatient unit (58.8%), multiple settings (33.3%), and the emergency department (13.7%). Individuals administering screeners included social workers (35.5%), nurses (34.2%), and physicians (4.0%). The most frequently reported method used to administer the screener was via oral interview (38.2%), followed by paper (10.5%), and electronic device (7.9%). Screener type included institution-specific (30.3%), "other" (15.8%), and the Hunger Vital Sign (2.6%). Interventions and responses to address identified FI included placing a social work consultation (51.3%), providing connections to community resources (47.4%), and/or offering food or meals (43.4%) (Table 2).

Addressing Inpatient Food Insecurity

Most respondents (84.2%) reported administering food/meals to some

TABLE 2 Survey Assessing Food Provision and Food Insecurity Screening for Caregivers of Admitted Pediatric Patients: Screening Administration and Follow-up ($N = 76$)

	n	(%)
Screens for food insecurity[a]		
Yes	51	(67.1)
No	20	(26.3)
Screened person[b]		
Everyone admitted to the hospital	26	(34.2)
Conditional		
Per medical team discretion	14	(18.4)
Unit-based	12	(15.8)
Location of screening[c]		
Inpatient unit	30	(58.8)
In multiple settings	17	(33.3)
In the emergency department	7	(13.7)
Other	7	(13.7)
Survey administrator or screener[d]		
Social worker	27	(35.5)
Nurse	26	(34.2)
Medical assistant or similar	9	(11.8)
Physician	3	(4.0)
Food services	3	(4.0)
Method of screener administration[e]		
Oral interview	29	(38.2)
Electronic medical record	21	(27.6)
On paper	8	(10.5)
On electronic device	6	(7.9)
Food insecurity screener used[f]		
Own institutional screener	23	(30.3)
Other	12	(15.8)
Not sure	10	(13.2)
Hunger Vital Sign[22]	2	(2.6)
Result of positive screen[g]		
Social work consult placed	39	(51.3)
Community resources given	36	(47.4)
Food or meals offered	33	(43.4)
Food insecurity added to problem list	17	(22.8)

[a] Five had no response.
[b] Eight had no response, participants could select >1 answer.
[c] Six had no response, participants could select >1 answer.
[d] Six had no response, participants could select >1 answer.
[e] Nine had no response, participants could select >1 answer.
[f] Six had no response, participants could select >1 answer.
[g] Seven had no response, participants could select >1 answer.

caregivers. Conditional qualifications for food or meals included need-based determination (31.6%) and presence of a breastfeeding mother (30.3%) (Table 3, Fig 2). Need-based was further defined by participant free-text responses and included food insecurity (25.0%), medical team assessment (18.4%), and being out of town (11.8%).

TABLE 3 Survey Assessing Food Provision and Food Insecurity Screening for Caregivers of Admitted Pediatric Patients: Qualifications, Type of Food, and Funding Sources (*N* = 76)

	n	%
Provides free or subsidized food or meals		
Yes	64	(84.2)
No	12	(15.8)
Qualifications for meals[a]		
All caregivers	21	(27.6)
Conditional		
Need-based	24	(31.6)
Breastfeeding mothers	23	(30.3)
1 caregiver	19	(25.0)
COVID-19 positive patient	2	(2.6)
2 caregivers	2	(2.6)
Out of town	2	(2.6)
Definitions for need-based[b]		
Financial insecurity	19	(25.0)
Health care team assessment	14	(18.4)
Out of town	9	(11.8)
Caregiver request or self-identified	5	(6.6)
Uses Medicaid	3	(4.0)
Other	3	(4.0)
Lack of resources	2	(2.6)
Food insecurity	2	(2.6)
Types of meals or food offered[c]		
Food voucher	30	(39.5)
Common area with snacks	28	(36.8)
3 meals per day	25	(32.9)
Food pantry	24	(31.6)
1 meal per day	14	(18.4)
Gift card or debit card	10	(13.2)
Ronald McDonald House meals	8	(10.5)
Bagged meal	6	(7.9)
Other	3	(4.0)
2 meals per day	1	(1.3)
Funding for meals or food[d]		
Hospital funding	28	(36.8)
Hospital cafeteria or food services	27	(35.5)
Monetary donations	20	(26.3)
Community organization	14	(18.4)
Other	5	(6.6)
State funding	4	(5.3)

[a] Six had no response, participants could select >1 answer.
[b] Twenty-six had no response.
[c] Seven had no response, participants could select >1 answer.
[d] Twelve had no response, participants could select >1 answer.

DISCUSSION

In this cross-sectional survey of representatives of United States children's hospitals, we found that, although many hospitals screened for FI, the majority did not conduct universal screening. Screening practices and interventions for identified FI varied among institutions. Most hospitals provided some food or meals to the caregivers of admitted pediatric patients, but there were often conditional qualifications.

Although the majority of institutions performed some FI screening, universal screening was conducted at one-third of institutions. In hospitals that did not perform universal screening, conditional qualifications for screening included admission to certain units and/or medical team discretion. These results are consistent with the previous study of 4 large United States children's hospitals, in which it was found that universal screening was less common than screening for FI when deemed clinically relevant.[32] As one-fourth of recently hospitalized children experience household FI and around 40% of pediatric caregivers experienced inpatient FI, transitioning from a conditional to a universal screening approach may present an opportunity for practice change to address unmet needs.[11,33]

We found that FI screening was conducted in multiple clinical settings, with the majority completed on inpatient units. Other studies have similarly found that screening for social stressors occurs in multiple clinical settings such as inpatient units, emergency departments, and primary care clinics.[32,34–36] Within these various clinical settings, we found that social workers and nurses accounted for the majority of individuals who administered screeners, whereas physicians made up a minority of screening. In 1 analysis of 4 large academic United States children's hospitals, it was found that nurses were the most common providers to screen for social stressors, although hospitalists also conducted many of the screens.[32] This variation in findings of physician-administration of screeners may be related to survey methodology (our respondents did not include physicians),

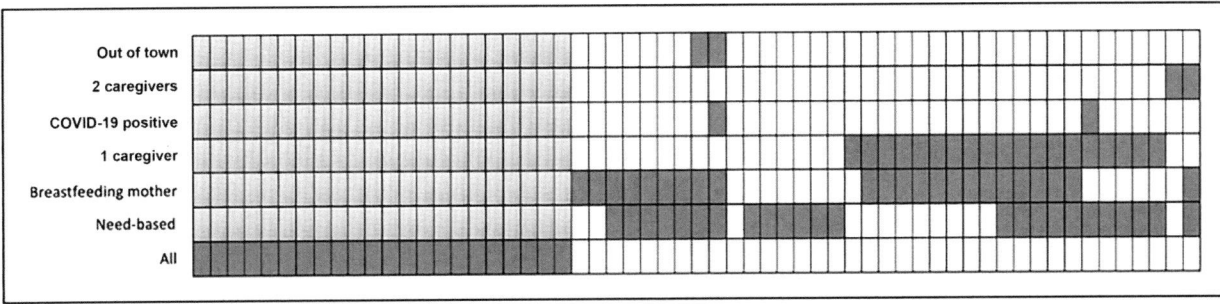

FIGURE 2 The types of conditional food provisions provided to the caregivers of admitted pediatric patients. [a] Each column represents a different hospital.

the breadth of institutions included, and/or the type of screeners administered.

Respondents identified that an oral interview was the most common screening method used, whereas few reported administering screeners with paper or electronic devices. Most hospitals used their own institutional screener, with only a small proportion using the Hunger Vital Sign, a validated tool.[37] Screened individuals have been found to be more likely to disclose health related social needs when using electronic tablets or written questionnaires, compared to oral interview.[38–40] Hospitals could consider refining screening practices by selecting validated, standardized screening tools and implementing evidence-based modalities of administration.

When there was a positive screen for FI, study participants shared that some hospitals provided caregivers with food or meals. Other hospitals provided food or meals to caregivers without specific FI screening but had conditional qualifications such as need-base and/or presence of a breastfeeding mother. These findings are similar to a 2007 study of United States and Canadian children's hospitals that found that 39% of institutions provided some caregivers with food or meals and 14% provided provisions without conditional qualifications.[18] These collective findings indicate that hospitals may meet the needs of some caregivers experiencing inpatient FI, but, because of conditional qualifications, others may be missed. Past research has shown that the caregivers of

admitted pediatric patients may not only experience exacerbations of household FI, but also encounter isolated inpatient FI.[11–12] Our results present a potential opportunity for institutions to target food or meal provisions to those who are in need but may be missed currently, allowing caregivers to fully engage in their child's care.

There were several limitations to this study. Most hospitals (91%) had 1 representative respondent who may not have had a complete knowledge of all screening protocols and interventions. Our study workflow did attempt to identify the key stakeholder with knowledge about food insecurity screening and interventions at each institution. Of note, the most frequent response provided to identified FI was "social work consult." Social workers, who made up the majority of survey respondents, thus may represent a key stakeholder group to evaluate institutional screening and food provision practices. Respondents may have been affected by social desirability bias, although an online survey platform offered an opportunity for confidential responses that may have helped to mitigate bias. We had a 40% response rate; thus, the reported results may reflect a response bias with participants being more likely to respond if their institutions had practices for screening for FI and providing food. It is also possible that institutions with fewer resources, specifically without dedicated social workers, may have been more represented in the nonrespondents, and thus, we may be underrepresenting available services especially in areas with limited resources. We were not able

to connect with an initial contact at 30% of hospitals; thus, our results may not represent all institutional practices. Although components of the survey were not validated, we field tested and refined the instrument with content and survey experts. Despite the discussed limitations, our results still highlight areas where many hospitals can make improvements to FI screening practices and interventions to identified needs.

CONCLUSIONS

In this survey of inpatient United States children's hospital representative, we found that the majority of respondents reported at least some institutional inpatient screening for FI. A lack of universal screening may lead to missed opportunities to address needs. Institutions had variable screening practices and interventions to address both inpatient and household FI, and there are opportunities to improve screening protocols and interventions to ensure that families in need receive support, especially during and around hospital admission.

Acknowledgments

We thank Drs Eugene Shapiro, Magna Dias, Mona Sharifi, Adam Berkwitt, Melissa Langhan, and Marc Auerbach and for their feedback on our survey. We would like to thank Drs Kristin Reese and Nishant Pandya for help with data collection. We would like to thank Denine Baxter MHA, BSN, RN, CNML and Drs Jaspreet Loyal and Magna Dias for working to improve food provisions for families admitted to our children's hospital. Finally, we would like to thank the parents and caregivers who inspired this work.

REFERENCES

1. Coleman-Jensen A, Rabbitt MP, Gregory CA, Sing A. Household food security in the United States in 2019. Available at: https://www.ers.usda.gov/publications/pub-details/?pubid=99281. Accessed November 13, 2021

2. Economic Research Service, US Department of Agriculture. Definitions of food security. Available at: https://www.ers.usda.gov/topics/food-nutrition-assistance/food-security-in-the-us/definitions-of-food-security.aspx. Accessed November 13, 2021

3. Coleman-Jensen A, Rabbitt MP, Gregory CA, Singh A. Economic Research Service UsS. Available at: Available at: https://www.ers.usda.gov/webdocs/publications/102076/err-298_summary.pdf?v=5234.3. Accessed January 28, 2022

4. Council on Community Pediatrics; Committee on Nutrition. Promoting food security for all children. *Pediatrics.* 2015;136(5): e1431–8

5. Cook JT, Black M, Chilton M, et al. Are food insecurity's health impacts underestimated in the U.S. population? Marginal food security also predicts adverse health outcomes in young U.S. children and mothers. *Adv Nutr.* 2013;4(1):51–61

6. Kirkpatrick SI, McIntyre L, Potestio ML. Child hunger and long-term adverse consequences for health. *Arch Pediatr Adolesc Med.* 2010; 164(8):754–762

7. Skalicky A, Meyers AF, Adams WG, Yang Z, Cook JT, Frank DA. Child food insecurity and iron deficiency anemia in low-income infants and toddlers in the United States. *Matern Child Health J.* 2006;10(2):177–185

8. Jyoti DF, Frongillo EA, Jones SJ. Food insecurity affects school children's academic performance, weight gain, and social skills. *J Nutr.* 2005;135(12):2831–2839

9. Melchior M, Chastang J-F, Falissard B, et al. Food insecurity and children's mental health: a prospective birth cohort study. *PLoS One.* 2012;7(12):e52615

10. Whitaker RC, Phillips SM, Orzol SM. Food insecurity and the risks of depression and anxiety in mothers and behavior problems in their preschool-aged children. *Pediatrics.* 2006;118(3):e859–e868

11. Lee AM, Lopez MA, Haq H, et al. Inpatient food insecurity in caregivers of hospitalized pediatric patients: A mixed methods study. *Acad Pediatr.* 2021;21 (8):1404–1413

12. Makelarski JA, Thorngren D, Lindau ST. Feed first, ask questions later: alleviating and understanding caregiver food insecurity in an urban children's hospital. *Am J Public Health.* 2015;105(8):e98–e104

13. Vessey JA, DiFazio RL, Strout TD, Snyder BD. Impact of non-medical out-of-pocket expenses on families of children with cerebral palsy following orthopaedic surgery. *J Pediatr Nurs.* 2017;37:101–107

14. Shields L, Tanner A. Costs of meals and parking for parents of hospitalised children in Australia. *Paediatr Nurs.* 2004;16(6):14–18

15. Callery P. Paying to participate: financial, social and personal costs to parents of involvement in their children's care in hospital. *J Adv Nurs.* 1997;25(4):746–752

16. Mumford V, Baysari MT, Kalinin D, et al. Measuring the financial and productivity burden of paediatric hospitalisation on the wider family network. *J Paediatr Child Health.* 2018;54(9):987–996

17. Chang LV, Shah AN, Hoefgen ER, et al; H2O Study Group. Lost earnings and nonmedical expenses of pediatric hospitalizations. *Pediatrics.* 2018;142(3):e20180195

18. Stremler R, Wong L, Parshuram C. Practices and provisions for parents sleeping overnight with a hospitalized child. Available at: https://academic.oup.com/jpepsy/article/33/3/292/902703. Published September 28, 2007. Accessed February 12, 2021

19. Ashbrook A, Essel K, Montez K, Bennett-Tejes D. Screen and intervene: a toolkit for pediatricians to address food insecurity. Available at: https://frac.org/aaptoolkit. Published March 2021. Accessed January 2021

20. Garg A, Boynton-Jarrett R, Dworkin PH. Avoiding the unintended consequences of screening for social determinants of health. *JAMA.* 2016;316(8):813–814

21. Finkelhor D. Screening for adverse childhood experiences (ACEs): Cautions and suggestions. *Child Abuse Negl.* 2018;85:174–179

22. Hager ER, Quigg AM, Black MM, et al. Development and validity of a 2-item screen to identify families at risk for food insecurity. *Pediatrics.* 2010;126(1):e26–e32

23. Garg A, Butz AM, Dworkin PH, Lewis RA, Thompson RE, Serwint JR. Improving the management of family psychosocial problems at low-income children's well-child care visits: the WE CARE Project. *Pediatrics.* 2007;120(3):547–558

24. Dubowitz H, Feigelman S, Lane W, Kim J. Pediatric primary care to help prevent child maltreatment: the Safe Environment for Every Kid (SEEK) Model. *Pediatrics.* 2009;123(3):858–864

25. Sokol R, Austin A, Chandler C, et al. Screening children for social determinants of health: A systematic review. *Pediatrics.* 2019;144(4):e20191622

26. Lindau ST, Makelarski JA, Abramsohn EM, et al. CommunityRx: A real-world controlled clinical trial of a scalable, low-intensity community resource referral intervention. *Am J Public Health.* 2019;109(4):600–606

27. Berry C, Paul M, Massar R, Marcello RK, Krauskopf M. Social needs screening and referral program at a large US public hospital system, 2017. *Am J Public Health.* 2020;110(S2):S211–S214

28. Gottlieb LM, Hessler D, Long D, et al. Effects of social needs screening and in-person service navigation on Child

health. *JAMA Pediatr.* 2016;170(11): e162521

29. The Children's Hospital Association. Available at: https://www. childrenshospitals.org. Accessed November 15, 2021

30. United States Census Bureau. Census regions and divisions of the United States. Available at: https://www2. census.gov/geo/pdfs/maps-data/maps/ reference/us_regdiv.pdf. Accessed November 13, 2021

31. County Health Rankings & Roadmaps. Children in poverty. Available at: https:// www.countyhealthrankings.org/explore-health-rankings/measures-data-sources/ county-health-rankings-model/health-factors/social-and-economic-factors/ income/children-in-poverty. Accessed November 14, 2021

32. Schwartz B, Herrmann LE, Librizzi J, et al. Screening for social determinants of health in hospitalized children. *Hosp Pediatr.* 2020;10(1):29–36

33. Banach LP. Hospitalization: Are we missing an opportunity to identify food insecurity in children? *Acad Pediatr.* 2016;16(5):438–445

34. Fraze TK, Brewster AL, Lewis VA, Beidler LB, Murray GF, Colla CH. Prevalence of screening for food insecurity, housing instability, utility needs, transportation needs, and interpersonal violence by US physician practices and hospitals. *JAMA Netw Open.* 2019;2(9):e1911514

35. Gonzalez JV, Hartford EA, Moore J, Brown JC. Food insecurity in a pediatric emergency department and the feasibility of Universal screening. *West J Emerg Med.* 2021;22(6):1295–1300

36. Meyer D, Lerner E, Phillips A, Zumwalt K. Universal screening of social determinants of health at a large US academic medical center, 2018. *Am J Public Health.* 2020;110(S2):S219–S221

37. Makelarski JA, Abramsohn E, Benjamin JH, Du S, Lindau ST. Diagnostic accuracy of two food insecurity screeners recommended for use in health care settings. *Am J Public Health.* 2017;107(11): 1812–1817

38. Palakshappa D, Goodpasture M, Albertini L, Brown CL, Montez K, Skelton JA. Written versus verbal food insecurity screening in one primary care clinic. *Acad Pediatr.* 2020;20(2): 203–207

39. Knowles M, Khan S, Palakshappa D, et al. Successes, challenges, and considerations for integrating referral into food insecurity screening in pediatric settings. *J Health Care Poor Underserved.* 2018;29(1):181–191

40. Cullen D, Woodford A, Fein J. Food for thought: A randomized trial of food insecurity screening in the emergency department. *Acad Pediatr.* 2019;19(6):646–651

BRIEF REPORT

Food Insecurity Screening of Hospitalized Patients: A Descriptive Analysis

Samantha L. Hanna, MD, MPH,[a] Chang L. Wu, MD, MSCR,[b] Cassi Smola, MD,[b] Tamera Coyne-Beasley, MD, MPH,[b] Mary Orr, MD, MPH,[b] Alexandra Healy, MD,[c] Adolfo L. Molina, MD, MSHQS[b]

A B S T R A C T

OBJECTIVES: The purpose of this study is to describe an advocacy effort to implement a food insecurity (FI) screening during hospital admission and describe characteristics of hospitalized patients with household FI.

METHODS: This is a descriptive study after the implementation of FI screening at a quaternary-care children's hospital in the Southeastern United States between August 2020 and April 2021. The Hunger Vital Sign, a 2-question screening tool for FI, was added to the intake questionnaire performed on inpatient admissions. A positive screen triggered a social work consult to connect patients with resources. Chart review and statistical analyses were performed on patients with household FI.

RESULTS: There were 7751 hospital admissions during the study period, of which 4777 (61.6%) had an FI screen completed. Among those with a completed screen, 233 patients (4.9%) were positive for household FI. Patients with household FI were more likely to be Black (P <.001) and have Medicaid (P <.001). Social work documented care specific to FI in 125 of the 233 (56%) FI patients, of which 39 (31%) were not enrolled in the Women, Infants, and Children Program/Supplemental Nutrition Assistance Program.

CONCLUSIONS: This initiative highlights hospitalization as an opportunity to screen for FI using a multidisciplinary approach. Our findings underscore the importance of identifying FI with the goal of reducing FI and mitigating the adverse effects of FI on child health outcomes.

www.hospitalpediatrics.org

DOI:https://doi.org/10.1542/hpeds.2022-006549

Copyright © 2022 by the American Academy of Pediatrics

[a]Department of Pediatrics, Saint Louis University, St. Louis, Missouri; [b]Department of Pediatrics, University of Alabama at Birmingham, Birmingham, Alabama; and [c]Department of Pediatrics, Children's Hospital of Philadelphia, Philadelphia, Pennsylvania

Address correspondence to Samantha L. Hanna, MD, MPH, Department of Pediatrics, Saint Louis University, 1465 South Grand Blvd, St. Louis, MO 63104. E-mail: samantha.hanna@health.slu.edu

HOSPITAL PEDIATRICS (ISSN Numbers: Print, 2154-1663; Online, 2154-1671).

FUNDING: No external funding.

CONFLICT OF INTEREST DISCLAIMER: The authors have indicated they have no conflicts of interest relevant to this article to disclose.

Dr Hanna conceptualized and designed the study, and drafted the initial manuscript; Drs Smola and Orr conceptualized and designed the study; Drs Coyne-Beasley and Healy contributed to interpretation of data; Drs Wu and Molina conceptualized and designed the study, and conducted the analyses; and all authors reviewed and revised the manuscript, approved the final manuscript as submitted, and agree to be accountable for all aspects of the work.

Food insecurity (FI), defined as limited or uncertain access to enough food for a healthy and active lifestyle, is a complex social problem.[1] Children that live in households with FI have been shown to have poorer health outcomes, including more frequent illness and hospitalization, increased risk of chronic disease, and higher rates of depression and anxiety.[1–4] Before the COVID-19 pandemic, 1 in 7 children in the United States lived in a household experiencing FI.[1] The pandemic caused rising unemployment and poverty rates, and FI rates also increased with as many as 20% to 25% of US children estimated to be living in FI households in 2020.[1,5,6] Similarly, in our local population, even before the pandemic, we experienced FI rates in children as high as 20%.[7] It is also important to note the role of racial discrimination and racism in FI because the pandemic has also highlighted the prominence of racial disparities in social determinants of health (SDOH).[8]

The American Academy of Pediatrics recommends pediatricians screen for FI.[1] However, limited data exist regarding FI in the inpatient pediatric population.[9] In response to rising FI rates, a hospitalwide inpatient FI screening was implemented to connect patients with appropriate resources as an advocacy initiative. The purpose of this study is to describe the implementation of a SDOH screening tool and describe the characteristics of hospitalized pediatric patients with a positive screen for household FI.

METHODS

The Hunger Vital Sign,[10] a validated 2-question screening tool for FI, was added to the intake questionnaire at a quaternary-care children's hospital in August 2020. The intake questionnaire is embedded within the electronic medical record (EMR) and is completed by bedside nursing with the patient's family/guardian at admission. The Hunger Vital Sign consists of the following 2 statements:

1. "Within the past 12 months, we worried whether our food would run out before we got money to buy more"; and

2. "Within the past 12 months, the food we bought just didn't last and we didn't have money to get more."[10]

Responses to each statement were: "never true," "sometimes true," "often true," and "don't know/refused." A positive screen for FI was defined as a response of often true or sometimes true to 1 or both statements. A negative screen for FI was defined as a response of never true. A screen that was not completed with the provided answer choices or completed as don't know/refused was considered as an incomplete screen. A screen that was completed with an answer of don't know/refused to 1 question and never true to the other question was also considered an incomplete screen. The screening was not a mandatory function in the EMR.

A positive screen for FI triggered a social work (SW) consult via the EMR. SW would perform an assessment specific to FI (Fig 1). Interventions for FI included providing the family with meal tickets to obtain food from the hospital cafeteria during the hospitalization, providing local food bank information for the patient's county of residence, and providing information on enrollment to the Supplemental Nutrition Assistance Program (SNAP) and/or the Women, Infant, and Children (WIC) Program if the family was not already enrolled.

Demographics were collected on admitted patients hospitalized from August 2020 to April 2021.

Further chart review was performed on patients with a positive screen for FI. Statistical analyses included 1-way analysis of variance in comparison of continuous data. For categorical data, Fisher's exact testing was used as the low incidence in FI observed as associated with very low expected values. To assist with the calculation of significance values, Monte Carlo simulation ($n = 50\,000$) was used. All statistical analyses were performed with SAS 9.4 (Cary, NC). This study was approved as exempt by the institutional review board.

RESULTS

There were 7751 admissions during the study period of August 2020 to April 2021, of which 4777 (61.6%) had an FI screen completed. There were 2974 (38.4%) admissions with a screen considered

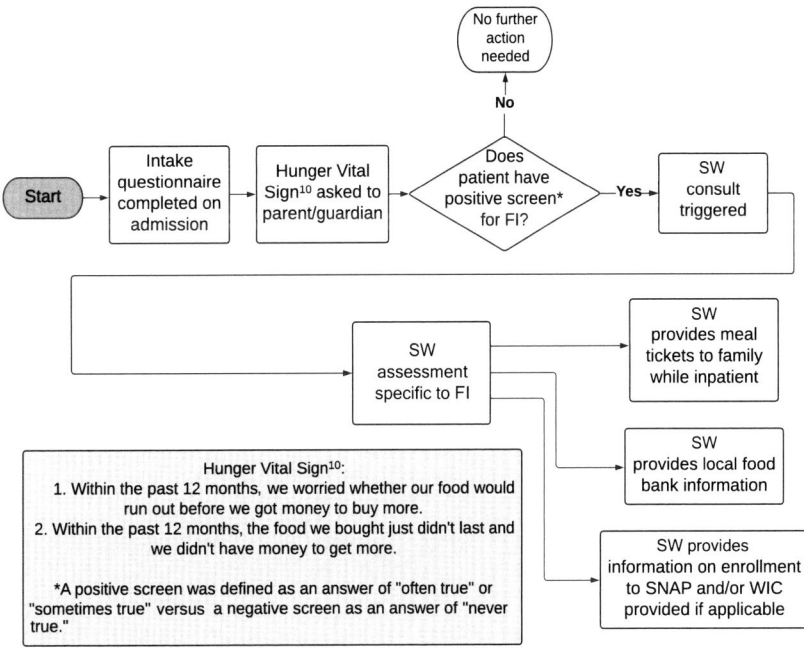

FIGURE 1 FI assessment.

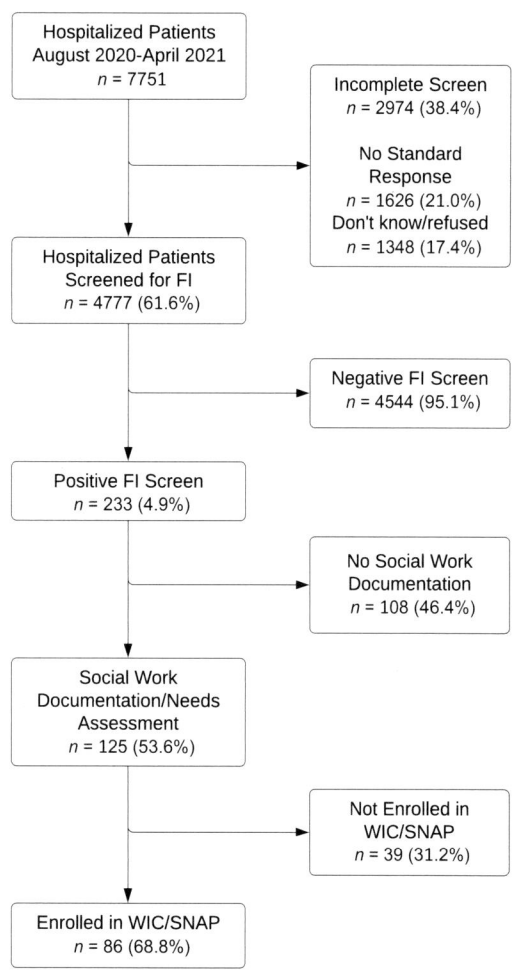

FIGURE 2 Flow diagram of screened patients.

incomplete (1348 [17.4%] with a response of don't know/refused and 1626 [21.0%] with no standard response to the screen documented). Among those with a completed screen, 233 patients (4.9%) were positive for household FI (Fig 2). Patients with household FI had an age range from 15 days to 22 years (mean age 8.7 years, interquartile range [IQR] 2–14 years) and were admitted to 17 unique service lines. Mean age was similar in patients with household FI and patients who had a negative screen for FI (mean age 8.3 years, IQR 2–14). Patients with an incomplete screen were younger with mean age of 7.7 years (IQR 1–13 years, $P < .001$). Patients with household FI were more likely to be Black ($P < .001$) and have Medicaid ($P < .001$). Additional demographics

can be found in Table 1. Of the positively screened FI patients, at least 1 previous medical diagnosis and at least 1 admission at our institution within the previous year was documented for 166 (74%) and 85 (36%) patients, respectively. SW documentation specific to FI was recorded for 125 of the 233 (54%) FI patients, of which 39 (31%) were not enrolled in WIC or SNAP.

DISCUSSION

This initiative highlights acute hospitalization as an opportunity to screen for FI using a multidisciplinary approach. Our findings are in line with previously described racial and insurance disparities related to FI.[5,6,9,11,12] The high proportion of existing medical diagnoses and previous hospitalization to our institution among

patients with FI underscores how often health care providers may interact with these patients. This furthers the importance of screening for FI and other SDOH in all health care settings. Similar practices could be implemented at other children's hospitals to identify FI and connect families to local and federal resources such as WIC and SNAP.

The proportion of patients with FI at our hospital was lower than expected on the basis of initial FI rates in our community before the COVID-19 pandemic. At the time of implementation, we anticipated a higher observed rate on the basis of reports of increasing FI rates.[7] This finding could be explained by the limitation that the screening tool was not a mandatory function of the admission intake questionnaire. Therefore, we may have missed patients living in food-insecure households in which the screen was not completed. Additionally, the screening was performed either verbally or written, which could lead to underreporting given the potentially sensitive nature of these questions and social desirability. Patient profile questionnaires are to be conducted in the preferred language of the patient; however, this study is limited in that we did not assess the language spoken, which may have led to underreporting of FI in non-English speaking populations. The pandemic also brought additional challenges with providing education to the bedside providers who performed the screening because the typical in-person education sessions had been postponed. This may have led to an answer response of don't know/refused to be used in situations where the bedside provider did not know the answer rather than the family reporting this answer, such as if a family was not at bedside. Though patients with an incomplete FI screen had a significantly lower mean age of 7.7 years as opposed to 8.7 years for patients who were FI and 8.3 years for patients who were not FI, it is unclear if this has clinical significance. Further investigation could be done to better characterize why this difference was seen, which could also help inform how best to address incomplete screens.

TABLE 1 Demographics of Children Screened for FI

	Food Insecure (n = 233)	Not Food Insecure (n = 4544)	Incomplete Screen (n = 2974)	P
Mean age, y (IQR)	8.7 (2–14)	8.3 (2–14)	7.7 (1–13)	<.001[a]
Sex, n (%)				.27[b]
Male	124 (53.2)	2365 (52.0)	1604 (53.9)	
Female	109 (46.8)	2179 (48.0)	1370 (46.1)	
Race/ethnicity				<.001[b]
White	103 (44.2)	2838 (62.5)	1662 (55.9)	
Black	123 (52.8)	1621 (35.7)	1244 (41.8)	
Asian American	0 (0)	45 (1.0)	22 (0.7)	
Hispanic	1 (0.4)	8 (0.2)	8 (0.3)	
Unknown	2 (0.9)	12 (0.3)	31 (1.0)	
Other	4 (1.7)	20 (0.4)	7 (0.2)	
Insurance type				<.001[b]
Medicaid	217 (93.1)	3345 (73.6)	2287 (76.6)	
Non-Medicaid	16 (6.9)	1199 (26.4)	687 (23.18)	

[a] One-way analysis of variance.
[b] Fisher's exact analysis, $P \leq .05$.

While FI and poverty are associated, they are not synonymous.[8] Literature has endorsed the relationship between racism and FI given the connection between racism on differences in socioeconomic status (SES) and in turn, FI.[8] In our population, patients with FI were more likely to be Black, and this association is consistent with previous research.[12] Although poverty and low SES are associated with FI, there are racial disparities in SES, and structural racism can contribute to these disparities.[8,13] One example of this may include hesitation to obtain government assistance because of concern for racial stereotypes.[8] Beyond economic disadvantage, social disadvantage among people of color should also be considered. In a study among African-American households in South Carolina, severity of household FI was associated with lifetime racial discrimination.[14]

We also hypothesize a potential relationship between FI and poor health care outcomes not addressed in this study. Appropriate nutrition is considered critical for physical health and neurodevelopment, especially from the time of conception through the first 2 years of life,[15] and FI can be associated with decreased quantity, as well as quality of available food. FI can also be a form of toxic stress.[1,16] Households experiencing FI may face difficult choices regarding how money is spent.[17] This exposure to FI and thus toxic stress affects the neuroendocrine-immune network, which could account for differences in health outcomes.[16] Although FI remains a complex issue and root causes should be addressed, screening and identifying FI can allow the medical team to intervene and mitigate the effects of FI. Future areas of study include evaluating FI as a potential high-yield screening tool for assessing risk of worse health care outcomes.

In response to initial findings and feedback, quality improvement methods have been implemented to standardize and improve the screening and resource provision process. This has included improving the education to providers regarding FI, screening flow, and resources. Future steps include follow-up with the family to determine if resources were obtained and used. If successful, there is opportunity to expand inpatient screening to include other SDOH to assess for risk of disparate hospital outcomes and connect patients to needed resources

with the ultimate goal of mitigating the effects of SDOH, including FI on child health.

REFERENCES

1. Ashbrook A, Essel K, Montez K, Bennett-Tejes D. American Academy of Pediatrics and the Food Research & Action Center. Screen and intervene: a toolkit for pediatricians to address food insecurity. 2021. Available at: https://frac.org/wp-content/uploads/FRAC_AAP_Toolkit_2021.pdf. Accessed January 21, 2022

2. Cook JT, Frank DA, Levenson SM, et al. Child food insecurity increases risks posed by household food insecurity to young children's health. *J Nutr.* 2006; 136(4):1073–1076

3. Kirkpatrick SI, McIntyre L, Potestio ML. Child hunger and long-term adverse consequences for health. *Arch Pediatr Adolesc Med.* 2010;164(8):754–762

4. Thomas MMC, Miller DP, Morrissey TW. Food insecurity and child health. *Pediatrics.* 2019;144(4):e20190397

5. Hake M, Dewey A, Engelhard E, et al. Feeding America. The impact of the coronavirus on food insecurity in 2020 & 2021. 2021. Available at: https://www.feedingamerica.org/sites/default/files/2021-03/National%20Projections%20Brief_3.9.2021_0.pdf. Accessed August 18, 2021

6. Hake M, Dewey A, Engelhard E, et al. Feeding America. The impact of coronavirus on food insecurity in 2020. Available at: https://www.feedingamerica.org/sites/default/files/2020-10/Brief_Local%20Impact_10.2020_0.pdf. Accessed August 19, 2021

7. America F. Child food insecurity in Alabama before COVID-19. Available at: https://map.feedingamerica.org/county/2018/child/alabama. Accessed August 19, 2021

8. Bowen S, Elliott A, Hardison-Moody A. The structural roots of food insecurity: how racism is a fundamental cause of food insecurity. *Sociol Compass.* 2021;15:e12846

9. Banach LP. Hospitalization: are we missing an opportunity to identify food

insecurity in children? *Acad Pediatr.* 2016;16(5):438–445

10. Hager ER, Quigg AM, Black MM, et al. Development and validity of a 2-item screen to identify families at risk for food insecurity. *Pediatrics.* 2010;126(1):e26–e32

11. Peltz A, Garg A. Food insecurity and health care use. *Pediatrics.* 2019;144(4): e20190347

12. Coleman-Jensen A, Rabbitt MP, Gregory CA, Singh A. U.S. Department of Agriculture Economic Research Service. Household food security in the United States in 2020. Available at: https://www. ers.usda.gov/webdocs/publications/102076/err-298.pdf?v=5134.6. Accessed January 24, 2022

13. Gundersen C, Kreider B, Pepper J. The economics of food insecurity in the United States. *Appl Econ Perspect Policy.* 2011;33(3):281–303

14. Burke MP, Jones SJ, Frongillo EA, Fram MS, Blake CE, Freedman DA. Severity of household food insecurity and lifetime racial discrimination among African-American households in South Carolina. *Ethn Health.* 2018;23(3):276–292

15. Schwarzenberg SJ, Georgieff MK. Committee on Nutrition. Advocacy for improving nutrition in the first 1000 days to support childhood development and adult health. *Pediatrics.* 2018;141(2): e20173716

16. Franke HA. Toxic stress: effects, prevention and treatment. *Children (Basel).* 2014;1(3):390–402

17. Fram MS, Frongillo EA, Jones SJ, et al. Children are aware of food insecurity and take responsibility for managing food resources. *J Nutr.* 2011;141(6):1114–1119

BRIEF REPORT

Evaluating Screening to Assess Endorsement of Food Insecurity in the Inpatient Setting

Kerry A. Tepe, BS,[a] Katherine A. Auger, MD, MSc,[a,b,c] Sonia Rodas Marquez, MD,[d] Denise Atarama, RD,[e] Hadley S. Sauers-Ford, MPH, CCRP[a]

A B S T R A C T

OBJECTIVE: Rates of food insecurity (FI) from screening in the inpatient setting is often not reflective of community prevalence, indicating that screening likely misses families with FI. We aimed to determine the combination of FI screening questions and methods that would result in identifying a percentage of FI families that matched or exceeded our area prevalence (approximately 20%).

METHODS: Research staff approached eligible English- and Spanish-speaking families across 4 inpatient units once weekly and screened for FI using a randomly selected method (face-to-face, phone, paper, and tablet). We asked questions from the 6-Item USDA Survey, Hunger Vital Sign screener, and questions utilized by our social workers.

RESULTS: We screened 361 families; 19.4% ($N = 70$) endorsed FI. Differences in rates were not significant by method. Differences in FI rates based on screening questions were: 17.7% for the 6-item USDA survey, 16.0% for Hunger Vital Sign, and 3.1% for the social work questions. When considering method and screening questions together, the 6-Item USDA on paper had the highest positivity rate of 20.9%. A higher percentage of Spanish-speaking families endorsed FI (61.1%) compared to 17.2% of English-speaking families ($P < .01$). Positivity also varied significantly by self-identified race ($P < .01$). Caregivers that identified as Hispanic or Latino were significantly more likely to endorse FI than those that did not ($P < .01$).

CONCLUSIONS: The positivity rate for FI while screening inpatient families using the 6-Item screening questions on paper matched our community prevalence of FI (approximately 20%).

www.hospitalpediatrics.org

DOI: https://doi.org/10.1542/hpeds.2023-007164

Copyright © 2024 by the American Academy of Pediatrics

Address correspondence to Kerry A. Tepe, BS, Cincinnati Children's Hospital Medical Center, 3333 Burnet Ave MLC 9016, Cincinnati, OH 45229. E-mail: Kerry.Tepe@cchmc.org

HOSPITAL PEDIATRICS (ISSN Numbers: Print, 2154-1663; Online, 2154-1671).

[a]*Division of Hospital Medicine,* [c]*James Anderson Center, and* [e]*Division of Nutritional Therapy, Cincinnati Children's Hospital Medical Center, Cincinnati, Ohio;* [b]*University of Cincinnati College of Medicine, Cincinnati, Ohio; and* [d]*Huntsville Hospital, Huntsville, Alabama*

Ms Tepe screened patients, assisted with acquisition and interpretation of data, and drafted the initial manuscript; Dr Auger conceptualized and designed the study, assisted in data interpretation, and reviewed and revised the manuscript; Ms Sauers-Ford conceptualized and designed the study, assisted in data interpretation, and reviewed and revised the manuscript; Dr Rodas Marquez and Ms Atarama screened patients and reviewed the manuscript; and all authors approved the final manuscript as submitted, and agree to be accountable for all aspects of the work.

FUNDING: This study was funded by the Place Outcomes Research Award at Cincinnati Children's Hospital Medical Center. All statements in this report, including findings and conclusions, are solely those of the authors and do not necessarily represent the views of the funding organization.

CONFLICT OF INTEREST DISCLOSURES: Ms Tepe, Dr Auger, and Ms Sauers-Ford's efforts were funded by the Place Outcomes Award. The other authors have indicated they have no conflicts of interest relevant to this article to disclose.

Of US households with children, 17% are food insecure,[1] defined as lacking access to enough food to fully meet nutritional needs. Adequate food among households is critical for proper development and growth of children, therefore food insecurity (FI) poses a major public health problem. FI can have negative effects on children, as it is associated with behavioral, academic, and emotional problems, and is a significant stressor for parents and caregivers.[2–4] Childhood hunger is associated with lower ratings of overall child health and wellbeing, worse outcomes from chronic illness, including mental illness,[5] and poor pediatric quality of life.[6]

Although many pediatric hospitals screen for FI,[7] often positivity rates are low.[8] This phenomenon has been seen at our own institution where positivity rates on routine FI screening by clinical staff were <10%; whereas our area prevalence of FI is much higher, between 19% and 31%.[9] Although prior research has shown nonverbal self-disclosure is more sensitive, these studies have been conducted in outpatient and emergency department settings.[10–12] We hypothesized that healthcare providers miss a significant number of families with FI because of either the wrong screening tool or a suboptimal screening method. Therefore, we sought to determine which combination of FI screening questions and methods resulted in a positivity rate that approximated or exceeded our area prevalence of 20%.

METHODS
Context

We surveyed caregivers across 4 inpatient units at both the main and satellite campuses of a freestanding children's hospital located in the Midwest. We screened caregivers on (1) a surgical short stay unit (SSS), (2) the transitional care center (TCC) unit, which admits children assisted mechanical ventilation outside of the intensive care unit, (3) the neuroscience unit (NNS), which includes both neurology and neurosurgery patients, and (4) the hospital medicine unit (HM) located at our satellite campus.

Study Design

We conducted a prospective study using a combination of 3 surveys and 4 methods to measure FI rates across our 4 study units. We approached all eligible caregivers of children hospitalized on a single unit 4 days a week (1 unit per day) using a screening method that was randomly-selected for each day; the order of the units was random such that a single unit was not always approached on the same day of the week. We used random number generation to randomize the unit and the method within week-long blocks. A research assistant and 2 Spanish-speaking qualified bilingual staff members conducted surveys. The survey was introduced to families as a tool for us to learn more about hospitalized patients and families.

We asked each caregiver questions from 3 surveys: (1) US Household Food Security Survey Module: 6-Item Short Form[13] (6-Item), (2) the Children's Health Watch Hunger Vital Sign[14] (a 2-item survey recommended by the American Academy of Pediatrics as a method to screen for FI),[15] and (3) questions currently utilized by our social workers (Supplemental Fig 2). Furthermore, we screened families

via 4 methods: face-to-face, phone, paper, and tablet. The face-to-face method consisted of a study team member approaching a caregiver at bedside and reading questions to them. For the phone call method, the study team called families, either on the in-hospital phone or the phone number listed in the electronic medical record. For the paper method, a study team member provided caregivers present in the hospital with a paper copy of the survey. The study team member then left the room and came back to collect the survey? 15 to 20 minutes later. Finally, for the tablet method, caregivers were given a tablet on which to complete the survey in REDCap. The study team member waited in the room while the caregiver completed the tablet survey.

Study Population

We included all English and Spanish speaking caregivers of children hospitalized on 1 of the study units from February to April 2022. We also included patients >18 years who lived independently, except those hospitalized for treatment of an eating disorder. We excluded caregivers of patients who lived in a skilled nursing facility, patients who had been hospitalized since birth, and those in the custody of child protective services. We classified patients as "unavailable" if the family was not in the room for medical reasons (ie, imaging, surgery, etc) or if the medical or nursing team was with the family while the study team was recruiting. Patients were classified as "no caregiver" if a caregiver was not present when the study team was on the unit or if there was no answer on either phone (phone call method). Patients were classified as "declined" when a caregiver declined to complete the survey. Each day we attempted to approach all eligible caregivers and patients on the unit (including those previously missed). Caregivers who had previously completed the survey or declined to do so were not approached again. This study was deemed exempt by Institutional Review Board review.

Defining positivity for FI: if a caregiver endorsed any FI item on any of the 3 surveys, the survey was considered positive. If any of the 3 surveys were positive, we classified the caregiver as endorsing FI (overall positive). For the caregivers that screened positive, we asked if they would like to speak with a social worker and provided them with a resource sheet.

Analysis

For bivariate analyses, we conducted chi square tests using STATA version 14 to examine for differences in overall positivity by survey method, clinical unit, race, ethnicity, language, and receipt of Supplemental Nutrition Assistance Program (SNAP) or Special Nutrition Assistance Program for Women, Infants, And Children (WIC) benefits. We also conducted a sensitivity analysis using multivariable logistic regression examining the association between method and overall positivity while accounting preferred language and unit. We selected these 2 covariates as it is reasonable that caregivers who prefer different languages may interpret the questions differently, making language an important covariate to include. Further, the method offered was not balanced across all hospital units but was balanced across all other

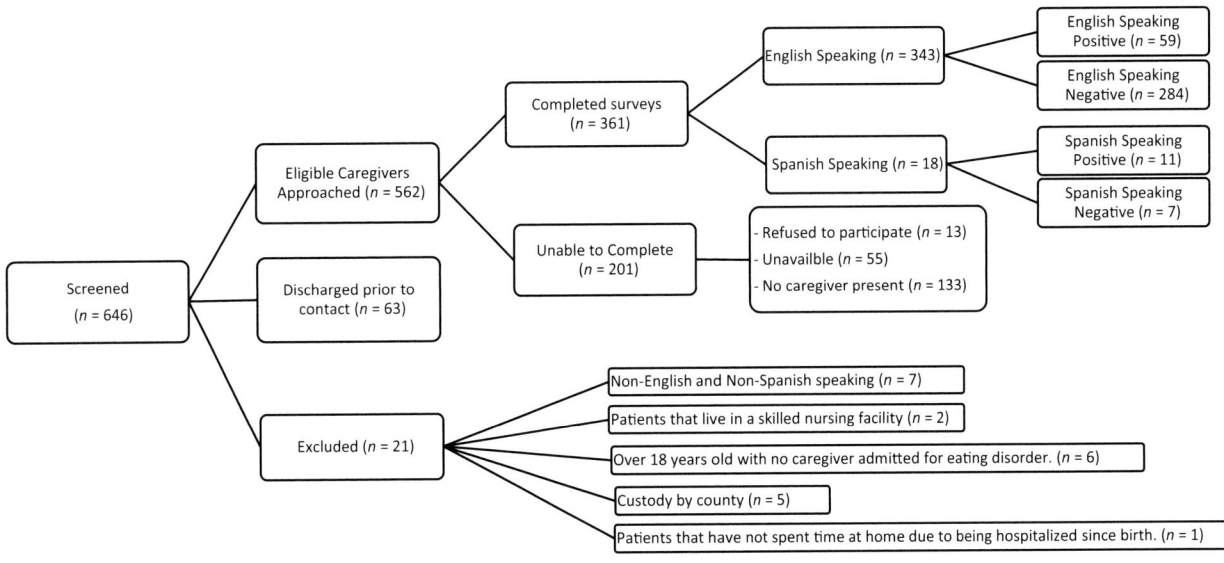

FIGURE 1 Breakdown of screening and approach numbers.

potential covariates. (Supplemental Table 3). We considered $P < .05$ statistically significant.

RESULTS

We assessed eligibility in 646 patients, and of those, 562 were eligible to be approached. We completed 361 surveys (64% of all eligible), 343 in English and 18 in Spanish. Of families unable to complete surveys, 55 patients were unavailable, 133 patients had no caregiver, and 13 patients declined (2.3% of eligible) (Fig 1). Overall, of the 361 caregivers who completed surveys, 19.4% ($N = 70$) endorsed FI.

Survey Questions and Methods

The 6-Item survey had 17.7% positivity rate, Hunger Vital Sign questions had a 16.0% positivity rate, and the social work questions had a 3.1% positivity rate. Regarding the method of screening, face-to-face had a positivity of 16.0%, paper 25.6%, tablet 17.2%, and phone 18.1%. The overall positivity rate did not vary significantly by method. (Table 1). In sensitivity analyses, the method of

screening was not statistically associated with positivity when accounting for language and hospital unit in multivariable analyses. When method and survey question were considered together, the 6-Item survey administered via paper had the highest positivity rate of 20.9%. The Hunger Vital Sign administered on paper had a very similar positivity rate of 19.8%.

Other Factors

The rates of FI did not vary significantly across the different hospital units; the TCC had a 31.43% positivity rate, the SSS had a 13.25% positivity rate, the NNS unit had a 17.88% positivity rate, and the satellite HM unit had a 22.83% positivity rate ($p = .10$) (Table 2).

Rates of FI varied significantly by preferred language, with 61.1% Spanish-speaking caregivers endorsing FI compared with only 17.2% of English-speaking caregivers ($P < .01$), despite a small number of caregivers who spoke Spanish ($n = 18$). The positivity rate also varied significantly by self-identified race ($P < .01$); 16.5% of caregivers who identified as white endorsed FI compared to 26.7% of caregivers

Method[a]	6-Item[b] $n = 360$ n (%, 95% CI)	HVS[c] $n = 360$ n (%, 95% CI)	SW[d] $n = 360$ n (%, 95% CI)	Overall Positivity Rate[a] n (%, 95% CI)
Face-to-face ($n = 81$)	12 (14.8, 7.9–24.4)	11 (13.6, 7.0–23.0)	1 (1.2, 0.03–6.7)	13 (16.0, 8.8–25.9)
Paper ($n = 86$)	18 (20.9, 12.9–31.0)	17 (19.8, 12.0–29.8)	6 (7.0, 2.6–14.6)	22 (25.6, 16.8–36.1)
Tablet ($n = 99$)	16 (16.2, 9.5–24.9)	15 (15.2, 8.7–23.8)	1 (1.0, 0.03–5.5)	17 (17.2, 10.3–26.1)
Phone ($n = 94$)	17 (18.1, 10.9–27.4)	14 (14.9, 8.4–23.7)	2 (2.1, 0.3–7.5)	17 (18.1, 10.9–27.4)

TABLE 1 Positivity by Method

[a] Positivity did not vary significantly by method of screening (chi-square, $P = .37$).
[b] 6-Item: US Household Food Security Survey Module: 6-Item Short Form.
[c] HVS: Children's Health Watch Hunger Vital Sign.
[d] SW: Questions utilized by social work across the institution.

TABLE 2 Positivity by Unit, Race, Ethnicity, and Language

	All Patients	Positive Patients
	N	N (%, 95% CI)
Total	361	
Unit [unit]		70 (19.4, 15.4–23.9)
SSS	83	11 (13.3, 6.8–22.5)
TCC	35	11 (31.4, 16.9–49.3)
NNS	151	27 (17.9, 12.1–24.9)
HM	92	21 (22.8, 14.7–32.8)
Race[ab]		48 (16.5, 12.4–21.3)
White	291	
Black or African American	30	8 (26.7, 12.3–45.9)
Asian or Pacific Islander	4	0 (0)
More than 1 race	16	3 (18.8, 0.0–37.9)
Other	18	11 (61.1, 38.6–83.6)
Ethnicity[ab]		
Non-Hispanic, Spanish, or Latino	326	54 (16.6, 12.7–21.1)
Hispanic, Spanish, or Latino	33	16 (48.5, 30.8–66.5)
Language[a]		
English	343	59 (17.2, 13.4–21.6)
Spanish	18	11 (61.1, 35.7–82.7)
Receives SNAP or WIC[a]		
Yes	92	31 (33.7, 24.2–44.3)
No	269	39 (14.5, 10.5–19.3)

[a] Indicates statistically significant variation in reporting food insecurity by group (chi square, all $P < .01$).
[b] Indicates 2 values were missing (not answered) for race and ethnicity.

who identified as Black; 61.1% of caregivers who selected other race on the survey also endorsed food insecurity. Significantly more caregivers that identified as Hispanic, Spanish, or Latino ethnicity endorsed FI (48.5%) compared with caregivers that did not identify as these ethnicities ($P < .01$). A total of 33.7% of respondents that receive SNAP or WIC benefits endorsed FI compared with only 14.5% of those that do not receive these benefits ($P < .01$) (Table 2).

DISCUSSION

Almost 20% of the families across our 4 study units endorsed FI. Screening using paper and the 6-Item had the highest positivity rate at 20.9%, though screening using paper and Hunger Vital Sign was also nearly identical. The highest rates of FI were seen in families whose primary language was Spanish, those identifying as nonwhite, those identifying as Hispanic, and those who receive SNAP or WIC benefits.

Overall, we found higher rates of FI (~20%) than most previously completed studies, including our own internal institutional screening.[16,17] The overall rate of FI in this work is consistent with the rate of FI in the community surrounding the hospital. Our study contrasts

to prior screening efforts in that screenings were completed by research staff unaffiliated with the medical team and at a different time than medical intake questions. Often FI screening questions are asked by clinical staff (usually nursing) upon admission. In another study that also used research staff for screening in an emergency department documented a FI rate similar to ours, 17.5%.[18] Importantly, our study also had a very low refusal rate (2.3% of those approached); this rate contrasts to previous studies with as many as 17% refusing screening.[17] Therefore, having an individual who is not affiliated with the clinical team completing screening separated from clinical care may be critical for families to feel comfortable endorsing FI. Although there are expenditures associated with having a dedicated individual to screen for FI and other social needs, hospitals may find hiring a dedicated care navigator to screen and offer resources a worthwhile investment. At minimum, this work offers an evidence-based intervention to improve FI screening rates to mirror community rates through a dedicated individual offering these screening questions.

We demonstrate disparities in FI rates across self-identified race as well as between Hispanic and non-Hispanic families. This finding is similar to prior research in the emergency department.[18] The intersection between social determinants of health, like FI, and structural racism has been well documented[19,20]; further work is needed to reduce these disparities and understand contextual factors that may exacerbate differences. Additionally, our study demonstrated that families at our hospital who receive supplemental food services, like SNAP and WIC, are still food insecure.

Our study has several limitations that should be noted. It was performed at a single hospital across 2 campuses. Further, the majority of caregivers in this population identified as white and had a preferred language of English, limiting generalizability. Second, all screening was done by a research team member; therefore, our rates could be difficult to replicate in a clinical environment without dedicated personnel; although, this may be needed to accurately identify families with FI. Third, as is inherent in all prospective studies, we do not know the rates of FI in nonresponders. Fourth, we did not pilot the survey as a whole, though both the 6-Item Survey and the Hunger Vital Sign are validated instruments. The additional social work questions were administrated after the other 2 surveys and should not threaten validity of either instrument. Additionally, although we screened over 360 families for FI, it is possible that we were underpowered to detect small differences in positivity by modality. Finally, our statistical analyses did not account for all possible confounders, including age, insurance, diagnosis, and medical complexity. Although some of these attributes may impact a child's risk for FI (eg, children with significant medical complexity are known to have increased medical expenses that may lead to or worsen FI[21]), it is unlikely that these attributes impacted the caregivers' understanding of the questions or the preferred modality.

CONCLUSIONS

The 6-Item Survey, when administered on paper, had a positivity rate of at least 20%, the a priori threshold that was established by the research team as it approximated our area prevalence. The Hunger Vital Sign administered on paper had a similar positivity rate (19.8%). Both surveys could be considered for future use. Future studies should evaluate interventions available to improve FI as it affects a significant proportion of inpatient families.

Acknowledgements

We want to acknowledge the following study team members who contributed to the success of this project: Dr Anita Shah, Dr Andrew Beck, Dr Ndidi Unaka, Stacey Litman, Samantha Ingham, Ericka Fortson, Stephanie Powers, and Dr Megan Smith. The use of REDCap was provided via grant support (UL1TR001425).

REFERENCES

1. Food Security in the U.S. Key statistics & graphics. Available at: https://www.ers.usda.gov/topics/food-nutrition-assistance/food-security-in-the-u-s/key-statistics-graphics/#foodsecure. Accessed December 5, 2023

2. Shankar P, Chung R, Frank DA. Association of food insecurity with children's behavioral, emotional, and academic outcomes: a systematic review. *J Dev Behav Pediatr.* 2017;38(2):135–150

3. Drennen CR, Coleman SM, Ettinger de Cuba S, et al. Food insecurity, health, and development in children under age four years. *Pediatrics.* 2019;144(4):e20190824

4. Lee AM, Lopez MA, Haq H, et al. Inpatient food insecurity in caregivers of hospitalized pediatric patients: a mixed methods study. *Acad Pediatr.* 2021;21(8):1404–1413

5. Weinreb L, Wehler C, Perloff J, et al. Hunger: its impact on children's health and mental health. *Pediatrics.* 2002;110(4):e41

6. Moafi F, Kazemi F, Samiei Siboni F, Alimoradi Z. The relationship between food security and quality of life among pregnant women. *BMC Pregnancy Childbirth.* 2018;18(1):319

7. Markowitz MA, Tiyyagura G, Quallen K, Rosenberg J. Food insecurity screening and intervention in United States children's hospitals. *Hosp Pediatr.* 2022;12(10):849–857

8. Hanna SL, Wu CL, Smola C, et al. Food insecurity screening of hospitalized patients: a descriptive analysis. *Hosp Pediatr.* 2022;12(6):e196–e200

9. Interact for Health. Community health status survey: 1 in 4 adults in our region report being food insecure. Available at: https://www.interactforhealth.org/upl/media/1_in_4_adults_in_our_region_report_being_food_insecure.pdf. Accessed September 7, 2021

10. Palakshappa D, Goodpasture M, Albertini L, Brown CL, Montez K, Skelton JA. Written versus verbal food insecurity screening in one primary care clinic. *Acad Pediatr.* 2020;20(2):203–207

11. Cullen D, Attridge M, Fein JA. Food for thought: a qualitative evaluation of caregiver preferences for food insecurity screening and resource referral. *Acad Pediatr.* 2020;20(8):1157–1162

12. Gottlieb L, Hessler D, Long D, Amaya A, Adler N. A randomized trial on screening for social determinants of health: the iScreen study. *Pediatrics.* 2014;134(6):1611–1618

13. U.S. Household Food Security Survey Module. U.S. household food security survey module: six-item short form. Available at: https://www.ers.usda.gov/media/8282/short2012.pdf. Accessed September 26, 2021

14. Hager ER, Quigg AM, Black MM, et al. Development and validity of a 2-item screen to identify families at risk for food insecurity. *Pediatrics.* 2010;126(1):e26–32

15. American Academy of Pediatrics. Food insecurity. Available at: https://www.aap.org/en/patient-care/food-insecurity/. Accessed December 14, 2022

16. Hardy R, Boch S, Keedy H, Chisolm D. Social determinants of health needs and pediatric health care use. *J Pediatr.* 2021;238:275–281.e1

17. Hanna SL, Wu CL, Smola C, et al. food insecurity screening of hospitalized patients: a descriptive analysis. *Hosp Pediatr.* 2022;12(6):e196–e200

18. Gonzalez JV, Hartford EA, Moore J, Brown JC. Food insecurity in a pediatric emergency department and the feasibility of universal screening. *West J Emerg Med.* 2021;22(6):1295–1300

19. Johnson TJ. Intersection of bias, structural racism, and social determinants with health care inequities. *Pediatrics.* 2020;146(2):e2020003657

20. Bailey ZD, Krieger N, Agénor M, Graves J, Linos N, Bassett MT. Structural racism and health inequities in the USA: evidence and interventions. *Lancet.* 2017;389(10077):1453–1463

21. Thomson J, Shah SS, Simmons JM, et al. Financial and social hardships in families of children with medical complexity. *J Pediatr.* 2016;172:187–193.e1

RESEARCH ARTICLE

Quality Improvement to Identify and Address Food Insecurity During Pediatric Hospitalizations

Cristin Q. Fritz, MD, MPH,[a,b] Gabrielle C. Lyons,[b] Amber R. Monaghan, RN, MSN, CPN,[a] Joseph R. Starnes, MD, MPH,[a] Sarah Hart, MSN, APRN, CPNP-AC,[a] Caroline B. Khanna,[b] David P. Johnson, MD[a,b]

OBJECTIVES: Hospitalized children represent a vulnerable population with high rates of unidentified food insecurity (FI). We aimed to improve FI screening for eligible families from 0% to 60%. Secondarily, we sought to provide location-based food resources to families that screened positive.

METHODS: In February 2021, we developed a multidisciplinary team and used the Model for Improvement to improve routine FI screening for eligible children on 1 inpatient unit at a single institution. Our primary measure was the overall percentage of eligible families screened for FI. Our secondary measure was the percentage of families with FI who received food resource information. Statistical process control charts were used to analyze the impact of our interventions.

RESULTS: A total of 8850 families were eligible for screening during the project period. The percentage of eligible families screened for FI increased from 0 to a mean of 77%, exceeding our goal, with special cause variation noted by 5 centerline shifts. The most impactful interventions were expansion of screening to patients admitted to all services and making FI screening questions required nursing admission documentation. Eleven percent of families screened positive for FI. Provision of resources increased from 56% with manual resource insertion into the after-visit summary to 100% with special cause variation associated with automated resource provision for positive screens.

CONCLUSIONS: Integrating FI screening into the nursing admission workflow with automated resource provision for positive screens is a feasible approach to integrating FI screening into routine clinical practice during pediatric hospitalizations.

www.hospitalpediatrics.org

DOI:https://doi.org/10.1542/hpeds.2024-007926

Copyright © 2024 by the American Academy of Pediatrics

Address correspondence to Cristin Q. Fritz, MD, MPH, Monroe Carell Jr. Children's Hospital at Vanderbilt, Pediatric Hospital Medicine, 2200 Children's Way, Nashville, TN 37232. E-mail: cristin.fritz@vumc.org

HOSPITAL PEDIATRICS (ISSN Numbers: Print, 2154-1663; Online, 2154-1671).

Dr Fritz conceptualized and designed the study, conducted and supervised data collection, analyzed the data, and drafted the initial manuscript; Ms Khana, Ms Hart, Ms Monaghan, and Dr Starnes collected data; Ms Lyons collected data and drafted the initial manuscript; Dr Johnson coordinated data collection and analyzed data; and all authors critically reviewed and revised the manuscript, approved the final manuscript as submitted, and agree to be accountable for all aspects of the work.

[a]Vanderbilt University Medical Center, Nashville, Tennessee, and [b]Vanderbilt University School of Medicine, Nashville, Tennessee

FUNDING: Dr Starnes is supported by grant T32 HS026122 from the Agency for Healthcare Research and Quality. The content is solely the responsibility of the authors and does not necessarily represent the official views of the Agency for Healthcare Research and Quality.

CONFLICT OF INTEREST DISCLOSURES: The authors have indicated they have no conflicts of interest relevant to this article to disclose.

Food insecurity (FI), the lack of consistent access to enough food to lead active and healthy lives,[1] occurred in 12.5% of US households with children in 2021.[2] FI is associated with adverse health outcomes including increased rates of diabetes, hypertension, anxiety, depression, and behavioral dysregulation.[3–6] Additionally, FI disproportionately impacts families who are low-income, immigrants, nonwhite, and single-parent households, thereby contributing to disparities in health outcomes.[7–9] Connection to food resources improves family food security and child health outcomes.[10,11] Thus, the American Academy of Pediatrics recommends screening to identify FI and intervene as soon as possible.[12]

Screening for social needs such as FI during inpatient admission is acceptable to families.[13,14] It is important to identify and address FI in hospitalized children because of higher rates of FI in this population,[15] the increased financial stress hospitalization places on low socioeconomic status families,[16,17] and lack of consistent medical home among many children.[18] The importance of addressing social needs as part of inpatient care is supported by recent mandates to screen for health-related social needs, including FI, by the Centers for Medicare and Medicaid Services and the Joint Commission.[19,20] However, this is not yet done as part of routine clinical care at children's hospitals across the country.[21,22]

Lacking social needs screening at our own institution, we applied quality improvement (QI) methodology to develop and implement FI screening as part of routine clinical care. We aimed to improve FI screening for eligible families from 0% to 60% within 2 years of initial screening implementation (July 2023).

METHODS
Context

Monroe Carell Jr. Children's Hospital at Vanderbilt is a 343-bed academic tertiary care pediatric hospital located in Nashville, Tennessee.[23] The hospital's patient population includes children from urban, suburban, and rural areas. In 2022 to 2023, 54.3% of admitted patients were insured by Medicaid. English (87.6%), Spanish (9.1%), and Arabic (1.4%) were the 3 most common preferred languages. The prevalence of FI in Tennessee at the time of this project was 11.5%.[24] This QI project took place on the 42-bed pediatric medicine acute care (PMAC) unit, a general pediatric inpatient unit with patients on medical or surgical services. The unit is staffed by attending physicians, advanced practice providers, residents, medical students, and pediatric nurses. Among pediatric nurses, the admission/discharge/transfer (ADT) nursing team on the PMAC unit is primarily responsible for patient intake between 11 AM and 9 PM on weekdays. Bedside nurses perform intake outside of these hours and during times of high admission volume. Previously, there was no routine screening for FI or other social needs occurring at any time during hospitalization. In the absence of routine screening, FI was only addressed if needs identified by a patient's care team prompted a social work (SW) consult. Our hospital system utilizes EPIC (Verona, Wisconsin) as its electronic health record (EHR).

Intervention

We used the Model for Improvement as a framework to guide this project.[25] The interprofessional QI team included unit physician and nursing leadership, attending pediatric hospital medicine (PHM) physicians, a PHM advanced practice provider, ADT nurses, social workers, pediatric residents, and medical students. Bedside nursing champions and SW leadership were also involved in key meetings and decisions. The team developed a key driver diagram to guide development of a FI screening process and referral to resources (Fig 1). Primary drivers included:

1. routine screening that accurately identifies FI;

2. clear communication between care team members and families;

3. buy-in from providers, nursing, SW, and families on the importance of addressing FI in the hospital;

4. availability of user-friendly food resources; and

5. documentation of screening results and response in the EHR.

Plan-Do-Study-Act (PDSA) cycles were used to identify, implement, and assess interventions targeting these key drivers.

Our hospital has a well-established family advisory council. This project's team leader worked with the council and developed a subcommittee focused on providing insight into FI screening and resource provision. The team leader partnered with them throughout the project to codesign interventions and receive feedback about the process from the caregiver perspective.

Plan-Do-Study-Act Cycles

In February 2021, PDSA cycles began for families cared for by the PHM service on PMAC. In the initial tests of change, ADT nurses provided families a paper screening form that included the hunger vital sign questions[26] at the time of nursing admission intake. See Fig 2 for full process maps of initial and current screening processes. Admission was chosen as the time to conduct screening for the following reasons:

1. ability to integrate into an existing nursing workflow;

2. hypothesized increased likelihood of caregiver presence during admission; and

3. to allow time to address positive screens.

A paper screening form completed by the family was intentionally prioritized over verbal screening on the basis of evidence of improved social risk disclosure when families do not have to discuss them aloud.[27,28] The paper form was available in the 3 most preferred languages at the hospital: Arabic, English, and Spanish. Families were considered to have a positive FI screen if they answered "sometimes" or "often" to at least 1 question. Screens were considered high risk if they answered often to at least 1 question, implying the experience of chronic

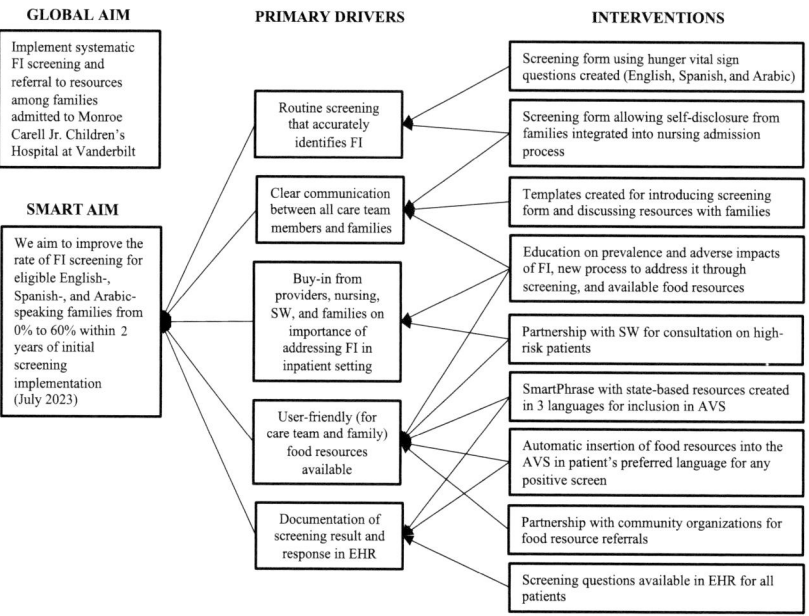

FIGURE 1 Key driver diagram.

FI. For positive screens, the physician team manually inserted an Epic SmartPhrase listing state-based food resources in the patient's preferred language into the after-visit summary (AVS) (Supplemental Information). Nurses reviewed this resource handout with families along with other discharge paperwork. In response to a high-risk screen, the physician team placed an SW consult to review available food resources with the family and assess for and address cooccurring social risks. Bedside nurses could also place an order for 1 daily, free guest tray at the family's request.

Subsequent interventions included standardizing our screening process, sending audit and feedback e-mails to PMAC nursing, integrating screening questions into the nursing admission history in the EHR and automating AVS resource provision for positive screens (Supplemental Information, AVS Food Resources and SmartText), expanding screening to patients on all services, making screening questions required documentation, and providing education to clinical team members throughout the project. Each PDSA cycle and its associated key driver(s) and lessons learned are described in Table 1.

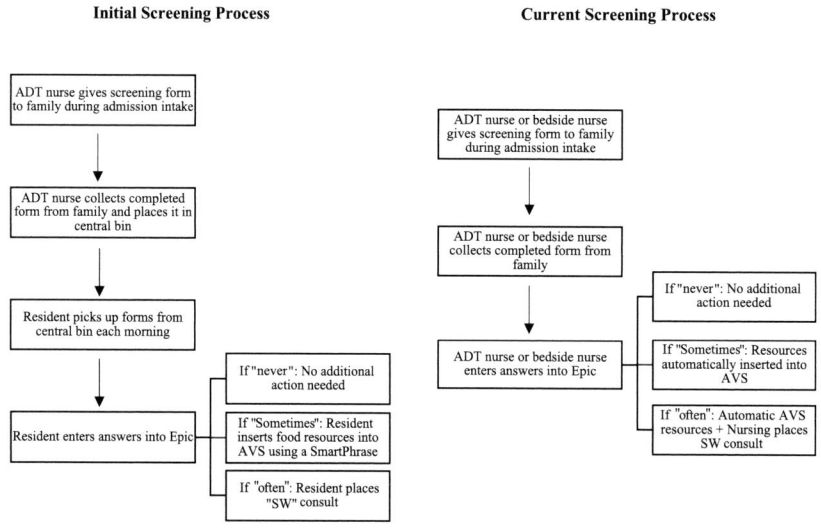

FIGURE 2 Initial and current FI screening processes.

TABLE 1 PDSA Cycle Interventions and Lessons Learned

PDSA Cycle	Date	Description	Lessons Learned
Initial PDSA cycle	February 2021	FI screening was performed by ADT nurses caring for PHM patients on the PMAC.	Implementing FI screening within an established nursing workflow allowed for rapid introduction of the process.
		ADTs placed completed forms in central location to be picked up daily by residents rotating on the PHM service.	Requiring handoffs of a paper screening form was an unreliable process.
		For positive screens, residents inserted food resource information into AVS using a SmartPhrase and placed an SW consult for high-risk screens.	Frequent turnover of residents on PHM service led to unreliable form pickup.
			A SmartPhrase for resource provision was convenient, but still relied on the discharging provider's recognition of a positive FI screen and knowledge of the screening process.
Bedside nurse screening expansion	November 2021	FI screening was performed by PMAC bedside nurses in addition to ADT nurses, expanding the reach of screening.	ADT nurses who were already familiar with the process were able to coach and support bedside nurses as they were introduced to the process.
Standardization of form pickup	January 2022	FI screening forms were picked up daily, Monday–Friday, by a designated PHM advanced practice nurse.	Consistency of form pickup responsibility created a more reliable process.
Audit and feedback	Biweekly from April 2022 to June 2022; November 2022	Audit of FI screening rates, as well as information on reason for the FI screening, the screening process, and the eligible patient population was provided to ADT and bedside nursing through e-mail.	Providing reminders of the screening initiative and evidence of underperformance improved fidelity to the process.
Resource provision enhancements	July 2022	The health information technology team built EHR logic so that a food resource information handout in the family's preferred language was automatically inserted into the AVS for any positive response to FI screening (Supplemental Information).	Eliminating the need for the physician team to manually add the SmartPhrase into the AVS increased reliability of resource provision.
		Nursing placed an SW consult for high-risk screens at time of admission.	Nursing responsibility for consulting SW increased promptness of consult placement.
EHR integration	August 2022	FI screening questions were added to the nursing admission intake form in Epic. Though paper forms continued to be used to preserve caregiver privacy, nurses were able to input responses from paper forms directly into Epic during the admission intake process (Fig 2).	Eliminating a paper form handoff increased reliability of the process.
			Medical receptionist team assumed they no longer needed to print screening forms with questions in the nursing admission intake, leading to a decline in screening rates. This misconception was successfully addressed with unitwide education.
Scaling	January 2023	Data from PDSA cycles of screening among PHM patients were used to gain institutional approval to scale FI screening to all patients on PMAC unit, regardless of primary service.	Evidence of success within the initial population supported expansion of a screening process within the institution.
			Broadening screening eligibility prompted greater adherence to the process by eliminating the need to identify eligible patients.
Key stakeholder interviews	May 2023	Semistructured interviews with 10 PMAC bedside nurses and 10 caregivers on PMAC who completed FI screening were completed. Questions gathered nurses' perspectives on successes and challenges of conducting screening and families' perspectives on how to improve the screening experience and how to best discuss resources available (Supplemental Information).	Interviews guided continued process improvements including additional nursing education on available food resources and advocacy for additional food resources during admission for families experiencing FI.

TABLE 1 Continued			
PDSA Cycle	Date	Description	Lessons Learned
Documentation requirement	May 2023	FI screening fields became a required component of intake documentation. The status of required indicates to the nursing team that this is an expected component of documentation and is indicated by a green checkmark when complete, but it does not confer a hard stop on the admission process if left incomplete.	FI screening could not be a hard stop admission documentation requirement given a variety of scenarios when form completion is not possible.
			The visual reminder of achieving a green checkmark for completing required documentation was an effective tool.
SW consult BPA	June 2023	Health information technology team built EHR logic so that a best practice alert appears with suggestion for SW consult using new consult indication of FI screening when an answer of often is documented in response to an FI screening question during the nursing admission process.	Standardized consult indication helped SW team appropriately identify who will respond to the consult.
Education	Throughout	During the initial screening process, education about FI and FI screening targeted ADT nurses and pediatric residents.	Standardized scripts for introducing FI screening, responding to a positive FI screen, and reviewing food resource information increased nursing comfort with the new process.
		Later, education focused on bedside nurses.	
BPA, best practice alert.			

To gauge nursing buy-in and parent perceptions of the screening process, we also conducted stakeholder interviews with a subset of 10 randomly selected PMAC nurses and 10 screened families. Each stakeholder was approached by a team member and completed a short questionnaire (Supplemental Information, Interviews) in a private location.

Eligible patients initially included Arabic-, English-, and Spanish-speaking families admitted to a PHM team on PMAC, then families preferring those same languages admitted to any team on PMAC, and finally all patients on PMAC. Once all patients on the unit were eligible, families that preferred languages other than English, Spanish, or Arabic had their screening form completed and resource handout information reviewed with the assistance of an interpreter. Screening was conducted once during each admission for any patient with multiple admissions during the study time frame.

Measures

Data, including screening results and social work consult (yes/no), were collected for eligible patients prospectively throughout the project via a report generated within the EHR by a member of the improvement team.

Primary Measure

The primary measure was the percentage of eligible families with FI screening documented during their admission. Data from each unique admission were included in analyses. To monitor for inequity in the screening process, the percentage of eligible families with documented FI screening was also stratified by preferred language (ie, number of screened families who prefer Spanish/number of eligible families who prefer Spanish).

Secondary Measure

We measured the percentage of screened patients who reported FI. To ensure resource information was being provided to families, our secondary measure was the percentage of families with a positive FI screen documented who received food resource information. Inclusion of food resource information in the AVS was determined through chart review for each patient with a positive screen.

Balancing Measure

The balancing measure was the percentage of families screened for FI with an SW consult ordered during their admission. This measure was included to monitor for a substantial increase in SW consults because of the screening process.

Analysis

Descriptive statistics were calculated for insurance status and preferred language overall, and by FI screening result.

Study of the Interventions

Data for all measures were grouped weekly except for the Arabic language stratification, which was grouped into consecutive groups of 5 given the small sample. Appropriate statistical process control p-charts were used to analyze the impact of interventions on process, outcome, and balancing measures and to identify special cause variation.[29] For the secondary measure of food resource provision in the AVS, the team followed the data prospectively in a p-chart but transitioned to a g-chart for the purposes of the manuscript given the abundance of weekly data points at 100%. Statistical process control charts were generated using QI charts (Process Improvement Products, San Antonio, Texas).

Ethical Considerations

The Vanderbilt University institutional review board approved this QI project as a nonresearch study. This manuscript was written according to the Standards for Quality Improvement Reporting Excellence 2.0 guidelines.[30]

RESULTS

A total of 8850 admissions between February 15, 2021, and August 6, 2023, were eligible for FI screening. Among the 2801 patients screened, 1% preferred Arabic, 91% preferred English, 7.5% preferred Spanish, and 0.5% preferred another language. Over half (56.1%) were insured by Medicaid. A total of 5.1% of screened patients had >1 admission during the study period.

Primary Measure

Five instances of special cause variation resulted in centerline shifts with cumulative improvement from 0% to 77% during the study period. Key interventions included testing of the FI screening process, standardization of daily screening form collection, audit and feedback e-mails to the nursing team, expansion of screening to patients admitted to all services, and making FI screening questions required, but not "hard-stop," nursing admission documentation (Fig 3). There was 1 point outside the control limits associated with the initial testing of EHR-based screening questions conducted among the ADT nursing team in preparation for implementing the new screening process with all PMAC nurses.

Improvements were observed in screening percentages for English-, Spanish-, and Arabic-speaking families. However, the means for families who preferred Spanish (59.4%) and Arabic (30.8%) were lower than the English-speaking (78.0%) families at the end of the data period (Supplemental Figs 5a–5c).

Secondary Measure

Among families screened, 11% (310) screened positive for FI, with 1.5% (42) reporting chronic FI. Among those screening positive, 1.3% preferred Arabic, 73.4% preferred English, 24.9% preferred Spanish, and 0.3% preferred another language. The majority (82.9%) were publicly insured. Special cause variation on the g-chart was associated with the automated EHR resource provision for positive FI screens, with the study concluding with 234 consecutive successful information provisions for families with a positive screen, well above the upper control limit (Fig 4).

Balancing Measure

The rate of SW consults among screened patients remained stable at a mean of 13% throughout the study period (Supplemental Fig 6), indicating that the FI screening process did not meaningfully impact SW consult volume. Two observed instances of special cause variation were separated by over a year, but investigation into these weeks did not reveal any insight into the potential causes of the increased SW consults.

Stakeholder Interviews

Interviews with bedside nurses revealed support for screening and appreciation for the paper screening form, as well as the opportunity to play a role in helping families get needed resources.

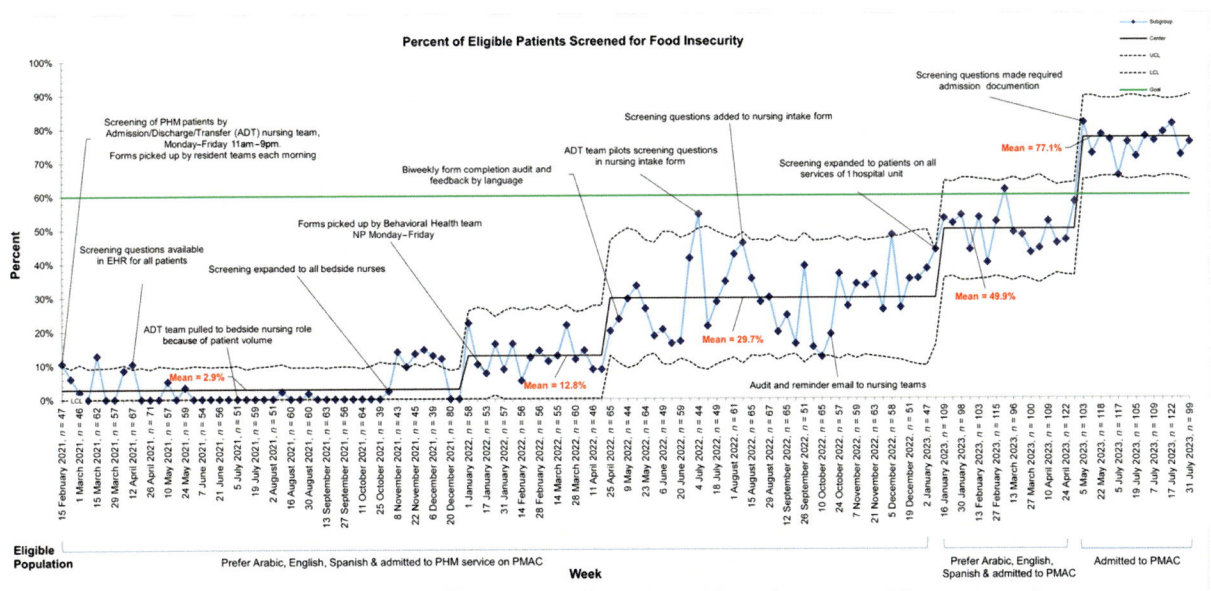

FIGURE 3 Percentage of eligible families with FI screening documented. Eligible families: February 2021 to December 2022: Prefer Arabic, English, or Spanish and admitted to PHM service on PMAC; January to April 2023: Prefer Arabic, English, or Spanish and admitted to any service on PMAC; May to July 2023: All patients admitted to PMAC.

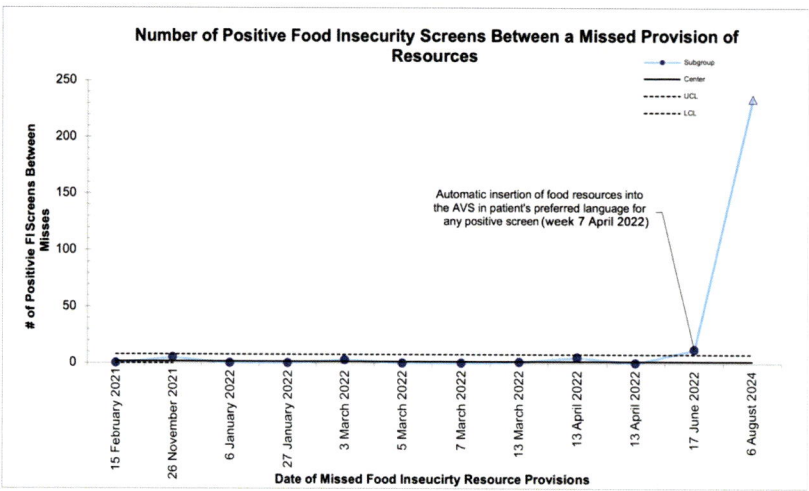

FIGURE 4 G-chart representing the number of positive FI screens between missing FI resources in the AVS. The open triangle as the last data point represents the end of the data set and not a missed opportunity to provide resources.

Families reported being receptive to, and even appreciative of, being asked the screening questions (Supplemental Information, Interviews).

DISCUSSION

Our multidisciplinary team successfully implemented FI screening at the time of hospital admission as part of routine clinical care in a tertiary, freestanding children's hospital. Using QI methodology and PDSA ramps, we scaled screening conducted by a specialized nursing team on a single unit among Arabic-, English-, and Spanish-speaking patients on PHM teams to all patients admitted to the hospital unit. We achieved our Specific, Measurable, Achievable, Relevant, Time-bound (SMART) aim by screening 77% of eligible patients. Using EHR automation, we provided food resource information to 100% of families (234 consecutive families) with a positive screen without a significant increase in SW consults among screened patients. This work demonstrates that FI screening can be completed routinely as part of hospital care with reliable resource provision.

Despite growing interest, limited reports exist describing efforts to integrate FI screening into routine clinical care for all patients on a general inpatient unit that can be used to guide hospitalwide FI screening. QI efforts focused on comprehensive social risk screening that included FI as 1 of the domains that have been implemented on specialized units, but these only screened English-speaking families via research assistants or residents.[31,32] Another QI initiative aimed to identify and address caregiver hunger during admission, with screening and interventions provided by a research assistant.[33] One freestanding academic children's hospital in the Southeast initiated hospitalwide screening for FI by incorporating the hunger vital sign questions into nursing admission intake. A positive screen triggered an SW consult to connect families with resources. During their study period, 61.6% of eligible admissions had an FI screen completed, with 4.9% of screened patients reporting FI.[34]

We began our screening pilot on a small scale using an approach similar to Hanna et al,[34] while also expanding on their work by including patients who prefer languages other than English and employing QI methodology to develop and test our approach. Because it was built using existing infrastructure, our initial screening approach involved a convoluted process with many steps reliant on multidisciplinary, rotating care team members integrating new tasks into their workflow (Fig 2a). This complexity is reflected in the low screening rates throughout the duration of this process. However, these initial data were instrumental in demonstrating feasibility, nursing buy-in, and the need for a more streamlined process to leadership. This ultimately resulted in our ability to integrate screening questions into the EHR nursing admission intake.

EHR integration represented a notable improvement in the reliability of our process but did not result in a sustained increase in screening rates like we had anticipated. Our most impactful interventions were expanding screening to patients on all services on PMAC and making screening questions required admission documentation. This highlights the benefit of decreasing the cognitive load required to identify eligible patients by making screening part of the standard admission process for every patient. Additionally, the use of a visual reminder (green checkmark) that accompanies the required documentation workflow, even without the questions being a true hard stop to the admission process, is an effective tool to remind and motivate staff to complete tasks. Early buy-in from nursing leadership and longitudinal support from nursing champions were also key components of successfully implementing and expanding this process. Other teams aiming to change behavior may consider incorporating these intervention approaches.

We saw a lower screening rate among families who prefer Spanish when examining data across the full study period (Supplemental Fig 7). There were sustained improvements with the Spanish population associated with adding screening questions to the EHR and making them required documentation and the Arabic population when screening expanded to all nurses, but not in response to other interventions that resulted in special cause among the full cohort and families who prefer English (Fig 3, Supplemental Fig 5 A–C). Possible explanations for this disparity were provided by patient and bedside nurse feedback throughout the project and are a focus for future interventions. These include limited introduction to why the forms are being provided when using an interpreter to complete an admission, unclear translation, inaccurate documentation of preferred language (ie, actually prefer Chuj instead of Spanish), or team difficulty in transcribing responses into the EHR. Importantly, this discrepancy in screening rates highlights the need for constant monitoring to ensure disparities do not develop as a result of interventions that lead to success within the overall cohort.

To improve screening rates among patients who prefer languages other than English, and to get closer to universal screening completion in general, additional measures such as better understanding of how to introduce screening forms in a culturally acceptable manner, additional translation services, and EHR reminders to circle back to complete unanswered questions outside of the admission period for patients with parents who are not at bedside during admission are likely needed.

Eleven percent of screened families reported FI, within the range of 5% to 38% in the existing literature[15,34,35] and similar to the local prevalence of 11.5%.[24] Our system of automated resource insertion into the AVS for patients screening positive resulted in consistent provision of food resource information for families experiencing FI. Because of limited ability for our SW team to support an increased consult volume, we developed a triage system to address positive screens that involved flagging only high-risk patients for an SW consult. Anecdotally, team members were entering consults for these high-risk patients, though our system does not allow us to capture whether an SW consult was placed specifically for FI. Although the most effective and desirable method of connecting families to resources from the hospital remains unknown, there is evidence from the acute care setting that provision of targeted resource handouts is noninferior to navigator assistance in decreasing social risks and improving child health.[36] Despite serving a population across a wide geographic area, we tried to ensure all families had relevant resource information by including quick-response codes that allow families to search for resources by zip code.

Limitations of this work include possible missing data during the time frame of our initial screening process that required transfer of screening forms between team members before entry into the EHR. We would expect this to result in an underestimation of our screening rate during that time, and there are clear trends toward improvement associated with specific interventions after transition to a more reliable, EHR-based screening process. Because this study was conducted on 1 unit at a single academic, freestanding children's hospital with an ADT nursing team, our specific process may not be generalizable to other institutions with different nursing infrastructure. Additionally, our most reliable interventions were designed within Epic, which may not translate directly to other EHRs. Nevertheless, this approach can be adapted to the specific nursing workflow and EHR infrastructure within any institution. Finally, following up with patients after discharge to determine who used the provided information to access resources was outside the scope of this QI project, but is an important focus for future research to guide effective inpatient social resource interventions.

CONCLUSIONS

We used QI methodology to test and implement FI screening as part of routine clinical care during nursing admission intake. Building this screening process has supported ongoing work to create a more robust response to positive screens including hiring an inpatient resource specialist. Health care systems with limited SW support may consider automated inclusion of food resource information in a family's preferred language in their discharge papers as an initial step toward addressing needs within their population. This is a feasible approach for hospitals to consider as they develop systems to screen for and address social risks in response to Centers for Medicare and Medicaid Services and Joint Commission mandates.

Acknowledgments

We thank bedside champions Dr Courtney Svenstrup, Shelby Gunther, Beth Loats, and the PMAC ADT and bedside nursing team; Julie Garcia, Brittany Davis, and Nyah Cade for assistance developing patient resources and SW support throughout the project; and Karen Wilson and the health information technology team that built our EHR-related interventions.

COMPANION PAPER: A companion to this article can be found online at www.hosppeds.org/cgi/doi/10.1542/hpeds.2024-008061.

REFERENCES

1. USDA. Food security in the United States: overview. Available at: https://www.ers.usda.gov/topics/food-nutrition-assistance/food-security-in-the-u-s/. Accessed January 26, 2022

2. Coleman-Jensen A, Rabbitt MP, Gregory CA, Singh A. Household Food Security in the United States in 2020, ERR-298. US Department of Agriculture, Economic Research Service; 2021

3. Cook JT, Frank DA, Berkowitz C, et al. Food insecurity is associated with adverse health outcomes among human infants and toddlers. *J Nutr.* 2004;134(6):1432–1438

4. Kirkpatrick SI, McIntyre L, Potestio ML. Child hunger and long-term adverse consequences for health. *Arch Pediatr Adolesc Med.* 2010;164(8):754–762

5. Melchior M, Chastang JF, Falissard B, et al. Food insecurity and children's mental health: a prospective birth cohort study. *PLoS One.* 2012;7(12):e52615

6. Rose-Jacobs R, Black MM, Casey PH, et al. Household food insecurity: associations with at-risk infant and toddler development. *Pediatrics.* 2008;121(1):65–72

7. USDA Economic Research Service. Food security in the United States: key statistics and graphics. Available at: https://www.ers.usda.gov/topics/food-nutrition-assistance/food-security-in-the-u-s/key-statistics-graphics/#:~:text=10.5%20percent%20(13.8%20million)%20of,from%2010.5%20percent%20in%202019. Accessed January 21, 2022

8. The Vanderbilt Center for Child Health Policy. Available at: https://www.vumc.org/childhealthpolicy/child-health-poll. Accessed February 10, 2022

9. Palakshappa D, Garg A, Peltz A, Wong CA, Cholera R, Berkowitz SA. Food insecurity was associated with greater family health care expenditures in the United States, 2016–2017. *Health affairs (Project Hope).* 2023;42(1):44–52

10. Black MM, Cutts DB, Frank DA, et al. Children's Sentinel Nutritional Assessment Program Study Group. Special Supplemental Nutrition Program for Women, Infants, and Children participation and infants' growth and health: a multisite surveillance study. *Pediatrics.* 2004;114(1):169–176

11. Center on Budget and Policy Priorities. SNAP is linked with improved nutritional outcomes and lower health care costs. Available at: https://www.cbpp.org/research/food-assistance/snap-is-linked-with-improved-nutritional-outcomes-and-lower-health-care. Accessed August 8, 2019

12. Council on Community Pediatrics; Committee on Nutrition. Promoting food security for all children. *Pediatrics.* 2015;136(5): e1431–e1438

13. Colvin JD, Bettenhausen JL, Anderson-Carpenter KD, Collie-Akers V, Chung PJ. Caregiver opinion of in-hospital screening for unmet social needs by pediatric residents. *Acad Pediatr.* 2016;16(2): 161–167

14. Leary JC, Rijhwani L, Bettez NM, et al. Parent perspectives on screening for social needs during pediatric hospitalizations. *Hosp Pediatr.* 2022;12(8):681–690

15. Lee AM, Lopez MA, Haq H, et al. Inpatient food insecurity in caregivers of hospitalized pediatric patients: a mixed methods study. *Acad Pediatr.* 2021;21(8):1404–1413

16. Beck AF, Solan LG, Brunswick SA, et al. H2O Study Group. Socioeconomic status influences the toll pediatric hospitalizations take on families: a qualitative study. *BMJ Qual Saf.* 2017;26(4): 304–311

17. Chang LV, Shah AN, Hoefgen ER, et al. H2O Study Group. Lost earnings and nonmedical expenses of pediatric hospitalizations. *Pediatrics.* 2018;142(3):e20180195

18. Data Resource Center for Child and Adolescent Health. Child and adolescent health measurement initiative. 2019 National Survey of Children's Health (NSCH) data query. Available at: https://www.childhealthdata.org/browse/survey/archive2021

19. The Joint Commission. New requirements to reduce health care disparities. Available at: https://www.jointcommission.org/-/media/tjc/documents/standards/r3-reports/r3_disparities_july2022-6-20-2022.pdf. Accessed June 6, 2024

20. American Medical Association. Quality ID #487 screening for social drivers of health. Available at: https://qpp.cms.gov/docs/QPP_quality_measure_specifications/CQM-Measures/2023_Measure_487_MIPSCQM.pdf. Accessed September 28, 2023

21. Markowitz MA, Tiyyagura G, Quallen K, Rosenberg J. Food insecurity screening and intervention in US children's hospitals. *Hosp Pediatr.* 2022;12(10):849–857

22. Krugman SD, Auger KA. Inadequacies of supporting families with food insecurity in the hospital setting. *Hosp Pediatr.* 2022;12(10): e377–e378

23. VUMC. Monroe Carell Jr. Children's Hospital at Vanderbilt. Available at: https://www.childrenshospitalvanderbilt.org/. Accessed August 28, 2023

24. Hake M, Engelhard E, Dewey A. *Map the Meal Gap 2023: An Analysis of County and Congressional District Food Insecurity and County Food Cost in the United States in 2021.* Feeding America; 2023

25. Langley GLMR, Nolan KM, Nolan TW, Norman CL, Provost LP. *The Improvement Guide: A Practical Approach to Enhancing Organizational Performance,* 2nd ed. Jossey-Bass Publishers; 2009

26. Hager ER, Quigg AM, Black MM, et al. Development and validity of a 2-item screen to identify families at risk for food insecurity. *Pediatrics.* 2010;126(1):e26–e32

27. Gottlieb L, Hessler D, Long D, Amaya A, Adler N. A randomized trial on screening for social determinants of health: the iScreen study. *Pediatrics.* 2014;134(6):e1611–e1618

28. Palakshappa D, Goodpasture M, Albertini L, Brown CL, Montez K, Skelton JA. Written versus verbal food insecurity screening in one primary care clinic. *Acad Pediatr.* 2020;20(2):203–207

29. Provost LPMS. *The Health Care Data Guide: Learning from Data for Improvement.* Jossey-Bass; 2011

30. Ogrinc G, Davies L, Goodman D, Batalden P, Davidoff F, Stevens D. SQUIRE 2.0 (Standards for QUality Improvement Reporting Excellence): revised publication guidelines from a detailed consensus process. *BMJ Qual Saf.* 2016;25(12):986–992

31. Fortin K, Vasan A, Wilson-Hall CL, Brooks E, Rubin D, Scribano PV. Using quality improvement and technology to improve social supports for hospitalized children. *Hosp Pediatr.* 2021;11(10):1120–1129

32. Cordova-Ramos EG, Jain C, Torrice V, et al. Implementing social risk screening and referral to resources in the NICU. *Pediatrics.* 2023;151(4):e2022058975

33. Auger KA, Demeritt B, Beck AF, et al. Reducing caregiver hunger during pediatric hospitalization. *Pediatrics.* 2023;151(5): e2022058080

34. Hanna SL, Wu CL, Smola C, et al. Food insecurity screening of hospitalized patients: a descriptive analysis. *Hosp Pediatr.* 2022; 12(6):e196–e200

35. Fritz CQ, Thomas J, Brittan MS, Mazzio E, Pitkin J, Suh C. Referral and resource utilization among food insecure families identified in a pediatric medical setting. *Acad Pediatr.* 2021;21(3):446–454

36. Gottlieb LM, Hessler D, Long D, et al. Effects of social needs screening and in-person service navigation on child health: a randomized clinical trial. *JAMA Pediatr.* 2016;170(11):e162521

Progress and Potential: Addressing Food Insecurity in Caregivers of Hospitalized Children

Michael Lugo, MD,[a] Meghan Fanta, MD, MS,[a,b,c] Anita Shah, DO, MPH[a,b]

Health care regulatory and accrediting organizations, notably The Centers for Medicare and Medicaid Services[1] and The Joint Commission,[2] have recommended and incentivized that health care institutions address their populations' health-related social needs (HRSN), such as food insecurity (FI). Cognizant of the negative health impact these social needs may have on children,[3] particularly in historically marginalized communities, understanding optimal methods for screening and responding to HRSN is paramount. Implementation, however, has faced challenges including resource allocation, time constraints, lack of standardization surrounding workflow delivery, and provider comfort and training broadly such as navigating administration of screening tools, handling of positive screens, and provision of referrals.[4] Despite these struggles, health care institutions must strive toward an evidence-based, equitable, and multidisciplinary approach to the identification of needs while also considering cross-organizational involvement for resource provision to comprehensively assist children and their families.

In the current issue of *Hospital Pediatrics*, Fritz et al[5] demonstrate the success of FI screening and resource provision through quality improvement (QI) methods on a general pediatric inpatient unit. Their implementation led to impressive improvement in rates of screening for FI from 0% to 77% among their eligible patient population. They found rates of FI consistent with their statewide rates. The most impactful interventions included (1) the integration of screening into required nursing documentation upon admission and (2) the expansion to all medical and surgical patients on the inpatient unit, which simplified the process of determining eligibility for screening. Their work demonstrates overall feasibility and provides an implementation guide for hospital teams to successfully incorporate FI screening into a standard admission workflow while maintaining operational efficiency. Additionally, they leveraged an electronic health record (EHR) automated process that inserted food resource information into the after-visit summary for any positive response to FI screening, which created a more sustainable, reliable, and efficient workflow for the physician team while standardizing resource connection for families.

Integration with EHR is a key strength of their work. Using EHR to improve HRSN screening has been shown to increase efficiency and screening rates while reducing biases.[6,7] Automation capabilities have also been

[a]Division of Hospital Medicine, Cincinnati Children's Hospital, Cincinnati, Ohio; [b]Department of Pediatrics, University of Cincinnati College of Medicine, Cincinnati, Ohio; and [c]James M. Anderson Center for Health Systems Excellence, Cincinnati, Ohio

www.hospitalpediatrics.org

DOI:https://doi.org/10.1542/hpeds.2024-008061

Address correspondence to Michael Lugo, MD, Cincinnati Children's Hospital, 3333 Burnett Ave, MLC 9016, Cincinnati, OH 45229. E-mail: michael.lugo@cchmc.org

HOSPITAL PEDIATRICS (ISSN Numbers: Print, 2154-1663; Online, 2154-1671).

Dr Lugo drafted the initial commentary, reviewed, and revised the commentary, and approved the final submission; and Drs Fanta and Shah critically reviewed and revised the commentary and approved the final submission.

FUNDING: No external funding

CONFLICT OF INTEREST DISCLOSURES: The authors have indicated they have no potential conflicts of interest to disclose.

COMPANION PAPER: A companion to this article can be found online at www.hosppeds.org/cgi/doi/10.1542/hpeds.2024-007926.

previously leveraged for resource generation.[7] EHR-based screening has many promising advantages. Ideally, EHR would provide a seamless transition from screening to responding; this could include private disclosure of caregivers' needs on a tablet followed by an automated, personalized referral to a hospital unit–based social worker, community-based health service organizations, and/or to their medical home. This electronic referral process, if expanded, could create a closed-loop referral practice to ensure comprehensive communication, coordination, and care in addressing social needs from the community resource back to the medical home. Advantages of this integrated approach include respondent privacy, prompt recognition of families with identified HRSN, and immediate resource connection and allocation. This vision, however, is far from a current reality and challenges remain.

Understanding EHR shortcomings, especially within the scope of specific organizations' current capabilities, will ultimately guide improvement processes both now and in the future. The redundancy of screening remains a broad challenge within institutions considering the multiple "touchpoints" between primary care, subspecialists, and inpatient admissions.[8] In this scenario, the screening could inadvertently promote repetitive individual-level trauma[8] while inducing a negative perception of communication among the different health care teams, particularly if resource connection and follow-up are not prioritized. A challenge for our organization, and we suspect for others, is the optimization of tablets linked to the EHR for caregivers to complete HRSN screening. We face barriers to this technological utilization including poor connection to the internet, missing or broken tablets, and navigating individual-level difficulties. Additionally, tablets generally present information in English, creating barriers for families who prefer another language. The integration of available technologies is a viable, practical opportunity to advance HRSN screening and referral processes, but learning from national workgroups and EHR-related subcommittees will be key to materializing this vision.

As the authors noted, there was a notably lower screening rate among Spanish-speaking families when compared with English-speaking families. We applaud the team for stratifying their data, which showed an equity gap in their QI efforts. Conscious that even as we screen to eliminate disparities, paradoxically we can worsen existing gaps. This is evident from prior work accentuating disparities with race, ethnicity, and language within HRSN screening.[9] This relationship is especially notable considering national FI rates among Hispanic individuals outpace both the general rates of FI and FI rates in the non-Hispanic, White population.[10] Although previous research has established positive perceptions surrounding pediatric inpatient HSRN screening, these studies outline limitations with Spanish-speaking families.[11] Despite recent research highlighting Spanish-speaking families' approval of inpatient HSRN screening,[12] limitations in generalizability and understanding of these families' experiences while inpatient remain.

Communication and language gaps are barriers to screening, but the cultural competence of the medical team and families' perceptions of disclosure of social risks[13] including potential negative ramifications[14] are also likely contributors. Involving an interdisciplinary team of stakeholders including physicians, trainees, nurses, social workers, Epic-support staff, and the family advisory council undoubtedly enhanced this QI outcome. The inclusion of language-relevant interpreters could provide an expanded voice and perspective. In-person interpreter services are known to bridge the language barrier while empowering participation[15] and bridging cultural components while advocating on patients' behalf.[16] Broad representation specifically the caregiver's voice, including those who speak languages other than English, must inform and ideally, lead to the cocreation of these processes to ensure perspectives are heard and needs are met. We must continue to strive toward more inclusive teams to create an equity-focused approach that will aim to mitigate biases while ultimately improving health outcomes.

The automated resource insertion to the after-visit summary within the study provided families with brief information and web-based links to community-based organizations (CBOs) and federal nutrition assistance programs. Previous work has demonstrated that only small proportions of identified FI families are connected to community-based food resources following discharge.[17] Additionally, even despite exhibiting high rates of local resource knowledge, there were continued unmet food needs.[18] Through collaboration with caregivers experiencing FI in the hospital, our colleagues identified meaningful discharge options including grocery store gift cards, food delivery, and frozen meals that were deemed feasible, acceptable, and appropriate, while decreasing FI following hospital discharge.[19] Continuing to understand stakeholder perspectives and utilization of resources, as well as barriers to food support, especially within the context of regional variance, could promote success in addressing FI following hospitalizations as families desire longitudinal support for all HSRNs.[12]

In building the capacity for addressing FI, a key component includes engaging, understanding, and financially supporting CBOs that will provide aid both acutely and longitudinally for families after acute hospitalization. CBOs must be a prioritized stakeholder given their grassroots presence, direct connection with community members, and previous experience providing support. To create flexible financial support for resource provisions, Section 1115 waivers within Medicaid are being leveraged, which are federal-to-state partnerships that allow for the reallocation of funds toward nonmedical services that address HRSN. A pioneering instance is North Carolina's Healthy Opportunities Pilots program because it supports food-based initiatives with CBOs to increase access to community-based food sources, provide nutrition counseling, and improve SNAP and WIC enrollment for those eligible but not currently receiving benefits.[20]

Continued efforts to identify and address HRSN will require a comprehensive approach rooted in collaboration and interdisciplinary partnerships across sectors and organizations. As we move forward in optimizing local processes using various strategies such as EHR integration, the historically marginalized communities we are striving to help must be at the forefront of our decisions. The caregivers we aim to positively impact must be partners in coproduction from the start with their perspectives and lived experiences guiding our processes and interventions. This study demonstrates exciting progress in meaningfully identifying hospitalized FI families and the potential to expand our current scope to support the diverse social needs of the population we serve.

REFERENCES

1. CMS. CMS issues new roadmap for states to address the social determinants of health to improve outcomes, lower costs, support state value-based care strategies. Available at: https://www.cms.gov/newsroom/press-releases/cms-issues-new-roadmap-statesaddress-social-determinants-health-improve-outcomes-lowercosts. Accessed July 29, 2024

2. The Joint Commission. New requirements to reduce health care disparities. Available at: https://www.jointcommission.org/-/media/tjc/documents/standards/r3-reports/r3_disparities_july2022-6-20-2022.pdf. Accessed August 1, 2024

3. Gitterman BA, Flanagan PJ, Cotton WH, et al. COUNCIL ON COMMUNITY PEDIATRICS. Poverty and child health in the United States. *Pediatrics.* 2016;137(4):e20160339

4. Trochez RJ, Sharma S, Stolldorf DP, et al. Screening health-related social needs in hospitals: a systematic review of health care professional and patient perspectives. *Popul Health Manag.* 2023;26(3):157–167

5. Fritz CQ, et al. Quality improvement to identify and address food insecurity during pediatric hospitalizations. *Hosp Pediatr.* 2024;14(12):e2024007926

6. Beck AF, Klein MD, Kahn RS. Identifying social risk via a clinical social history embedded in the electronic health record. *Clin Pediatr (Phila).* 2012;51(10):972–977

7. Fortin K, Vasan A, Wilson-Hall CL, Brooks E, Rubin D, Scribano PV. Using quality improvement and technology to improve social supports for hospitalized children. *Hosp Pediatr.* 2021;11(10):1120–1129

8. Bouchelle Z, Vasan A, Cholera R. Mandates and incentives to support social needs screening—challenges and opportunities. *JAMA Pediatr.* 2024;178(2):105–106

9. Torres CIH, Gold R, Kaufmann J, et al. Social risk screening and response equity: assessment by race, ethnicity, and language in community health centers. *Am J Prev Med.* 2023;65(2):286–295

10. Feeding America. Food insecurity in Latino communities. Available at: https://www.feedingamerica.org/hunger-in-america/latino-hunger-facts. Accessed August 8, 2024

11. Colvin JD, Bettenhausen JL, Anderson-Carpenter KD, Collie-Akers V, Chung PJ. Caregiver opinion of in-hospital screening for unmet social needs by pediatric residents. *Acad Pediatr.* 2016;16(2):161–167

12. Luke MJ, Fernandes DM, Leon Rodriguez FD, Acholonu RG, Fiori K. Caregiver perspectives on social needs screening and interventions in an urban children's hospital. *Hosp Pediatr.* 2023;13(8):670–681

13. Ray KN, Gitz KM, Hu A, Davis AA, Miller E. Nonresponse to health-related social needs screening questions. *Pediatrics.* 2020;146(3):e20200174

14. Julliard K, Vivar J, Delgado C, Cruz E, Kabak J, Sabers H. What Latina patients don't tell their doctors: a qualitative study. *Ann Fam Med.* 2008;6(6):543–549

15. Velez T, Gati S, Batista CA, Nino de Rivera J, Banker SL. Facilitating engagement on family-centered rounds for families with limited comfort with English. *Hosp Pediatr.* 2022;12(5):439–447

16. Latif Z, Makuvire T, Feder SL, Crocker J, Quintero Pinzon P, Warraich HJ. Forgotten in the crowd: a qualitative study of medical interpreters' role in medical teams. *J Hosp Med.* 2022;17(9):719–725

17. Fritz CQ, Thomas J, Brittan MS, Mazzio E, Pitkin J, Suh C. Referral and resource utilization among food insecure families identified in a pediatric medical setting. *Acad Pediatr.* 2021;21(3):446–454

18. Asay S, Abramsohn EM, Winslow V, et al. Food insecurity and community-based food resources among caregivers of hospitalized children. *Hosp Pediatr.* 2024;14(7):520–531

19. Smith M, Tepe KA, Sauers-Ford H, et al. Addressing food insecurity in the inpatient setting: Results of a postdischarge pilot study. *J Hosp Med.* Published online June 4, 2024

20. North Carolina Healthy Opportunities Pilots. Available at: https://www.ncdhhs.gov/healthy-opportunities-pilot-fee-schedule-and-service-definitions/open. Accessed August 1, 2024

BRIEF REPORT

Disparities and Biases in Food Insecurity Screening Among Admitted Children

Mary M. Orr, MD, MPH,[a] Adolfo L. Molina, MD, MSHQS,[a] Cassandra N. Smola, MD,[a] Samantha L. Hanna, MD, MPH,[b] Ariel E. Carpenter, MD,[a] Chang L. Wu, MD, MSCR[a]

ABSTRACT

BACKGROUND AND OBJECTIVES: Food insecurity (FI) has increasingly become a focus for hospitalized patients. The best methods for screening practices, particularly in hospitalized children, are unknown. The purpose of the study was to evaluate results of an electronic medical record (EMR) embedded, brief screening tool for FI among inpatients.

METHODS: This was a cross-sectional study from August 2020 to September 2022 for all children admitted to a quaternary children's hospital. Primary outcomes were proportion of those screened for FI and those identified to have a positive screen. FI was evaluated by The Hunger Vital Sign, a validated 2-question screen verbally obtained in the nursing intake form in the EMR. Covariates include demographic variables of age, sex, race, ethnicity, primary language, and insurance. Statistical analyses including all univariate outcome and bivariate comparisons were performed with SAS 9.4.

RESULTS: There were 31 553 patient encounters with 81.7% screened for FI. Patients had a median age of 6.3 years, were mostly male (54.2%), White (60.6%), non-Hispanic (92.7%), English-speaking (94.3%), and had government insurance (79.8%). Younger (0–2 years), non-White, and noninsured patients were all screened significantly less often for FI (all $P < .001$). A total of 3.4% were identified as having FI. Patients who were older, non-White, Hispanic, non-English speaking, and had nonprivate insurance had higher FI (all $P < .001$).

CONCLUSIONS: Despite the use of an EMR screening tool intended to be universal, we found variation in how we screen for FI. At times, we missed those who would benefit the most from intervention, and thus it may be subject to implementation bias.

www.hospitalpediatrics.org

DOI: https://doi.org/10.1542/hpeds.2023-007602

Copyright © 2024 by the American Academy of Pediatrics

Address correspondence to Mary Orr, MD, MPH, Children's of Alabama, 1600 7th Ave South, Suite 108, McWane Building, Birmingham, AL 35233. E-mail: morr@uabmc.edu

HOSPITAL PEDIATRICS (ISSN Numbers: Print, 2154-1663; Online, 2154-1671).

Dr Orr contributed to the design of the study, drafted the initial manuscript, reviewed and revised the manuscript, and approved the final manuscript as submitted; Dr Molina conceptualized the study, supervised data collection and analysis, critically reviewed and revised the manuscript, and approved the final manuscript as submitted; Drs Smola, Carpenter, and Hanna contributed to the design of the study, reviewed and revised the manuscript, and approved the final manuscript as submitted; and Dr Wu conceptualized the study, analyzed and interpreted the data, critically reviewed and revised the manuscript, and approved the final manuscript as submitted.

FUNDING: No external funding.

CONFLICT OF INTEREST DISCLOSURES: The authors have indicated they have no potential conflicts of interest to disclose.

[a]Division of Pediatric Hospital Medicine, Department of Pediatrics, University of Alabama at Birmingham Heersink School of Medicine, Birmingham, Alabama; and [b]Section of Pediatric Hospital Medicine, Department of Pediatrics, Saint Louis University, Saint Louis, Missouri

Food insecurity (FI) is an important social determinant of health that has been shown to negatively impact numerous measures of the health of children.[1] According to the Centers for Disease Control and Prevention, in 2019–2020, 1 in 10 children lived in households affected by FI. Rates were almost 19% in non-Hispanic Black children and 15.7% in Hispanic children compared with 6.5% in non-Hispanic White children, with similar rates for different age groups.[2]

Although many FI screening tools include 10 to 20 questions, other, briefer, screening tools to identify FI have also been employed, such as the Hunger Vital Sign, a 2-question screening tool validated in the outpatient setting.[3] When implemented in the primary care setting and the emergency department for children, it had a sensitivity of 97% and specificity of 86%.[4] Higher rates of FI have been found in recently hospitalized patients,[5] and higher than expected rates of FI have been found in pediatric emergency departments.[4] Children's hospitals are increasingly using screening tools to identify FI in inpatients, with 67% of survey respondents in 1 study having some sort of screening tool in place and 34% having universal screening, but best practice methods in obtaining accurate results are not known.[6] We hypothesized that an electronic medical record (EMR) embedded tool would universally screen inpatients for FI, and we would not see a difference among groups.

METHODS

We performed a cross-sectional study of all inpatients admitted from August 1, 2020, to September 2022 after our hospital instituted FI screening by embedding The Hunger Vital Sign in the nursing intake form. There were no exclusion criteria. Primary outcomes were proportion of those screened for FI and those identified to have a positive screen. Covariates were collected from the EMR and included standard demographic variables of age, sex, race, ethnicity, primary language, and insurance type. Race and ethnicity are recorded on admission by administrative staff and are either asked verbally or observed. Patients were grouped into White, Black, and Other because of small sample sizes of other races. Statistical analyses consisting of t test or χ^2 testing were conducted as appropriate with SAS 9.4.

The Hunger Vital Sign identifies households as being at risk for FI if they answer that either or both of the following 2 statements is "often true" or "sometimes true" (vs "never true"):

1. Within the past 12 months, we worried whether our food would run out before we got money to buy more.
2. Within the past 12 months, the food we bought just didn't last and we didn't have money to get more.

Unit nurse educators were provided instructions regarding the screening process before implementation. Dissemination to unit nurses occurred through usual means (a combination of e-mail and conferences). Questions are administered to caregivers verbally on admission by nursing staff along with other social and demographic questions but are not mandatory. The vast majority of patients who do not use English as a primary language are Spanish speaking at our institution, and interpreter services are available at all times. Families with positive screens received an automatic social work consultation through a linked order in the EMR. Social workers would visit that family and ensure enrollment in Supplemental Nutrition Program for Women, Infants, and Children benefits if eligible and provide a list of food resources in their area. This study was deemed exempt by our institutional review board, record number IRB-300005776.

RESULTS

The study period included 31 553 inpatient patient encounters. FI screening was documented in 81.7% of them. Among those screened, patients had a median age of 6.3 years, were majority male, White, non-Hispanic, English speaking, and had government insurance (Table 1). Younger patients, non-White patients, and patients with government or other insurance were all screened significantly less often than their counterparts ($P < .001$). We detected no difference in screening rates based on sex, Hispanic ethnicity, or English vs non-English as the primary language.

Among those that were screened, 824 (3.2%) had a positive screen. Statistically significant higher rates of FI were detected among patients who were older, non-White race, Hispanic ethnicity, possessed a primary language other than English, and did not possess private insurance. FI was not significantly different between patient sex (Table 1).

DISCUSSION

In this pragmatic study of FI screening practices, we demonstrated an EMR embedded screening tool was able to identify FI in the inpatient population. However, although a majority of patients were successfully screened, the proportion of those who endorsed FI was lower than expected, and screening was not uniform across all populations as it was intended to be applied. Overall, the rates of FI occurred higher in school aged, non-White race, non-English speaking, and uninsured patients. We found significant overlap in those not screened with those that also possessed higher rates of FI; non-white patients and patients without insurance were both screened less often and had higher rates of FI when screened.

In context, our findings of identified FI are similar with previous efforts with similar methodology.[7] We chose the Hunger Vital Sign screening tool because of its brief nature and validation in the outpatient setting, but a survey of FI screening practices at pediatric hospitals reported a variety of screening methods used, with the majority being institution-specific screening tools administered orally in the inpatient setting.[6] Our state is the fifth poorest in the nation, with 17% of adults and 23% of children having inadequate access to enough nutritious food.[8] Recent hospitalization is associated with higher than expected rates of FI, and household FI among families of pediatric inpatients may be higher than the expected general population level.[9,10] This suggests that

TABLE 1 Comparison Among Those Screened for and Those Who Endorsed Food Insecurity		
Characteristic	Screened for Food Insecurity *n* (%)	Endorsed Food Insecurity *n* (%)
Age[a,b]		
0-2 y	7158 (76.62)	215 (3.00)
3-5 y	5153 (84.25)	163 (3.16)
6-12 y	6414 (84.22)	215 (3.35)
13+ y	7044 (83.08)	231 (3.28)
Sex		
Male	13 948 (81.59)	468 (3.36)
Female	11 812 (81.76)	356 (3.01)
Race[a,b]		
White	15 858 (82.92)	416 (2.62)
Black	9173 (79.84)	377 (4.11)
Other	738 (78.59)	31 (4.20)
Ethnicity[a]		
Non-Hispanic	23 906 (81.74)	689 (2.88)
Hispanic	1863 (80.82)	135 (7.25)
Primary language[a]		
Non-English	1434 (80.11)	125 (8.72)
English	24 335 (81.76)	699 (2.87)
Insurance[a,b]		
Government	20 491 (81.35)	764 (3.73)
Private	5002 (83.27)	46 (0.92)
Other	276 (77.31)	14 (5.07)

[a] Statistical difference among those screened, $P < .001$.
[b] Statistical difference among those who endorsed food insecurity, $P < .001$.

hospitalization is an acute stressor that may impact FI and is an important opportunity for intervention. The discrepancy in FI identified may suggest that our method may not detect those at highest risk for FI and is still subject to bias in real-life implementation.

Reasons why this tool was not applied universally may be multifactorial. Education of nursing staff took place during the pandemic, when fewer in-person meetings were occurring. No direct observations of screening implementation were made, and so it is possible that questions were not being asked and/or responses were recorded inaccurately. Specific reasons for disparate screening rates are currently unknown, but we hypothesize the following: negative screening logistics (eg, limited caregiver availability at admission, limitations on nursing time, patient acuity), responder participation, or discomfort with asking personal questions that may imply judgment or implicit bias. Health care providers have been shown to have negative implicit bias toward people of color at the level of the general population,[11] and this may contribute to the structural racism many non-White families face. Race is a social construct that is difficult to separate from other social factors. Lack of screening in this population may contribute to worse health outcomes. Although every effort was made to ensure the same level of care was provided to all patients screened on inpatient admission, the lack of uniformity in screening would suggest a missed opportunity for identification and intervention.

Reasons why responders may have endorsed FI at a lower than expected rate may also be multifactorial. Families may feel uncomfortable talking to a doctor or nurse about FI.[12] There could also be discordant responses by patients versus parents of FI, with adolescents experiencing FI differently.[13] Other studies have shown that 75% of families preferred to complete a written rather than verbal FI screening tool, and that lower rates of FI were detected using verbal questionnaires as compared with written.[5,14] Parents may answer "no" to screening questions because of feelings of guilt or shame, all of which may attribute to our lower detected rates and are limitations to this study.

This research project is part of a larger quality improvement initiative to identify and intervene in food insecure hospitalized children. The study is limited by its nature as a single-institution study but does include a large number of patients. Although the Hunger Vital Sign is a well-validated tool for outpatient use, its application in the inpatient setting has not yet been fully explored. Further research is needed to determine best practices for screening for social determinants of health, including FI, particularly in hospitalized children. Future directions include exploration of comparison between questions asked by a trained member not involved in the clinical care team versus written questionnaires by tablet so families can directly enter information into the medical record. In this cross-sectional study of FI screening for hospitalized children, we found that an EMR embedded screening intended to be universal was inequitable and susceptible to missing populations that are often vulnerable. For institutions interested in implementing similar programs, opportunity exists to improve screening practices and mitigate barriers to provide support to families that need it.

REFERENCES

1. Thomas MMC, Miller DP, Morrissey TW. Food insecurity and child health. *Pediatrics.* 2019;144(4):e20190397

2. Ullmann H, Weeks JD, Madans JH. *Children living in households that experienced food insecurity: United States, 2019–2020. NCHS Data Brief, no 432.* Hyattsville, MD: National Center for Health Statistics; 2021

3. Hager ER, Quigg AM, Black MM, et al. Development and validity of a 2-item screen to identify families at risk for food insecurity. *Pediatrics.* 2010;126(1):e26–e32

4. Gattu RK, Paik G, Wang Y, Ray P, Lichenstein R, Black MM. The hunger vital sign identifies household food insecurity among children in emergency departments and primary care. *Children (Basel).* 2019;6(10):107

5. Gonzalez JV, Hartford EA, Moore J, Brown JC. Food insecurity in a pediatric emergency department and the feasibility of universal screening. *West J Emerg Med.* 2021;22(6):1295–1300

6. Markowitz MA, Tiyyagura G, Quallen K, Rosenberg J. Food insecurity screening and intervention in United States children's hospitals. *Hosp Pediatr.* 2022;12(10):849–857

7. Gore E, DiTursi J, Rambuss R, Pope-Collins E, Train MK. Implementing a process for screening hospitalized adults for food insecurity at a tertiary care center. *J Healthc Qual.* 2022; 44(5):305–12.

8. Gundersen C, Strayer M, Dewey A, Hake M, Engelhard E. *Map the Meal Gap 2022: An Analysis of County and Congressional District Food Insecurity and County Food Cost in the United States in 2020.* Feeding America; 2022

9. Banach LP. Hospitalization: are we missing an opportunity to identify food insecurity in children? *Acad Pediatr.* 2016; 16(5):438–445

10. Lee AM, Lopez MA, Haq H, et al. Inpatient food insecurity in caregivers of hospitalized pediatric patients: a mixed methods study. *Acad Pediatr.* 2021;21(8):1404–1413

11. Hall WJ, Chapman MV, Lee KM, et al. Implicit racial/ethnic bias among health care professionals and its influence on health care outcomes: a systematic review. *Am J Public Health.* 2015;105(12):e60–e76

12. Barnidge E, LaBarge G, Krupsky K, Arthur J. Screening for food insecurity in pediatric clinical settings: opportunities and barriers. *J Community Health.* 2017;42(1):51–57

13. Harper K, Seligman H. A call for consistent screening and measurement of adolescent food insecurity. *JAMA Pediatr.* 2023;177(5):450–451

14. Palakshappa D, Goodpasture M, Albertini L, Brown CL, Montez K, Skelton JA. Written versus verbal food insecurity screening in one primary care clinic. *Acad Pediatr.* 2020;20(2):203–207

Food Insecurity and Experiences of Discrimination Among Caregivers of Hospitalized Children

Alexis M. Cacioppo, BA,[a] Victoria Winslow, MPH,[b] Emily M. Abramsohn, MPH,[b] Jyotsna S. Jagai, PhD, MPH, MS,[b] Jennifer A. Makelarski, PhD, MPH,[b] Elaine Waxman, PhD, MPP,[c] Kristen Wroblewski, MS,[d] Stacy Tessler Lindau, MD, MAPP[e]

BACKGROUND AND OBJECTIVES: Pediatric hospitals are adopting strategies to address food insecurity (FI), a stigmatizing condition, among families with children. We hypothesized that parents and other caregivers ("caregivers") from households with FI or marginal food security (MFS) are more likely to experience discrimination during their child's hospitalization.

METHODS: We analyzed data from 319 caregivers of children admitted to an urban, academic children's hospital and randomly assigned to the control arm of the double-blind randomized controlled CommunityRx-Hunger trial (November 2020 to June 2022, NCT R01MD012630). Household food security in the 30 days before admission and discrimination during hospitalization were measured with the US Household Food Security Survey and the Discrimination in Medical Settings Scale, respectively. We used logistic regression to model the relationship between food security status and discrimination, adjusting for gender, race, ethnicity, income, and partner status.

RESULTS: Most participants were African American or Black (81.5%), female (94.7%), and the parent of the hospitalized child (93.7%). FI and MFS were prevalent (25.1% and 15.1%, respectively). Experiences of discrimination during a child's hospitalization were prevalent (51.9%). Caregivers with FI had higher odds than caregivers with food security of experiencing discrimination (adjusted odds ratio = 2.0, 95% confidence interval 1.1–3.6, $P = .03$); MFS was not significantly associated with discrimination ($P = .25$). Compared with food secure caregivers, those with FI had higher odds of 5 of 7 experiences of discrimination assessed.

CONCLUSIONS: Among parents and other caregivers, household FI is associated with experiences of discrimination during a child's hospitalization.

[a]Pritzker School of Medicine, and [b]Departments of Obstetrics and Gynecology, and [c]The Urban Institute, Washington, District of Columbia, and [d]Public Health Sciences, [e]Medicine-Geriatrics, The University of Chicago, Chicago, Illinois

Ms Cacioppo conceptualized and designed the study, conducted the initial analyses, and drafted the initial manuscript; Ms Winslow coordinated and supervised the analyses and replicated the analyses; Ms Abramsohn conceptualized and designed the study and coordinated and supervised data collection; Dr Jagai and Ms Wroblewski coordinated and supervised the analyses; Dr Makelarski conceptualized and designed the study and coordinated and supervised the analyses; Dr Waxman conceptualized and designed the study; Dr Lindau conceptualized and designed the study and provided material support and supervised the study team; and all authors reviewed and revised the manuscript, approved the final manuscript as submitted, and agree to be accountable for all aspects of the work.

This trial has been registered at www.clinicaltrials.gov (identifier NCT04171999) and the NIH's RePORTER database (5R01MD012630-03, ST Lindau, 2021). Deidentified individual participant data (including data dictionaries) will be made available, in addition to study protocols, the statistical analysis plan, and the informed consent form. The data will be (Continued)

WHAT'S KNOWN ON THIS SUBJECT: Food insecurity is an especially stigmatizing condition for caregivers with dependent children. Accessing food assistance has been associated with experiences of discrimination. Recommendations from pediatric organizations have motivated the assessment of and intervention on food insecurity in children's hospitals.

WHAT THIS STUDY ADDS: This study reveals that caregivers from food-insecure households are at higher odds of experiencing discrimination in the children's hospital setting. Interventions to mitigate food insecurity should be delivered in a manner that optimizes the care experience and minimizes stigma.

To cite: Cacioppo AM, Winslow V, Abramsohn EM, et al. Food Insecurity and Experiences of Discrimination Among Caregivers of Hospitalized Children. *Pediatrics*. 2023;152(6): e2023061750

ARTICLE

Food insecurity (FI), defined as having limited or uncertain access to adequate foods for an active and healthy life,[1,2] poses a significant risk to the immediate and long-term health of children and their parents/caregivers ("caregivers").[3,4] It is a particularly stigmatizing condition, especially for caregivers with dependent children.[5] Households with children headed by a single woman, people who identify as non-Hispanic African American/Black or Hispanic, and people living in poverty have disproportionately high rates of FI.[6] These inequities have persisted and, for some groups, worsened throughout the coronavirus disease 2019 (COVID-19) pandemic.[6-9] As proposed in the Stigma and Food Inequity Conceptual Framework, stigma is linked to food inequities through mediating mechanisms that affect an individual's psychosocial processes and behavior, including discrimination.[5] For people with FI, the perception of discrimination by others in the food assistance setting is a known catalyst for feelings of shame that deter government nutrition program participation and community pantry use.[10-12] That said, little is known about the relationship between FI and experiences of discrimination while being connected to food assistance in the health care setting.

A child's hospitalization can trigger an episode of FI (particularly for families living in or near poverty), but it also provides a unique opportunity to intervene on FI, with frequent conversations about health between families and clinicians facilitating intervention.[13,14] A number of children's hospitals have implemented system-wide protocols for the routine assessment of FI and other common health-related socioeconomic risks,[15] as recommended by the American Academy of Pediatrics[16] and the Children's Hospital Association.[17] To inform calls for and the implementation of routine screening for FI and other health-related socioeconomic risks in pediatric inpatient settings, this study tested the hypothesis that caregivers from food insecure and marginally food-secure households were at higher odds than caregivers from food-secure households of experiencing discrimination during a child's hospitalization.

METHODS

Study Sample and Setting

This study was conducted at a 155-bed academic children's hospital in Chicago, Illinois. The population in the hospital's primary service area is predominantly African American or Black (74% of 626 264 in the hospital's service area) and more than one-quarter of people (27%) in this area live below the Federal Poverty Level.[18] The hospital has ~5300 admissions each year.[19]

Caregivers of children admitted to the hospital's general inpatient and ICUs and enrolled in the control arm ("usual care") of the CommunityRx for Hunger double-blind randomized controlled trial between November 2020 and June 2022 were included in this analysis.[20]

Eligible English- or Spanish-speaking caregivers lived in a 42-zip-code region, including the hospital's 12-zip-code primary service area, on Chicago's South and West sides and adjacent suburbs and self-identified as the primary caregiver of a hospitalized child. Eligible caregivers also consented to receive text messages from the research team. Caregivers of non-NICU newborns, children hospitalized <24 hours or >30 days, children with a diagnosed eating disorder, and those who recalled participating in a previous Community-Rx study were excluded from the study. Eligible caregivers were consented and enrolled after their child's hospital admission, before discharge. All caregivers provided written documentation of informed consent, documented electronically. During the consent process, participants were informed that the study was about food security and related needs. The study protocol was approved by the University of Chicago's Institutional Review Board (IRB20-0324).

The 319 caregivers enrolled in the control arm of the CommunityRx for Hunger trial and included in this analysis received usual clinical care at the time of admission. Usual clinical care included information in the standard "Caregiver FYI Admissions Packet" from hospital admission staff about all available retail food options in the hospital and self-serve food pantries operated by Feed1st, a longstanding 24/7/365 self-serve food pantry program operating at multiple sites in the children's hospital.[13,21] Usual clinical care also included a referral to social work at the discretion of the health care team. Usual clinical care did not include screening for FI.

Data Collection

Validated survey measures were used when possible. Sociodemographic characteristics were assessed in the baseline survey administered during the child's admission. Gender identity was assessed with the following item recommended by the 2014 Best Practices for Asking Questions to Identify Transgender and Other Gender Minority Respondents on Population-Based Surveys.[22] While the response options provided for this item were "Male" vs "Female", indicating sex, the item also included the following options: Trans male/Trans man, Trans female/trans woman, Genderqueer/gender non-conforming, and Different identity.[22] We also assessed sex as a biological variable in accordance with NIH policy, and found no significant differences in sex vs gender. Relationship with the hospitalized child was assessed with an item sourced from the 2016 Consumer Assessment of Healthcare Providers and Systems Child Hospital Survey.[23] Caregiver race, caregiver ethnicity, and partner status were assessed with items from the 2018 Behavioral Risk Factor Surveillance System (BRFSS).[24] Race and ethnicity were assessed with 2 items: "Which one or more of the following would you say your race is?" (American Indian or Alaskan

Native, Asian, Black or African American, Native Hawaiian or Pacific Islander, White, or other)" and "Are you Hispanic, Latino/a, or of Spanish origin?" (yes or no).[24] Because of small numbers, participants who selected American Indian or Alaskan Native, Asian, Native Hawaiian or Pacific Islander, other race, or multiple races were categorized as "Other."

Economic and household characteristics were also assessed in the baseline survey. Annual income, educational attainment, and insurance status were assessed with items from or adapted from the 2018 BRFSS.[24] The median number in the household was assessed with an item from the 2018 American Community Survey.[25] The median number of children <18 years old in the household was assessed with an item from the 2018 BRFSS.[24] Household receipt of Supplemental Nutritional Assistance Program (SNAP) and Special Supplemental Nutritional Program for Women, Infants, and Children (WIC) were assessed with items from the 2014 Hunger in America Survey.[26]

Household FI in the 30 days before the child's hospitalization was assessed in the baseline survey with the 18-item US Household Food Security Survey Module.[27] Affirmative responses were summed by using standard scoring to generate a raw score of 0 to 18.[27] Raw scores were first used to categorize households into 4 food security statuses as specified by the US Household Food Security Survey Module: food security (0 items endorsed), marginal food security (MFS; 1–2 items endorsed), low food security (3–5 items endorsed), and very low food security (≥6 items endorsed).[28] However, because of a small sample size of participants from households affected by very low food security, we collapsed households experiencing low and very low food security and categorized households into 3 food security statuses: food security (0 items endorsed), MFS (1–2 items endorsed), food insecure (≥3 items endorsed).[29]

Experiences of perceived discrimination in the children's hospital were assessed in the survey administered 7 days after the child's discharge. Experiences of discrimination were measured as a proxy for stigma by using the 7-item Discrimination in Medical Settings (DMS) Scale.[30] The DMS Scale was developed to assess the frequency of individual-level discrimination in the health care setting attributed to "race, ancestry, or national origin."[30] To capture discrimination during the child's hospitalization, the measure's introduction was adapted to say, "Now I'm going to ask you about your experiences during your child's hospitalization. Thinking about your experiences when you child was hospitalized last week, would you say … ". In this introductory statement, no reference was made to any specific reason for discrimination, such as race, ancestry, national origin, or other factors. Standard scoring with a 5-point Likert scale was used (1: never, 2: rarely, 3: sometimes, 4: most of the time, and 5: always).

Preliminary analyses revealed skewed distributions in responses to each DMS item, with 59% to 90% of participants responding "never," as consistent with findings from the 2011 validation study.[30] Therefore, responses were dichotomized according to whether caregivers had any experiences of discrimination (raw score >7) or no experiences of discrimination (raw score = 7) during their child's hospitalization, as outlined by Benjamins and Middleton et al.[31]

Data Analysis

Descriptive statistics were calculated for sample sociodemographic characteristics and responses to DMS items by food security status, including medians with interquartile ranges (IQRs; continuous variables with skewed distributions) and response frequencies (categorical variables). Bivariate analyses were performed to assess statistically significant differences in sample characteristics by food security status. Logistic regression, both unadjusted and adjusted, was used to test the relationship between food security status and discrimination in medical settings as reported overall (dichotomized any vs no experiences of discrimination during child's hospitalization) and per-item on the DMS scale. Analyses were repeated by using Poisson regression with robust standard errors to estimate adjusted and unadjusted relative risks. Models were adjusted for variables previously reported to be associated with FI and discrimination: gender ("female" vs "male"), race and ethnicity (non-Hispanic, African American or Black vs all others), partner status (married or in a relationship vs not), and income (<$50 000 vs ≥$50 000). These variables were selected because they are well-documented in the literature to be related to both FI[2] and experiences of discrimination.[5] Race and ethnicity were combined to create a single covariate in these models because caregivers who identified as non-Hispanic, African American or Black comprised the vast majority in our sample. Because a small percentage of participants identified as Hispanic, including ethnicity and race as separate covariates affected model convergence and decreased precision.

Participants who did not complete all relevant items were excluded from these models. The significance level was set at α = 0.05. All analyses were conducted with Stata version 16 (StataCorp LLC, College Station, TX).

RESULTS

The majority of participants were African American or Black, women, and the parent of the hospitalized child (Table 1). Participants had a median age of 33.5 years (IQR = 28.3–40.1). Most caregivers were insured through Medicare/Medicaid (74.4%) and lived in a household enrolled in government food assistance through SNAP and/or WIC (75.0%).

TABLE 1 Sociodemographic, Economic, and Household Characteristics of Caregivers in the Control Arm of the CommunityRx for Hunger Trial (n = 319)

	Overall (n = 319)	Food Secure (n = 191)	Marginally Food Secure (n = 48)	Food Insecure (n = 80)
		59.9%	15.1%	25.1%
Sociodemographic characteristics				
Age, median (IQR)	33.5 (28.3–40.1)	33.4 (28.1–39.6)	33.5 (27.5–39.1)	33.8 (29.0–42.2)
Gender, n (%)[a]				
Female	302 (94.7)	180 (94.2)	45 (93.8)	77 (96.3)
Relationship with hospitalized child, n (%)[b]				
Parent	299 (93.7)	180 (94.2)	42 (87.5)	77 (96.3)
Caregiver race, n (%)[c,d]				
African American or Black	259 (81.5)	155 (81.2)	39 (83.0)	65 (81.3)
White	27 (8.5)	21 (11.0)	2 (4.3)	4 (5.0)
Other	32 (10.1)	15 (7.9)	6 (12.8)	11 (13.8)
Caregiver ethnicity, n (%)[c]				
Hispanic	41 (12.9)	20 (10.5)	9 (18.8)	12 (15.0)
Partner status, n (%)[c]				
Partnered	170 (53.3)	103 (53.9)	26 (54.2)	41 (51.3)
Unpartnered	149 (46.7)	88 (46.1)	22 (45.8)	39 (48.8)
Economic characteristics				
Annual income, n (%)[e,f]				
<$50 000	245 (79.0)	131 (70.8)	42 (89.4)	72 (92.3)
≥$50 000	65 (21.0)	54 (29.2)	5 (10.6)	6 (7.7)
Educational attainment, n (%)[c]				
More than high school	180 (56.4)	110 (57.6)	25 (52.1)	45 (56.3)
High school or less	139 (43.6)	81 (42.4)	23 (47.9)	35 (43.8)
Insurance status, n (%)[c,g]				
Medicaid/Medicare	235 (74.4)	131 (69.0)	42 (89.4)	62 (78.5)
Private	73 (23.1)	55 (29.0)	4 (8.5)	14 (17.7)
No insurance	8 (2.5)	4 (2.1)	1 (2.1)	3 (3.8)
Household characteristics				
Number in household, median (IQR)[h]	4 (3–5)	4 (3–5)	4 (3–5)	4 (3–5)
Number of children <18, median (IQR)[c]	2 (1–3)	2 (1–3)	2 (1.5–3)	2 (1–4)
Household receipt of SNAP, n (%)[i]	220 (69.2)	132 (69.5)	33 (68.8)	55 (68.8)
Household receipt of WIC, n (%)[i]	70 (34.5)	44 (36.4)	14 (37.8)	12 (26.7)

Column percentages may not total 100% because of rounding.
[a] This item was sourced from the 2014 Best Practices for Asking Questions to Identify Transgender and Other Gender Minority Respondents on Population-Based Surveys.[22]
[b] This item was sourced from the 2016 Consumer Assessment of Healthcare Providers and Systems Child Hospital Survey.[23]
[c] This item was sourced from the 2018 Behavioral Risk Factor Surveillance System.[24]
[d] Participants who selected American Indian or Alaskan Native, Asian, Native Hawaiian or Pacific Islander, other race, or multiple races were categorized as "Other."
[e] This item was adapted from the 2018 BRFSS.[24]
[f] Bivariate analysis yielded a significant difference (P < .001).
[g] Two participants who reported insurance coverage through TRICARE or other sources were excluded because of small bin sizes; bivariate analysis yielded a significant difference (P = .03).
[h] This item was sourced from the 2018 American Community Survey.[23]
[i] This item was sourced from an item from the Hunger in America Survey.[26]

At baseline, >1 in 4 caregivers were food insecure in the 30 days before their child's hospitalization. An additional 15.1% were marginally food secure. Most sample characteristics were similar by food security status. Differences by food security status were observed for annual household income (overall P < .001), with caregivers from food-insecure households reporting annual incomes of <$50 000 at the highest rate (92.3% for caregivers from food-insecure households vs 89.4% from marginal food-secure households and 70.8% from food-secure households). Also, differences in

insurance status by food security status were observed (P = .03), with caregivers from marginal food-secure households reporting being insured with Medicaid/Medicare at the highest rate (89.4% for caregivers from marginally food-secure households vs 78.5% from food-insecure households and 69.0% from food-secure households).

More than one-half of caregivers reported experiencing discrimination in the medical setting during their child's hospitalization (Fig 1). Experiences of discrimination were highest for caregivers from food-insecure households, followed

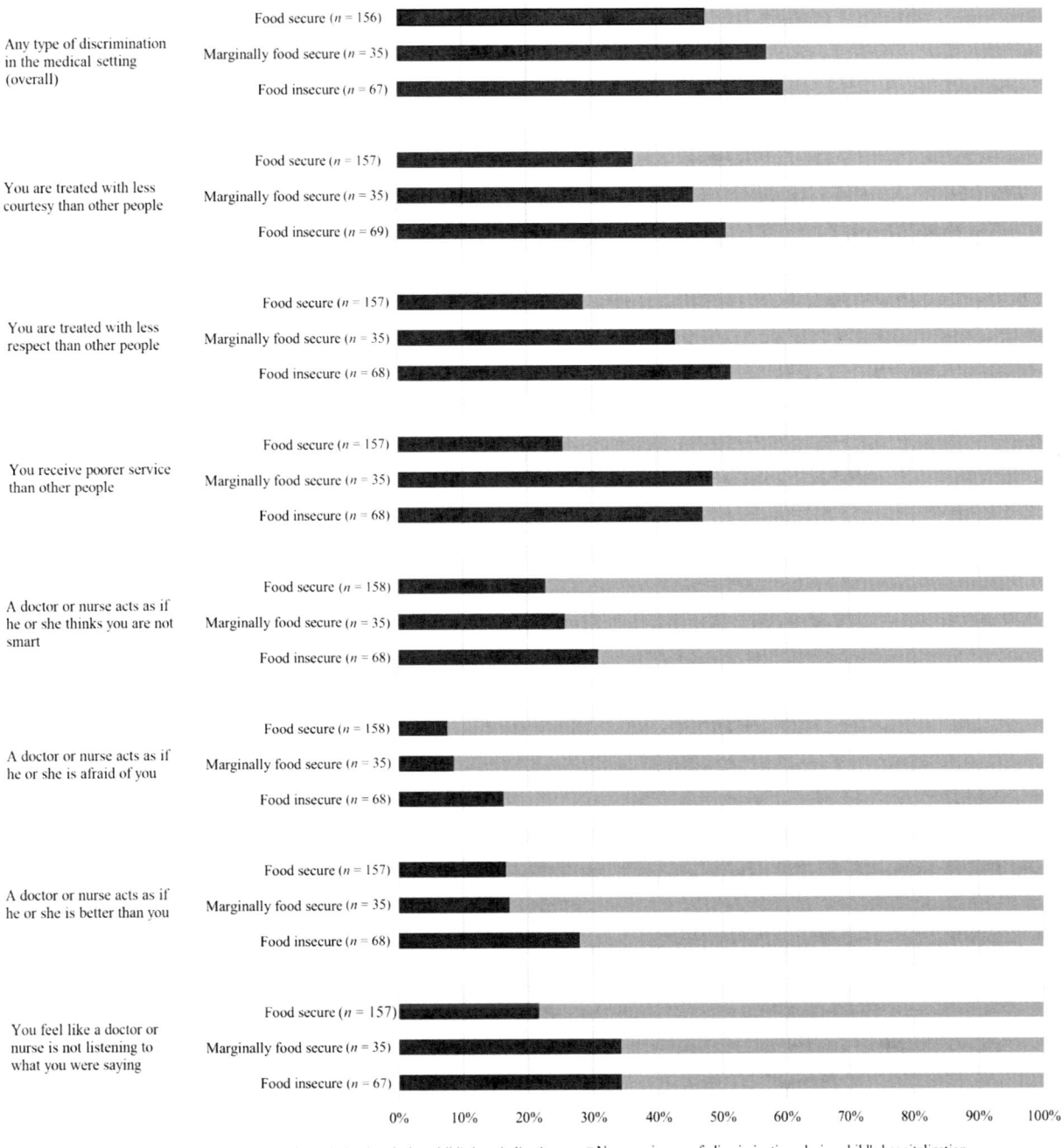

Any type of discrimination in the medical setting (overall)
- Food secure (*n* = 156)
- Marginally food secure (*n* = 35)
- Food insecure (*n* = 67)

You are treated with less courtesy than other people
- Food secure (*n* = 157)
- Marginally food secure (*n* = 35)
- Food insecure (*n* = 69)

You are treated with less respect than other people
- Food secure (*n* = 157)
- Marginally food secure (*n* = 35)
- Food insecure (*n* = 68)

You receive poorer service than other people
- Food secure (*n* = 157)
- Marginally food secure (*n* = 35)
- Food insecure (*n* = 68)

A doctor or nurse acts as if he or she thinks you are not smart
- Food secure (*n* = 158)
- Marginally food secure (*n* = 35)
- Food insecure (*n* = 68)

A doctor or nurse acts as if he or she is afraid of you
- Food secure (*n* = 158)
- Marginally food secure (*n* = 35)
- Food insecure (*n* = 68)

A doctor or nurse acts as if he or she is better than you
- Food secure (*n* = 157)
- Marginally food secure (*n* = 35)
- Food insecure (*n* = 68)

You feel like a doctor or nurse is not listening to what you were saying
- Food secure (*n* = 157)
- Marginally food secure (*n* = 35)
- Food insecure (*n* = 67)

0% 10% 20% 30% 40% 50% 60% 70% 80% 90% 100%

■ Any experiences of discrimination during child's hospitalization   ■ No experiences of discrimination during child's hospitalization

FIGURE 1
Participants who did not complete relevant items were excluded from this analysis. Caregivers' experiences of discrimination were dichotomized with any experiences of discrimination corresponding to raw scores >7 and no experiences of discrimination corresponding to raw scores = 7.

by those from marginally food secure and food-secure households (59.7% vs 57.1%, and 47.4%, respectively, *P* = .20). Caregivers from food-insecure households had the highest rate of discrimination for 5 of 7 DMS items, with feelings of "being treated with less respect than other people" being the most prevalent: 51.5% for caregivers from food-insecure households (P = .001) versus 42.9% from marginally food-secure households (P = .4), compared with 28.7% from food-secure households.

In logistic models adjusted for baseline characteristics, caregivers from food-insecure households had twice the odds of experiencing any discrimination during their

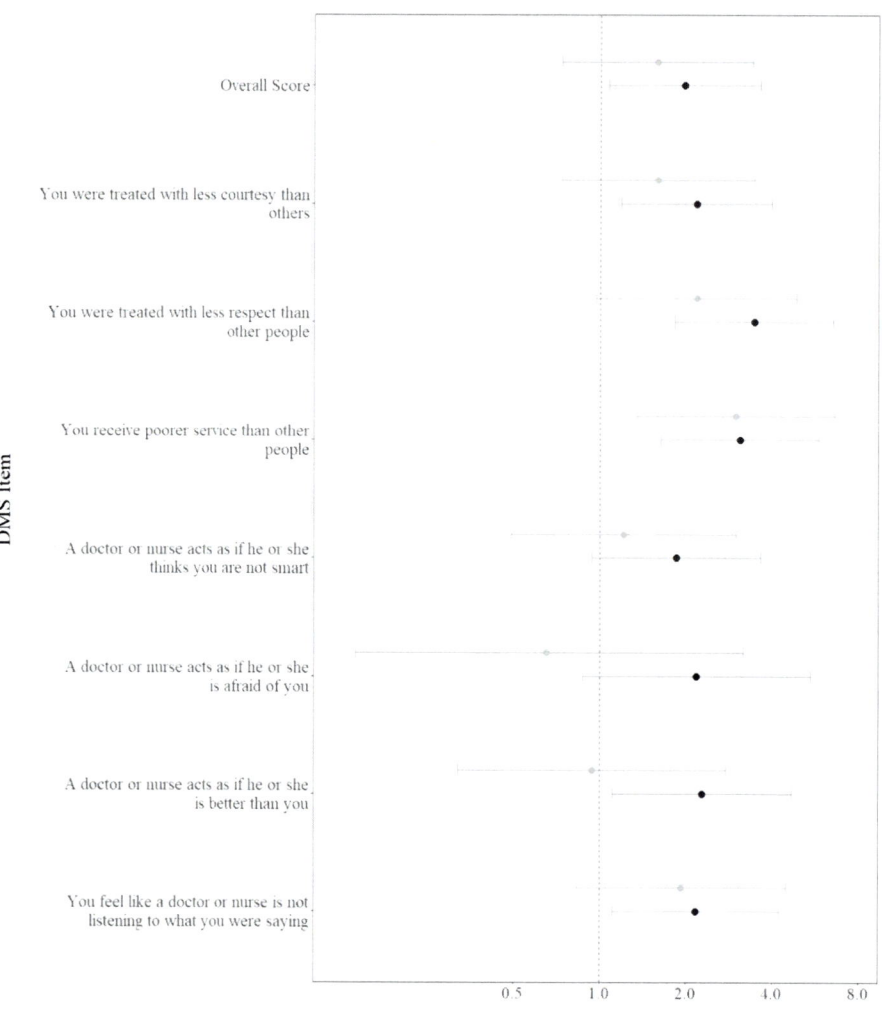

FIGURE 2
Participants who did not complete relevant items were excluded from this analysis. Covariates in adjusted models were sex, race and ethnicity, income, and partner status; an additional seven participants were excluded based on missing data for these covariates. X-axis uses a log2 scale.

child's hospitalization compared with those from food-secure households (adjusted odds ratio [aOR] = 2.0, 95% confidence interval [CI] 1.1–3.6, *P* = .03; Fig 2). The odds of experiencing discrimination during the child's hospitalization were not significantly higher among caregivers from marginally food-secure households compared with caregivers from food-secure households (aOR = 1.6, 95% CI 0.7–3.4, *P* = .25).

In adjusted logistic models, caregivers from food-insecure households had significantly higher odds of experiencing 5 of the 7 types of discrimination assessed during their child's hospitalization compared with caregivers from food-secure households. The adjusted odds of being "treated with less respect than other people" were

>3-fold higher (aOR = 3.4, 95% CI 1.8–6.5, *P* < .001; Fig 2). In addition, caregivers from marginally food-secure households had significantly higher odds than caregivers from food-secure households of reporting that they "receive[d] poorer service than other people" at the child's hospital (aOR = 3.0, 95% CI 1.3–6.6, *P* < .01). These results are consistent with adjusted relative risk estimates (Supplemental Fig 3).

DISCUSSION

More than 1 in 4 caregivers of a child hospitalized during the COVID-19 pandemic, mostly lower-income African American or Black women, lived in a household that was food insecure in the 30 days before their child's hospitalization.

Household FI, especially during a pandemic that has disproportionately impacted African American and Black people,[9] presents a major risk for poor outcomes after a child's hospitalization. Without access to a sufficient diet, a child may not be able to adhere to medication regimens, healing can be compromised by poor nutrition, and caregivers can struggle to make critical caregiving and other medical decisions for their child. As hypothesized, we found that household FI in the month before the child's hospitalization was a predictor of experiences of discrimination for caregivers during their child's hospitalization.

Our data were collected in parallel with unprecedented federal interventions to address a massive food security crisis in the United States throughout the COVID-19 pandemic.[32] Even with these interventions, the proportion of households experiencing MFS or FI in our sample during the pandemic (40.2%) was similar to the rate in a 2011 study at the same site (43.6%, using a 12-month recall period)[13] and were several-fold higher than national averages from mid-November to mid-December 2020 for households with children (7.2%) and with heads of households who identified as non-Hispanic, African American or Black (11.8%).[33] The high rates of FI among families with a hospitalized child can be attributed in part to hospitalization itself[13] and supports emerging policies and calls from the Centers for Medicare and Medicaid Services, the Joint Commission, the National Quality Forum, and others to move health systems toward integrating social with medical care.[34–36]

More than one-half of caregivers in this study reported experiencing discrimination in the medical setting during their child's hospitalization. In addition, caregivers from food-insecure households were at significantly higher odds of experiencing 5 of the 7 types of discrimination assessed compared with caregivers from food-secure households. In this study, participants were not asked to indicate the perceived cause of discrimination. It is possible that parents and other caregivers in our study would have attributed their experiences of discrimination to race, gender, socioeconomic, or other circumstances. As described in the Stigma and Food Inequity Conceptual Framework, manifestations of stigma (like the perception of discrimination) have harmful effects on the psychosocial processes and behavior of people with FI, ultimately worsening food inequities and health.[5] The link between experiences of discrimination and food assistance use is well-documented in the case of SNAP; perceived discrimination by SNAP caseworkers triggers feelings of stigma that deter eligible participants from accessing food assistance.[10–12] To our knowledge, the current study is the first to assess the relationship between food security status and caregivers' experiences of discrimination in the children's hospital setting.

The finding that caregivers from food-insecure households had twice the odds of experiencing discrimination during their child's hospitalization compared with caregivers from food-secure households has implications for efforts to intervene in FI in the children's hospital setting. As reported in a 2019 cross-sectional study, the majority of African American or Black patients and adult caregivers of pediatric patients (79%) saw health-care-based screening for social risks as appropriate.[37] At the same time, consistent with the current study findings, qualitative studies of adult patients and caregivers of pediatric patients highlight stigmatization, including discrimination, as a barrier to both the disclosure of need and the use of referral resources.[38–42] In settings in which FI is highly prevalent, the benefits of a screening-based approach to assistance versus a universal approach (for example, availing everyone in the clinical setting access to emergency food assistance and information about community-based food supports) ought to be weighed against risks. The authors of the CommunityRx-Hunger randomized controlled trial are evaluating the impact of a universal approach to intervention in a setting in which everyone has 24/7/365 access to emergency food support.[13,20,21]

In addition, this study sheds new light on experiences of discrimination in the hospital setting among caregivers from marginally food-secure households. Specifically, this group had significantly higher odds of reporting receiving poorer service than other people during their child's hospitalization. Households with MFS are regarded as similar to those with food security in most food security research and in practice.[43] However, the experience of MFS is increasingly being recognized in the literature as having a unique psychosocial profile.[29,44–46] This study offers more evidence for consideration of marginally food secure caregivers as a distinct group.

Findings should be interpreted in light of certain limitations. The informed consent process did explain to study participants that the study was about food security and related needs, a factor that could have affected or primed their responses regarding both FI and discrimination.[45] Preenrollment screening for health-related social risks for the purpose of randomization into the randomized controlled trial may have impacted perceptions of discrimination. Although, with this study, we find a relationship between FI and experiences of health care discrimination, we do not discern perceived causes of discrimination. The single-site design and focus on caregivers of hospitalized children may limit this study's generalizability to other populations. Rapid cycle temporal trends in food access and food support related to the COVID-19 pandemic likely contributed to observed rates of FI throughout the study period. In addition, contemporaneous increases in societal awareness and action on issues of racism (health care- and community-based) and increased rates of health care worker burnout[47] may have increased perceptions of discrimination during the study period.

CONCLUSIONS

Experiences of discrimination in the children's hospital setting were prevalent overall and were associated with household FI in the 30 days before a child's hospitalization. Interventions in the children's hospital setting to mitigate FI should be delivered in a manner that optimizes the care experience and minimizes stigma.

ACKNOWLEDGMENTS

We would like to thank Eva Shiu, MPH, for overseeing data collection and Charlie Fuller and Veera Anand for verifying our citations. We would like to acknowledge the Feed1st Community Advisory Board for their ongoing guidance, commitment and collaboration on this work.

ABBREVIATIONS

aOR: adjusted odds ratio
BRFSS: Behavioral Risk Factor Surveillance System
CI: confidence interval
COVID-19: coronavirus disease 2019
DMS: Discrimination in Medical Settings
FI: food insecurity
MFS: marginal food security
SNAP: Supplemental Nutritional Assistance Program
WIC: Special Supplemental Nutritional Program for Women, Infants, and Children

made available after publication to researchers who provide a methodologically sound proposal for use in achieving the goals of the approved proposal. Proposals should be submitted to eabramsohn@bsd.uchicago.edu.

DOI: https://doi.org/10.1542/peds.2023-061750

Accepted for publication Sept 6, 2023

Address correspondence to Alexis Cacioppo, BA, Department of Obstetrics and Gynecology, 5841 South Maryland Ave, MC2050, Chicago, IL 60637. E-mail: alexis.cacioppo@uchicagomedicine.org

PEDIATRICS (ISSN Numbers: Print, 0031-4005; Online, 1098-4275).

Copyright © 2023 by the American Academy of Pediatrics

FUNDING: Funded by the National Institutes of Health (NIH). Research reported in this publication was supported by the National Institute on Minority Health and Health Disparities of the NIH under award number R01MD012630 and the Center for Healthcare Delivery Science and Innovation at the University of Chicago. The content is solely the responsibility of the authors and does not necessarily represent the official views of the NIH or the University of Chicago.

CONFLICT OF INTEREST DISCLOSURES: Dr Lindau discloses that she is a contributor to UpToDate, Inc, which generated royalties <$100/year to her laboratory at the University of Chicago (2019, 2020). Dr Lindau is also an unpaid advisor to and holds stock in Unite USA Inc, and holds debt in another corporate entity unrelated to the content of this manuscript. Dr Lindau and her spouse hold stocks and mutual funds managed by third parties. All other co-authors report no conflicts of interest.

REFERENCES

1. Coleman-Jensen A, Rabbitt MP, Hales L, Gregory CA. Definitions of food security. Available at: https://www.ers.usda.gov/topics/food-nutrition-assistance/food-security-in-the-us/definitions-of-food-security/. Accessed December 15, 2021

2. Coleman-Jensen A, Rabbitt MP, Gregory CA, Singh A. Household food security in the United States in 2021. Available at: https://www.ers.usda.gov/webdocs/publications/104656/err-309.pdf. Accessed September 25, 2022

3. Gundersen C, Ziliak JP. Food insecurity and health outcomes. *Health Aff (Millwood)*. 2015;34(11):1830–1839

4. Shankar P, Chung R, Frank DA. Association of food insecurity with children's behavioral, emotional, and academic outcomes: a systematic review. *J Dev Behav Pediatr*. 2017;38(2):135–150

5. Earnshaw VA, Karpyn A. Understanding stigma and food inequity: a conceptual framework to inform research, intervention, and policy. *Transl Behav Med*. 2020;10(6):1350–1357

6. Coleman-Jensen A, Rabbitt M, Gregory C, Singh A; United States Department of Agriculture, Economic Research Service. Household food security in the United States in 2019. Available at: https://www.ers.usda.gov/webdocs/publications/99282/err-275.pdf?v=6115.7. Accessed June 15, 2021

7. Morales DX, Morales SA, Beltran TF. Racial/ethnic disparities in household food insecurity during the COVID-19 pandemic: a nationally representative study. *J Racial Ethn Health Disparities*. 2021;8(5):1300–1314

8. Waxman E, Gupta P; Urban Institute. Food insecurity fell nearly 30 percent between spring 2020 and 2021. Available at: https://www.urban.org/sites/default/files/publication/104286/food-insecurity-fell-nearly-30-percent-between-spring-2020-and-2021-pdf_0.pdf. Accessed June 15, 2021

9. Feeding America. The impact of the coronavirus on food insecurity in 2020 & 2021. Available at: https://www.feedingamerica.org/sites/default/files/2021-03/National%20Projections%20Brief_3.9.2021_0.pdf. Accessed June 15, 2021

10. Edin K, Boyd M, Mabli J, et al; United States Department of Agriculture. SNAP food security in-depth interview study. Available at: https://fns-prod.azureedge.us/sites/default/files/SNAPFoodSec.pdf. Accessed August 28, 2022

11. Gaines-Turner T, Simmons JC, Chilton M. Recommendations from SNAP participants to improve wages and end stigma. *Am J Public Health*. 2019;109(12):1664–1667

12. Guardia FPL, Policy FSN, Lacko RAA; Food Research & Action Center. To end hunger, we must end stigma. Available at: https://frac.org/blog/endhungerendstigma. Accessed August 28, 2022

13. Makelarski JA, Thorngren D, Lindau ST. Feed first, ask questions later: alleviating and understanding caregiver food insecurity in an urban children's hospital. *Am J Public Health*. 2015;105(8):e98–e104

14. Lee AM, Lopez MA, Haq H, et al. Inpatient food insecurity in caregivers of hospitalized pediatric patients: a mixed methods study. *Acad Pediatr*. 2021;21(8):1404–1413

15. Schwartz B, Herrmann LE, Librizzi J, et al. Screening for social determinants of health in hospitalized children. *Hosp Pediatr*. 2020;10(1):29–36

16. Ashbrook A, Essel K, Montez K, Bennett-Tejes D; American Academy of Pediatrics and Food Research & Action Center. Screen and intervene: a toolkit for pediatricians to address food insecurity. Available at: https://frac.org/wp-content/uploads/FRAC_AAP_Toolkit_2021.pdf. Accessed June 21, 2021

17. Biddinger S; Children's Hospital Association. Screening for social determinants of health. Available at: https://www.childrenshospitals.org/-/media/files/migration/pophlth_social_determinants_health_report.pdf. Accessed May 10, 2022

18. University of Chicago Medical Center. Community health needs assessment 2021–2022. Available at: https://issuu.com/communitybenefit-ucm/docs/ucmc-chna-2021-2022?fr=sNTc0NTE00Dc0MDM. Accessed February 3, 2022

19. Cunningham J. 2019 annual report. Available at: https://pediatrics.uchicago.edu/node/2056. Accessed December 20, 2021

20. National Institute on Minority Health and Health Disparities (NIMHD). CommunityRx-Hunger: a hospital-based intervention for primary caregivers of children admitted to the hospital. Available at: https://clinicaltrials.gov/ct2/show/NCT04171999. Accessed December 19, 2022

21. Frazier CRM, Pinkerton EA, Grana M, et al. Feed1st, no questions asked: how a hospital-based food pantry program grew its impact during the COVID-19 pandemic. *Am J Public Health*. 2022;112(10):1394–1398

22. Lee Badgett M, Baker KE, Conron K, et al; University of California, Los Angeles School of Law. Best practices for asking questions to identify transgender and other gender minority respondents on population-based surveys. Available at: https://williamsinstitute.law.ucla.edu/wp-content/uploads/Survey-Measures-Trans-GenIUSS-Sep-2014.pdf. Accessed July 3, 2023

23. Agency for Healthcare Research and Quality. The CAHPS child hospital survey. Available at: https://www.ahrq.gov/cahps/surveys-guidance/hospital/about/child_hp_survey.html. Accessed July 4, 2023

24. Centers for Disease Control and Prevention. The behavioral risk factor surveillance system (BRFSS). Overview: BRFSS 2018. Available at: https://www.cdc.gov/brfss/annual_data/2018/pdf/overview-2018-508.pdf. Accessed July 4, 2023

25. United States Census Bureau. American community survey (ACS). Available at: https://www.census.gov/programs-surveys/acs. Accessed August 11, 2021

26. Feeding America. Hunger in America 2014 executive summary. Available at: https://www.feedingamerica.org/sites/default/files/research/hunger-in-america/hia-2014-executive-summary.pdf. Accessed July 4, 2023

27. Bickel G, Nord M, Price C, et al; United States Department of Agriculture, Food and Nutrition Service, Office of Analysis, Nutrition, and Evaluation. Guide to measuring household food security revised 2000. Available at: https://naldc.nal.usda.gov/download/38369/PDF. Accessed February 7, 2022

28. Coleman-Jensen A, Rabbitt MP, Hales L, Gregory CAUS. Household food security survey module. Available at: https://www.ers.usda.gov/media/8279/ad2012.pdf. Accessed July 9, 2021

29. Cook JT, Black M, Chilton M, et al. Are food insecurity's health impacts underestimated in the U.S. population? Marginal food security also predicts adverse health outcomes in young U.S. children and mothers. *Adv Nutr*. 2013;4(1):51–61

30. Peek ME, Nunez-Smith M, Drum M, Lewis TT. Adapting the everyday discrimination scale to medical settings: reliability and validity testing in a sample of African American patients. *Ethn Dis*. 2011;21(4):502–509

31. Benjamins MR, Middleton M. Perceived discrimination in medical settings and perceived quality of care: a population-based study in Chicago. *PLoS ONE*. 2019;14(4):e0215976

32. Caspi C, Seligman H, Berge J, et al; Health Affairs. COVID-19 pandemic-era nutrition assistance: impact and sustainability. Available at: https://www.healthaffairs.org/do/10.1377/hpb20220330.534478/full/. Accessed July 4, 2022

33. Coleman-Jensen A, Rabbitt MP, Gregory CA, Singh A; Unites States Department of Agriculture, Economic Research Service. Statistical supplement to household food security in the United States in 2020. Available at: https://www.ers.usda.gov/webdocs/publications/102072/ap-091.pdf?v=5937.3. Accessed August 2, 2021

34. Tsai D. Additional guidance on use of in lieu of services and settings in Medicaid managed care. Available at: https://www.medicaid.gov/federal-policy-guidance/downloads/smd23001.pdf/. Accessed February 14, 2022

35. The Joint Commission. New requirements to reduce health care disparities. Available at: https://www.jointcommission.org/-/media/tjc/documents/standards/r3-reports/r3_disparities_july2022-6-20-2022.pdf. Accessed February 14, 2023

36. Committee on Integrating Social Needs Care into the Delivery of Health Care to Improve the Nation's Health, Board on Health Care Services, Health and Medicine Division, National Academies of Sciences, Engineering, and Medicine. *Integrating Social Care into the Delivery of Health Care: Moving Upstream to Improve the Nation's Health*. National Academies Press; 2019

37. De Marchis EH, Hessler D, Fichtenberg C, et al. Part I: a quantitative study of social risk screening acceptability in patients and caregivers. *Am J Prev Med*. 2019;57(6 Suppl 1):S25–S37

38. Hsu C, Cruz S, Placzek H, et al. Patient perspectives on addressing social needs in primary care using a screening and resource referral intervention. *J Gen Intern Med*. 2020;35(2):481–489

39. Knowles M, Khan S, Palakshappa D, et al. Successes, challenges, and considerations for integrating referral into food insecurity screening in pediatric settings. *J Health Care Poor Underserved*. 2018;29(1):181–191

40. Barnidge E, Krupsky K, LaBarge G, Arthur J. Food insecurity screening in pediatric clinical settings: a caregivers' perspective. *Matern Child Health J.* 2020;24(1):101–109

41. Cullen D, Woodford A, Fein J. Food for thought: a randomized trial of food insecurity screening in the emergency department. *Acad Pediatr.* 2019;19(6):646–651

42. Steeves-Reece AL, Totten AM, Broadwell KD, et al. Social needs resource connections: a systematic review of barriers, facilitators, and evaluation. *Am J Prev Med.* 2022;62(5):e303–e315

43. Economic Research Service, U.S. Department of Agriculture. Measurement. Available at: https://www.ers.usda.gov/topics/food-nutrition-assistance/food-security-in-the-u-s/measurement/#security. Accessed February 4, 2023

44. Children's Health Watch. Report card on food security among young children in 2015. Available at: http://childrenshealthwatch.org/wp-content/uploads/Hidden-Food-Stress-Report-Card.pdf. Accessed July 12, 2022

45. Bayoumi I, Birken CS, Nurse KM, et al. Screening for marginal food security in young children in primary care. *BMC Pediatr.* 2021;21(1):196

46. Men F, Tarasuk V. Classification differences in food insecurity measures between the United States and Canada: practical implications for trend monitoring and health research. *J Nutr.* 2022;152(4):1082–1090

47. Galanis P, Vraka I, Fragkou D, et al. Nurses' burnout and associated risk factors during the COVID-19 pandemic: a systematic review and meta-analysis. *J Adv Nurs.* 2021;77(8):3286–3302

Reducing Caregiver Hunger During Pediatric Hospitalization

Katherine A. Auger, MD, MSc,[a,b,c] Brenda Demeritt, MHA, RN, CPN,[d] Andrew F. Beck, MD, MPH,[a,c,e] Anita Shah, DO, MPH,[a,c] Stacey Litman, MSW,[d] Julie Pinson, RN,[d] Thomas Wright, BS,[f] Susan C. Cronin, PhD,[g] Carlos A. Casillas, MD, MPH,[a] Hadley Sauers-Ford, MPH,[a] Sarah Ferris, BA,[h] Calise Curry, BA,[a] Ndidi Unaka, MD, MEd[a,c]

BACKGROUND AND OBJECTIVES: Pediatric hospitalizations are costly, stressful events for families. Many caregivers, especially those with lower incomes, struggle to afford food while their child is hospitalized. We sought to decrease the mean percentage of caregivers of Medicaid-insured and uninsured children who reported being hungry during their child's hospitalization from 86% to <24%.

METHODS: Our quality improvement efforts took place on a 41-bed inpatient unit at our large, urban academic hospital. Our multidisciplinary team included physicians, nurses, social workers, and food services leadership. Our primary outcome measure was caregiver-reported hunger; we asked caregivers near to the time of discharge if they experienced hunger during their child's hospitalization. Plan-do-study-act cycles addressed key drivers: awareness of how to obtain food, safe environment for families to seek help, and access to affordable food. An annotated statistical process control chart tracked our outcome over time. Data collection was interrupted because of the COVID-19 pandemic; we used that time to advocate for hospital-funded support for optimal and sustainable changes to caregiver meal access.

RESULTS: We decreased caregiver hunger from 86% to 15.5%. A temporary test of change, 2 meal vouchers per caregiver per day, resulted in a special cause decrease in the percentage of caregivers reporting hunger. Permanent hospital funding was secured to provide cards to purchase 2 meals per caregiver per hospital day, resulting in a sustained decrease in rates of caregiver hunger.

CONCLUSIONS: We decreased caregivers' hunger during their child's hospitalization. Through a data-driven quality improvement effort, we implemented a sustainable change allowing families to access enough food.

[a]Division of Hospital Medicine, [b]James M. Anderson Center, [d]Department of Patient Services, and [e]Divisions of General Pediatrics and [g]Pulmonary Medicine, Cincinnati Children's Hospital Medical Center, Cincinnati, Ohio; [c]Department of Pediatrics, University of Cincinnati College of Medicine, Cincinnati, Ohio; [f]Sodexho Healthcare Services, Cincinnati, Ohio; and [h]Clinical Trials Support Unit, Michigan Medicine, University of Michigan, Ann Arbor, Michigan

Dr Auger conceptualized and designed the study, drafted the initial manuscript, carried out the initial analyses, and reviewed and revised the manuscript. Dr Unaka conceptualized and designed the study, drafted the initial manuscript, and reviewed and revised the manuscript. Drs Beck, Shah, Cronin, Casillas; Mss Demeritt, Litman, Pinson, and Sauers-Ford; and Mr Wright conceptualized and designed the study and reviewed and revised the manuscript. Mss Ferris and Curry coordinated and supervised data collection, and critically reviewed the manuscript for important intellectual content. All authors approved the final manuscript as submitted and agree to be accountable for all aspects of the work.

DOI: https://doi.org/10.1542/peds.2022-058080

Accepted for publication Jan 18, 2023

Address correspondence to Katherine A. Auger, MD, MSc, 3333 Burnet Ave, MLC 9016, Cincinnati, OH 45229. E-mail: Katherine.auger@cchmc.org

PEDIATRICS (ISSN Numbers: Print, 0031-4005; Online, 1098-4275).

Copyright © 2023 by the American Academy of Pediatrics

FUNDING: Dr Auger's research is supported through a grant from AHRQ (1K08HS024735). Early tests of change were supported through a gift from the Cooperative Society of Cincinnati Children's Hospital Medical Center.

CONFLICT OF INTEREST DISCLOSURES: The authors have indicated they have no potential conflicts of interest to disclose.

To cite: Auger KA, Demeritt B, Beck AF, et al. Reducing Caregiver Hunger During Pediatric Hospitalization. *Pediatrics.* 2023;151(5): e2022058080

One in 5 US households with children is food insecure,[1] lacking access to enough food to fully meet nutritional needs because of insufficient resources. Food insecurity is a major public health challenge and has significant implications for child health. Household food insecurity, and the hunger that often results, is associated with poor quality of life among children and families[2] and lower rating of overall child health and wellbeing.[3]

Food insecurity is unrelenting for many families and can extend into the hospital setting. Many families report an inability to pay for food during their child's hospitalization.[4] Hunger, resulting from an inability to afford food, may impair processing of new or complex information. Many caregivers report a feeling of "fog" during hospitalization,[5] which makes comprehension of new information about their child's illness more challenging. Addressing caregiver hunger may decrease this fog and

QUALITY REPORT

support caregivers' capacity to fully participate in their child's hospitalization.

We assessed hunger during hospitalization among parents/caregivers, hereafter caregivers, on 1 inpatient unit. Most caregivers of Medicaid-insured youth reported going hungry during their child's hospitalization. Therefore, our improvement aim was to decrease the mean percentage of caregivers of Medicaid-insured and uninsured children who reported being hungry during their child's hospitalization from a baseline of 86% in July 2019 to <24%.

METHODS

Context

Cincinnati Children's Hospital Medical Center (CCHMC) is a large, urban, academic, free-standing pediatric hospital located in metropolitan Cincinnati. Rates of food insecurity range from 19% to 31% across regional counties.[6] Our improvement efforts took place on a 41-bed general medical unit that serves as the primary unit for patients admitted to CCHMC's Hospital Medicine (HM) service. Annually, ~6500 patients are admitted to the HM service, with an average length of stay of 1.6 days. Approximately 60% of the patients admitted to HM are insured by Medicaid; <2% of patients are uninsured. The remainder of the patients have private insurance.

We focused on caregivers of children with Medicaid or no insurance because the difference in the rates of hunger between this group of caregivers was striking (86% of Medicaid/uninsured reported hunger from 96 surveys and 24% of private-pay caregivers reported hunger from 50 surveys; data were collected from August 22, 2019, to October 7, 2019). Even though nearly 1 in 4 caregivers

of children with private insurance reported hunger, potential interventions to address hunger in this population would have required developing a screening system to predict which families may need food support during hospitalization. We elected to focus on caregivers of children with Medicaid or no insurance because of the near-universal need for help in this population as well as the disparity. Therefore, 24% was set as the goal for caregivers of children with Medicaid/uninsured in an attempt to eliminate this disparity.

During hospitalizations, caregivers can purchase full meals (main course, 2 sides, and drink) delivered to their room for $6. Only caregivers with a credit card could order meals over the phone in the patient's room. Alternatively, caregivers could purchase meals with cash or credit card in the cafeteria, which is open 24 hours a day. It typically costs $8 to $10 in the cafeteria for the same amount of food that can be ordered through room delivery. Before initiating this improvement project, caregivers were eligible for meal assistance through a social work referral by physicians or nurses. With social work approval, a caregiver could pick up 2 meal cards per day, each worth $6, from the family resource center (located on the main floor of the hospital some distance from the unit and open only during the day). The caregiver had to go to the cafeteria to use the meal cards; a caregiver could not use the meal cards to purchase food through the room delivery option.

Interventions

We assembled a multidisciplinary team to assess the current state of caregiver hunger on the unit and to understand and improve processes to reduce hunger in this at-risk population. Our team consisted of nursing and physician unit leaders

and representation from bedside nursing, social work, HM attending and resident physicians, research assistants, and food services leadership.

We created a process map of the existing supports for caregivers who reported hunger (Supplemental Fig 5). We also created a key driver diagram (Fig 1) to highlight: (1) what needed to be in place to address caregiver hunger and (2) potential interventions to reduce hunger among caregivers. In addition, we created a Pareto chart to categorize and prioritize reasons for caregiver hunger during hospitalization (Fig 2).

Our key drivers and associated interventions follow.

Education for Staff and Providing a Safe Environment for Families to Seek Food Assistance (Intervention 1)

Our first test of change consisted of education provided to the unit's bedside nurses. We pursued this test to raise awareness of hunger as an issue for hospitalized families. Education was provided via presentations at staff meetings and through e-mail communication containing instructions on how to connect families with social work if they reported hunger. We also placed signs in patient rooms, instructing caregivers to ask a nurse for help with obtaining food (Supplemental Fig 6, Table 1).

Adequate Access to Affordable Food (Interventions 2-6)

We carried out multiple tests of change designed to enhance caregiver access to food (Table 1). Some interventions were designed to be temporary changes because of a lack of funding for sustainability. These temporary interventions allowed us to evaluate what support might decrease hunger if funds were to become available long term. Intervention 2 was a 1-week test in

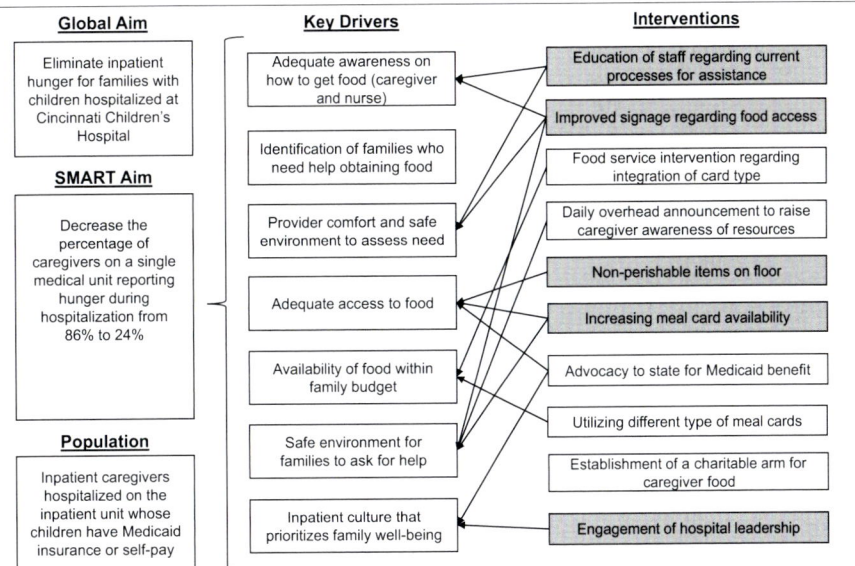

Reducing Inpatient Caregiver Hunger Key Driver Diagram

Global Aim

Eliminate inpatient hunger for families with children hospitalized at Cincinnati Children's Hospital

SMART Aim

Decrease the percentage of caregivers on a single medical unit reporting hunger during hospitalization from 86% to 24%

Population

Inpatient caregivers hospitalized on the inpatient unit whose children have Medicaid insurance or self-pay

Key Drivers

Adequate awareness on how to get food (caregiver and nurse)

Identification of families who need help obtaining food

Provider comfort and safe environment to assess need

Adequate access to food

Availability of food within family budget

Safe environment for families to ask for help

Inpatient culture that prioritizes family well-being

Interventions

Education of staff regarding current processes for assistance

Improved signage regarding food access

Food service intervention regarding integration of card type

Daily overhead announcement to raise caregiver awareness of resources

Non-perishable items on floor

Increasing meal card availability

Advocacy to state for Medicaid benefit

Utilizing different type of meal cards

Establishment of a charitable arm for caregiver food

Engagement of hospital leadership

FIGURE 1

Key driver diagram and potential interventions. Shaded interventions were part of quality improvement project. Interventions in white were listed as potential interventions but were not tested during this project.

which caregivers were offered a single meal voucher per day. Meal vouchers allowed families to receive a main course, 2 sides, and drink delivered to the bedside. Intervention 3 was a change to keep nonperishable food items on the unit for newly admitted patients and caregivers who arrived on the unit late at night. Intervention 4 was a temporary test of change to determine if hunger could be

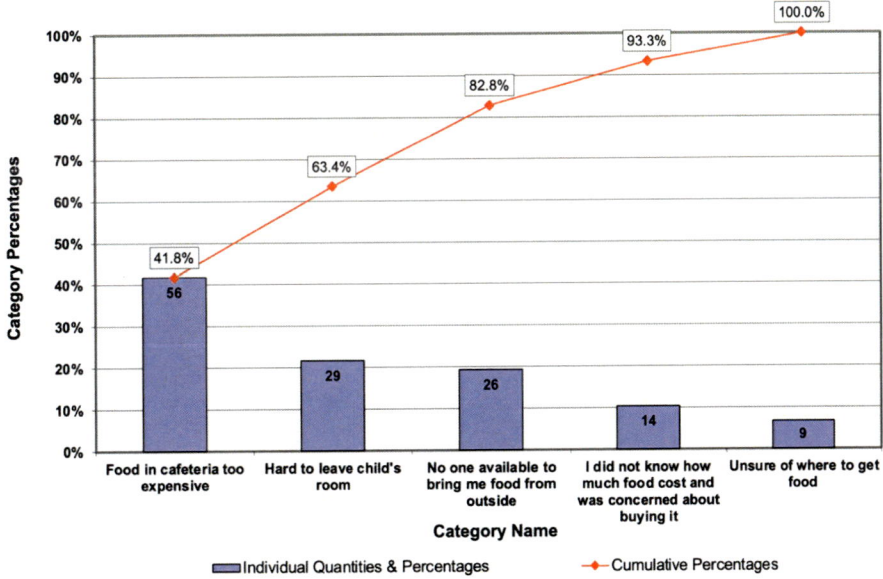

Reasons for Hunger (*n* = 134 reasons from 83 caregivers)

FIGURE 2

Pareto chart examining reasons that caregivers reported going hungry during their child's hospitalization. Caregivers could select more than 1 category. Data were collected during the baseline period (August 22, 2019–October 7, 2019).

TABLE 1 Interventions, Descriptions, and Population

Intervention	Description	Support Details	Period	Eligible Population
Preintervention	Meal card[a] available in family resource center	$6 cash equivalent to be redeemed in the cafeteria	Ongoing	Those for whom an order for a social work consult was placed
1	Signs placed in patient rooms raising awareness of food support	Sign instructed families to ask their nurse for help with food assistance	Ongoing	All families of children with Medicaid or who were uninsured
2	One meal voucher[a] per caregiver per day	Allowed caregivers to receive 1 full meal delivered to their room. Vouchers were distributed by research assistant	1 wk	All families of children with Medicaid or who were uninsured
3	Nonperishable food items stored on unit[b]		Ongoing	Only families with extenuating circumstances, such as a very late admission or if the caregiver could not go to cafeteria
4	Two meal vouchers[a] per caregiver per day	Allowed caregivers to receive 2 full meals per caregiver per day delivered to their room Vouchers were distributed by research assistant	2 wk	All families of children with Medicaid or who were uninsured hospitalized on half of unit
5	Two meal cards[a] per caregiver per day	$7.50 cash equivalent per card redeemable in the cafeteria. Cards were given to bedside nurses to distribute to families	Ongoing	All families of children with Medicaid or who were uninsured
6	Two meal cards[a] per caregiver per day	Same as intervention 5 but with a dedicated charge nurse distributing to all eligible families	Ongoing	All families of children with Medicaid or who were uninsured

[a] Meal cards are redeemable in the cafeteria for a cash-equivalent value. Meal vouchers allow for delivery of full meals (main course, 2 sides, and drink) to the patient room.
[b] Example food items include macaroni and cheese, instant soups, and snack bars.

addressed through meal vouchers. Intervention 4 ran for 2 weeks on half of the inpatient unit and provided up to 2 caregivers per patient with 2 meal vouchers per day. We list the half of the unit that received the cards as "intervention" and the half of the unit that did not as "control." Intervention 5 was an adaptation of intervention 4 using meal cards. In contrast to meal vouchers, meal cards are redeemable in the cafeteria for cash-equivalent value. Intervention 5 provided 2 caregivers per patient with 2 meal cards per day (each valued at $7.50). Intervention 6 was a change in the distribution method for these meal cards (from bedside nurse to charge nurse).

System-Level Advocacy: Leveraging an Inpatient Culture That Prioritizes Family Well-Being

We presented information to hospital leadership on the scope of the problem, our successes, and our challenges. Specifically, we presented our control charts updated through intervention 4, as well as the estimated costs of the program (detailed in the Results section). By providing evidence of the effectiveness of the proposed solution to hospital leadership, we obtained sustainable financial support from hospital administration, making it a permanent change on the unit (allowing us to implement intervention 5 described previously and in Table 1).

Study of the Intervention

We began collecting baseline data in August 2019. Each weekday, a research assistant reviewed the list of hospitalized patients on the intervention unit to determine insurance status for eligibility. Nurses routinely predict discharge timing for each patient.[7] If the patient was predicted to be discharged that day, the research assistant asked 1 caregiver per patient questions about experiencing hunger during their child's hospitalization. We chose to survey caregivers near to time of discharge to ensure caregivers could reflect on their hunger throughout the entire hospitalization. Questionnaires were available in English and Spanish and were administered on paper before the COVID-19 pandemic.

At the onset of the COVID-19 pandemic (March 2020), all research and quality improvement initiatives were paused. Our quality improvement project restarted in November 2020 with several system and logistical changes. Caregivers of patients who tested positive for COVID-19 or were awaiting COVID-19 test results were given free meals in their rooms. We included these caregivers in our data collection because we hypothesized that they may still experience hunger if they received meals for only part of their hospital stay. Data collection changed from in person to by phone to keep research assistants off the inpatient units.

Measures

Our primary outcome measure was the percentage of caregivers with self-reported hunger during their child's hospitalization. We adapted questions from the US Department of Agriculture's Food Security Survey Module.[8] Specifically, we defined hunger as a caregiver responding in the affirmative to any of the following questions:

- During this hospitalization, did you or other adults in your household ever cut the size of your meals or skip meals because there wasn't enough money for food?
- During this hospitalization, did you ever eat less than you felt you should because there wasn't enough money for food?
- During this hospitalization, were you ever hungry but didn't eat because there wasn't enough money for food?
- During this hospitalization, did you ever eat less than you felt you should for some other reason other than money?

These questions were asked on the day of discharge to assess hunger that may have occurred at any time during hospitalization. Additionally, the day-of-discharge questionnaire included questions on contributors to hunger (if present) (eg, food was too expensive) and whether the family received meal assistance during hospitalization (ie, meal vouchers, meal cards) (process measure).

We also estimated programmatic costs. For vouchers distributed by a research assistant, we tracked the number distributed to capture cost ($6 per voucher). For meal cards, we tracked the amount of money

redeemed in the cafeteria. For example, if the card had a $7.50 value on it, but the caregiver only purchased $7 worth of food, the cost captured was only $7.

Analysis

We analyzed our outcome (the percentage of caregivers who reported hunger during their child's hospitalization) and process measure (the percentage of caregivers who received meal assistance) using a statistical process control charts (P-charts). We tracked initial data with subgrouping of 8 caregivers to collect baseline data quickly (12 baseline points) before testing interventions. After the baseline data collection, we switched to tracking data weekly. Given that we changed our data collection procedures (paper to phone) and with the changes in food access for caregivers of children with COVID-19, we recalculated baseline hunger rates after the data collection restart in November 2020, before initiating further tests of change.

Centerline shifts were based on established rules for special cause variation; specifically, either points outside control limits or ≥8 points above or below the mean line.[9] Short interventions that ran for 1 to 2 weeks (interventions 2 and 4) were not included in calculation of means or toward or against midline shifts (ie, we skipped these weeks when counting for runs of 8 points) because these interventions were not intended to result in sustained system change.

Finally, we describe the financial cost of the interventions, presenting the average number of cafeteria cards redeemed per month and the average monthly cost.

Ethical Considerations

Our study was deemed exempt by the CCHMC institutional review board.

RESULTS

Initially, a mean of 86% of all caregivers of Medicaid-insured/uninsured hospitalized children reported that they were hungry during hospitalization (Fig 3). All the caregivers who indicated being hungry during the baseline data collection indicated that they were hungry because of financial reasons. Although many caregivers identified more than 1 factor contributing to their hunger during hospitalization, concern about costs of food was the most common factor identified (Fig 2). The mean line shifted to 94% of surveyed caregivers reporting hunger at the time of this change when signs to raise awareness about hunger were placed in patient rooms (intervention 1). Our tests of providing 1 meal voucher per caregiver per day (intervention 2) and the opening of a food closet with nonperishable food on the unit (intervention 3) were not associated with changes in our primary outcome.

Providing 2 meal vouchers per caregiver per day on half of the inpatient unit (intervention 4) resulted in special cause variation (2 points outside the statistical process control limits), reflecting a significant decrease in the number of caregivers reporting hunger. Of note, the other half of the unit in which meal cards were not provided continued to have high rates of reported hunger without evidence of a change. After intervention 4 concluded, the improvement project was paused because of the COVID-19 pandemic.

We recalculated baseline data after the 8-month pause. This recalculation revealed a new baseline of 81% of caregivers reporting hunger during hospitalization. After obtaining funding to provide 2 meal cards per caregiver per day, each worth

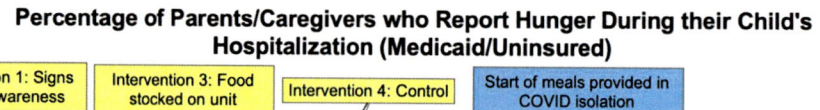

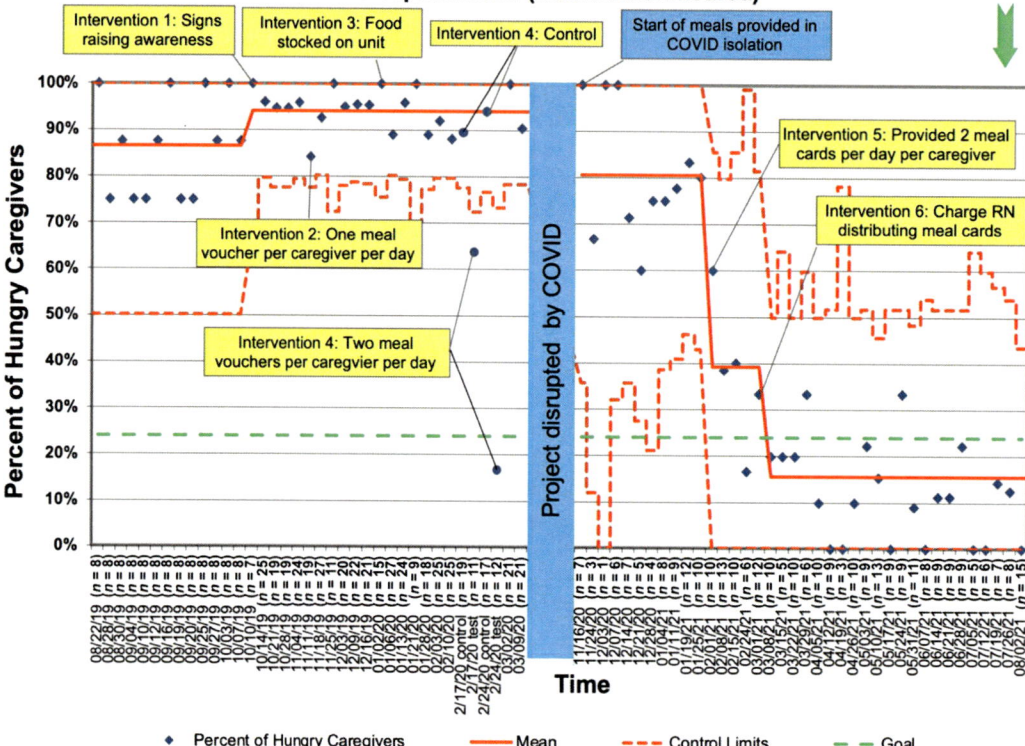

FIGURE 3

Statistical process control chart displaying the percentage of caregivers who reported hunger during their child's hospitalization (primary outcome measure). Data with circles indicate that the intervention was performed on only half of the unit, with the other half serving as a control. Interventions are highlighted in yellow. Other system changes not part of the intervention are highlighted in blue. The desired direction of change, indicated by the green arrow, is down. The solid red line represents the mean; the dashed red lines represent the control limits. Special cause was defined as 8 consecutive points above or below the mean or points outside the control limits. Temporary interventions (interventions 2 and 4) did not contribute to special cause rules (ie, excluded when counting)

$7.50, redeemable in the cafeteria (intervention 5), the rate of hunger fell to 39%. After changing the distribution to charge nurses (intervention 6), the unit's mean rate of caregiver hunger fell to 15.5%, a rate sustained for 7 months.

In regard to our process measure, the percentage of caregivers reporting meal assistance, the baseline rate of 48% remained stable before pausing because of COVID, with the exception of the period corresponding to tests 2 and 4. During this time, significantly more caregivers

reported receiving meal assistance during the distribution of meal vouchers (Fig 4). After restarting the data collection, the baseline rate of assistance was 28%. When the team began providing 2 meal cards per caregiver per day (interventions 5/6), the rate of caregivers reported receiving meal assistance rose to 99% and was sustained.

Cost Measures

During intervention 4, the research assistant distributed 234 meal cards to 51 families over a 2-week period, costing $1404. During interventions 5 and 6, an average of 685 cards per

month (standard deviation, 107) were redeemed in the cafeteria. The average cost was $4939 per month (standard deviation, $780).

DISCUSSION

Our multidisciplinary improvement team reduced reported hunger among caregivers of hospitalized children insured by Medicaid or uninsured from a baseline of 86% to 15.5%. The most impactful intervention was providing caregivers with vouchers or cash equivalent cards for 2 meals per day. This study underscores the importance of assessing and

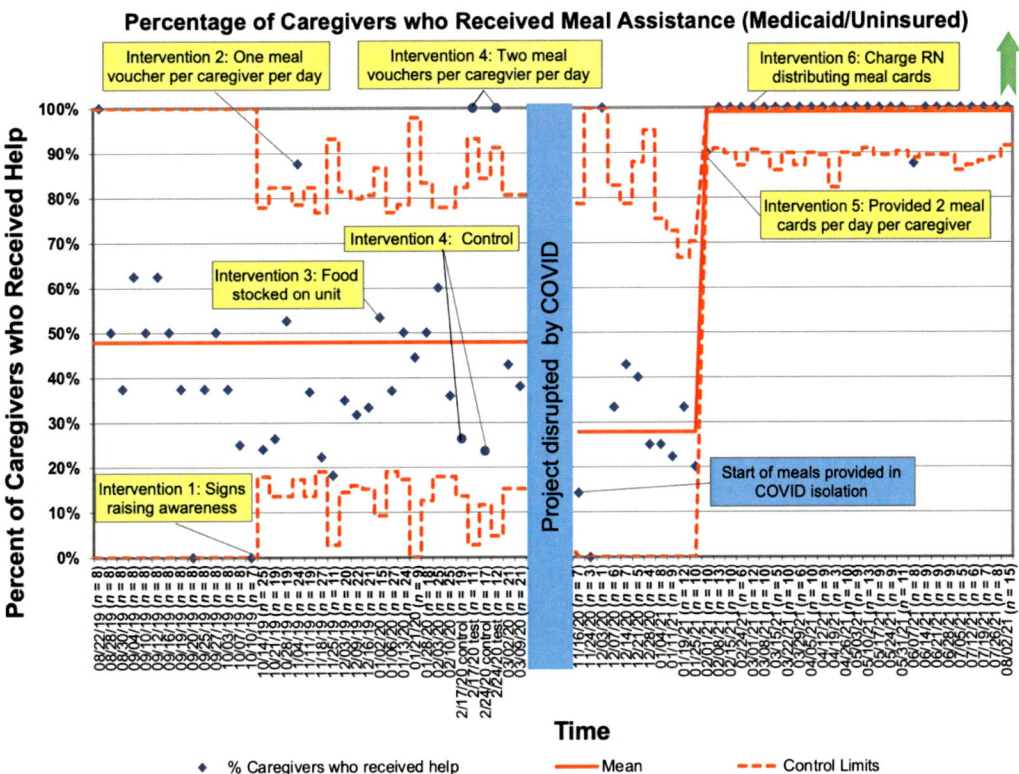

FIGURE 4

Statistical process control chart displaying the percentage of caregivers who reported receiving help with meals during their child's hospitalization (process measure). Data with circles indicate that the intervention was performed on only half of the unit, with the other half serving as a control. Interventions are highlighted in yellow. Other system changes not part of the intervention are highlighted in blue. The desired direction of change, indicated by the green arrow, is up. The solid red line represents the mean; the dashed red lines represent the control limits. Special cause was defined as 8 consecutive points above or below the mean or points outside the control limits.

addressing caregiver hunger during their child's hospitalization. Ensuring families have enough food to eat while their child is hospitalized may support caregivers' capacity to be at bedside, engage in and comprehend education, and, importantly, uphold basic human dignity.

Hospitalizations are stressful and can lead many families to incur significant financial costs.[10,11] The resulting financial strain almost certainly worsens food insecurity within the hospital and in the days following discharge. These costs disproportionately burden those with limited financial means and make transitions from hospital to home even more difficult. Screening

for food insecurity during health care encounters provides the opportunity to connect families to community resources.[12,13] Providing direct food support in the hospital may bolster the relationship with families and improve outcomes. For these reasons, the American Academy of Pediatrics recommends that pediatricians screen and identify children at risk for food insecurity and connect these families to resources.[14] The high rates of caregiver hunger highlight the importance of recognizing hospitalization as an important opportunity to discuss hunger and food insecurity. Our rates of caregiver hunger are higher than some other studies[4,15]; however,

we focused on families with Medicaid/uninsured who are more likely to be lower income and, therefore, experience hunger.

Our first intervention relied predominantly on education through staff communication via e-mail and staff meetings. We also placed signs in all patient rooms on the unit with instructions on how to obtain food and encouraged families to ask for help if they were experiencing hunger. Although education is generally a low reliability intervention,[16,17] we noted an increase in the number of caregivers reporting hunger. We hypothesize that the signs may have created an explicit invitation to caregivers to discuss hunger without shame and subsequently empowered families to report their hunger when surveyed by our research assistant.

The high frequency with which caregivers reported hunger before the initiation of our initiative likely reflected inadequacies of the meal support structure for caregivers. Before our work, hungry caregivers could receive a meal card worth $6 in the cafeteria by meeting with a social worker on the unit. The $6 card had to be picked up by the family each day in the family resource center (which is not located near the unit) and was redeemable only by going down to the cafeteria. The amount provided was often of insufficient value to purchase a full meal in the cafeteria. In contrast, families with access to credit cards could order a full meal (ie, main course, 2 sides, and drink) for $6 through the same room service that prepares patient meals. Conceptually, the most intuitive solution would be to provide these same in-room meals to all families for the same price; this approach would likely be preferred at institutions with the capability and capacity to provide bedside meals. However, food service leadership noted at the beginning of our project that we could not increase the number of caregivers receiving in-room meals without risking delays to patient meals. So, the large number of caregivers who required meal assistance could not be fed through the same room-service process. The main cafeteria, however, had adequate capacity to provide meals to caregivers with limited financial means. Without collaboration with food services leaders, we may not have been able to successfully identify ways to adapt interventions that were successful in our system; in this case, providing meal cards with enough money to purchase full meals.

We also benefited from the expertise of the bedside nurses on the study team. During intervention 5 (in which caregivers received 2 meal cards per day), the bedside nurses were excited to distribute cards and did so with excellent fidelity (nearly 100% of caregivers reported receiving meal assistance). However, there was ongoing confusion regarding eligibility and how to use the meal cards once they were received. Ultimately, changing the distribution to a single person per shift (charge nurse) improved efficiencies as well as consistency for families, resulting in a further decline in the number of caregivers reporting hunger.

Importantly, this work took place during the COVID-19 pandemic. Early data indicate that the pandemic has likely worsened food insecurity.[18] Thus, supporting food access to caregivers became even more important during the pandemic. That said, on our restart, the baseline rate of hunger was similar after we restarted data collection (86% vs. 81%). Despite our hospital providing meals to caregivers of children in COVID-19 isolation, fewer caregivers reported receiving meal assistance when we restarted data collection (48% vs 28%); this finding may reflect the impact of altered care processes and increased isolation due to COVID-19 precautions.

Finally, the ability to make this project sustainable required evidence and cost estimates for discussions with hospital leadership. Hospital leaders were motivated to support families and decrease disparities in experiences between our Medicaid and private-pay families. Presenting evidence on the prevalence of the problem, as well as the effectiveness of the intervention, and detailing costs of implementation, allowed us to

secure funding to implement a permanent change.

Our work is not without limitations. First, this project took place on 1 unit at a single children's hospital and may not be generalizable to other units, hospitals, or regions. However, key drivers and highlighted interventions would likely be relevant to other settings. Second, although the percentage of caregivers who reported hunger was extremely high, we may have missed some who did not feel comfortable reporting their experience with hunger during their child's hospitalization. Furthermore, we did not have a caregiver partner involved in the project, so we may have missed potential ways to mitigate this weakness. Third, we only surveyed caregivers and provided meal assistance to caregivers of children insured by Medicaid or who were uninsured. Although our interventions were successful in eliminating the Medicaid/uninsured to private disparity, the rate of baseline hunger in the group of private-pay caregivers was still close to 1 in 4. Fourth, although it is a strength that we administered surveys in both English and Spanish, several interventions (eg, signs in rooms) were in English. Future work should ensure information on assistance is equitably available regardless of language. Last, we did not examine if in-hospital food support meaningfully changes patient outcomes or parent experiences. Does having in-hospital food allow more caregivers to remain at the bedside? Is the "fog" that families report during hospitalization partially relieved by alleviating hunger? Answers to these questions, which we will consider as we spread our intervention, would add to an already strong case for widespread adoption, providing evidence that stretches beyond the humanitarian appeal of alleviating hunger.

CONCLUSION

Nearly all caregivers of children hospitalized with Medicaid insurance reported experiencing hunger during hospitalization. Providing support for 2 meals per caregiver per day drastically reduces caregiver hunger. Providing evidence of the prevalence of the problem, as well as the effectiveness of the solution, allowed us to implement sustainable change at our institution.

ABBREVIATIONS

CCHMC: Cincinnati Children's Hospital Medical Center
HM: Hospital Medicine

REFERENCES

1. Coleman-Jensen A, Gregory CA, Singh A. Household food security in the United States in 2013. Available at: https://www.ers.usda.gov/webdocs/publications/45265/48787_err173.pdf?v=8343.5. Accessed January 31, 2023

2. Moafi F, Kazemi F, Samiei Siboni F, Alimoradi Z. The relationship between food security and quality of life among pregnant women. BMC Pregnancy Childbirth. 2018;18(1):319

3. Drennen CR, Coleman SM, Ettinger de Cuba S, et al. Food insecurity, health, and development in children under age four years. Pediatrics. 2019;144(4):e20190824

4. Lee AM, Lopez MA, Haq H, et al. Inpatient food insecurity in caregivers of hospitalized pediatric patients: a mixed methods study. Acad Pediatr. 2021;21(8):1404–1413

5. Solan LG, Beck AF, Brunswick SA, et al; H2O Study Group. The family perspective on hospital to home transitions: a qualitative study. Pediatrics. 2015;136(6): e1539–e1549

6. Interact for Health. Community Health Status Survey: 1 in 4 adults in our region report being food insecure. Available at: https://www.interactforhealth.org/upl/media/1_in_4_adults_in_our_region_report_being_food_insecure.pdf. Accessed September 7, 2021

7. White CM, Statile AM, White DL, et al. Using quality improvement to optimise paediatric discharge efficiency. BMJ Qual Saf. 2014;23(5):428–436

8. U.S. Household Food Security Survey Module. Six-item short form. U.S. household food security survey module: six-item short form. Available at: https://www.ers.usda.gov/media/8282/short2012.pdf. Accessed September 26, 2021

9. Provost LP, Murray SK. The Health Care Data Guide: Learning from Data for Improvement. San Francisco, CA: Jossey-Bass; 2011

10. Chang LV, Shah AN, Hoefgen ER, et al; H2O Study Group. Lost earnings and nonmedical expenses of pediatric hospitalizations. Pediatrics. 2018;142(3):e20180195

11. Bassett HK, Coller RJ, Beck J, et al. Financial difficulties in families of hospitalized children. J Hosp Med. 2020;15(11): 652–658

12. Cullen D, Abel D, Attridge M, Fein JA. Exploring the gap: food insecurity and resource engagement. Acad Pediatr. 2021;21(3):440–445

13. Vasan A, Darko O, Fortin K, Scribano PV, Kenyon CC. Community resource connection for pediatric caregivers with unmet social needs: a qualitative study. Acad Pediatr. 2022;22(3):461–469

14. American Academy of Pediatrics. Food insecurity. Available at: www.aap.org/en/patient-care/food-insecurity/. Accessed October 11, 2022

15. Makelarski JA, Thorngren D, Lindau ST. Feed first, ask questions later: alleviating and understanding caregiver food insecurity in an urban children's hospital. Am J Public Health. 2015;105(8): e98–e104

16. Luria JW, Muething SE, Schoettker PJ, Kotagal UR. Reliability science and patient safety. Pediatr Clin North Am. 2006;53 (6):1121–1133

17. Nolan T, Resar R, Haraden C, Griffin F. Improving the reliability of health care. Available at: www.ihi.org:80/resources/Pages/IHIWhitePapers/Improvingthe ReliabilityofHealthCare.aspx. Accessed January 31, 2023

18. Feeding America. Hunger in America. Available at: https://www.feedingamerica.org/hunger-in-america. Accessed April 20, 2022

Food Insecurity and Community-Based Food Resources Among Caregivers of Hospitalized Children

Spencer Asay, BS,[a] Emily M. Abramsohn, MPH,[b] Victoria Winslow, MPH,[b] Jyotsna S. Jagai, MS, MPH, PhD,[b] Elaine Waxman, PhD,[c] Jennifer A. Makelarski, PhD, MPH,[b] Stacy Tessler Lindau, MD, MAPP[b,d,e]

ABSTRACT

OBJECTIVE: Children's hospitals are implementing interventions to connect families to community-based resources. This study describes food insecurity (FI) and food resource knowledge, need, and use among families with a hospitalized child.

METHODS: Between November 2020 and June 2022, 637 caregivers of hospitalized children in an urban 42-ZIP-code area were surveyed as part of a randomized controlled trial. The United States Department of Agriculture 18-item Household Food Security Survey was used to evaluate 12-month food security (food secure [score of 0 = FS]; marginally secure [1–2 = MFS]; insecure [3–18 = FI]). Food resource knowledge, need, and use were described by food security status and examined using Cochran-Armitage tests. The distribution of local resources was obtained from a database and mapped by ZIP code.

RESULTS: Comparing FI (35.0%) with MFS (17.6%) and FS (47.4%) groups, the rates of resource knowledge were lower (70.2% vs 78.5%, 80.5%), and the rates of need (55.1% vs 30.6%, 14.2%) and use (55.3% vs 51.4%, 40.8%) were higher. Rates of food resource knowledge increased linearly with increasing food security (FI to MFS to FS; $P = .008$), whereas the rates of resource need ($P < .001$) and use ($P = .001$) decreased with increasing food security. There were 311 community-based organizations across 36 ZIP codes with participants (range/ZIP code = 0–20, median = 8).

CONCLUSIONS: Half of families with a hospitalized child experienced FI or MFS. Although families exhibited high food resource knowledge, nearly half of families with FI had unmet food needs or had never used resources.

www.hospitalpediatrics.org

DOI: https://doi.org/10.1542/hpeds.2023-007597

Copyright © 2024 by the American Academy of Pediatrics

Address correspondence to Spencer Asay, BS, University of Chicago Pritzker School of Medicine, 924 E 57th St #104, Chicago, IL 60637. E-mail: spencer.asay@uchicagomedicine.org

HOSPITAL PEDIATRICS (ISSN Numbers: Print, 2154-1663; Online, 2154-1671).

Mr Asay contributed to conceptualization, methodology, formal analysis, writing the original draft, and visualization; Ms Abramsohn contributed to conceptualization, methodology, investigation, writing, review, and editing, supervision, project administration, and funding acquisition; Ms Winslow contributed to conceptualization, validation, data curation, writing, review, and editing, and visualization; Dr Jagai contributed to conceptualization, validation, data curation, and writing, review, and editing; Dr Waxman contributed to writing, review, and editing and supervision; Dr Makelarski contributed to conceptualization, methodology, funding acquisition, validation, data curation, and writing, review, and editing; Dr Lindau contributed to conceptualization, methodology, resources, writing, review, and editing, supervision, and funding acquisition; and all authors approved the final manuscript as submitted and agree to be accountable for all aspects of the work.

The CommunityRx-Hunger randomized controlled trial is registered on ClinicalTrials.gov (NCT04171999).

[a]University of Chicago Pritzker School of Medicine, [b]Department of Obstetrics and Gynecology, [d]Department of Medicine-Geriatrics and Palliative Medicine, and [e]Comprehensive Cancer Center, University of Chicago, Chicago, Illinois; and [c]Urban Institute, Washington, District of Columbia

Food insecurity (FI), the condition of limited or uncertain access to adequate food, is a prevalent health-related social risk factor in the United States.[1,2] In 2019, 13.6% of households with children were food insecure.[3] The coronavirus disease 2019 pandemic exacerbated FI nationwide,[4,5] even despite major policy interventions intended to mitigate pandemic-related hardship.[6,7] Historically marginalized populations were disproportionately impacted by pandemic-associated FI.[5] In 2021, rates of FI were highest among African American and Black (22.7%) and Hispanic (18.0%) households with children.[1]

Studies link the lack of food security to poor child health outcomes[2,8–13] and increased risk for hospitalization.[2,14] In turn, hardship arising from lost caregiver wages and costs associated with child hospitalization[15–19] can precipitate or exacerbate FI.[20,21] Prepandemic studies revealed increased FI prevalence among families with a hospitalized child (19% to 38%).[20–23] In one study, 21% of families experienced FI as a consequence of the hospitalization itself.[20] Food security is a dynamic state, not a trait,[24] that fluctuates over time in relation to family (eg, a child's unexpected hospitalization) and exogenous (eg, the coronavirus disease 2019 pandemic, job loss) factors.[2,4,8,20,21,23,25] Because new or worsening FI can compromise the health of a hospitalized child[2,8,13,25] and a child's caregiver,[2,10,13,26] the transition from hospital to home is a critical opportunity to optimize household conditions for the child's recovery through preemptive screening and intervention.[20,21,23,27,28]

Bolstered by initiatives from the Centers for Medicare & Medicaid Services,[29] the Joint Commission,[30] the National Quality Forum,[31] and even *U.S. News and World Report* hospital rankings,[32] social risk screening and referral interventions are being widely adopted in health care settings.[23,33] The American Academy of Pediatrics recommends routine FI screening and intervention in pediatric settings[25] and, in collaboration with the Food Research and Action Center, has developed a toolkit to aid providers in addressing FI.[34] Among other strategies, this toolkit recommends referring families to community-based food resources, such as food pantries, community meal programs and food delivery services.

Consistent with American Academy of Pediatrics and Food Research and Action Center recommendations, many pediatric hospital-based food security interventions include risk-based FI screening on admission followed by the provision of resource information to households that screen positive.[33] Importantly, qualitative studies of such interventions indicate a need to assess not only social risk factors like FI but also a perceived need for resources to address such risk factors.[35–37] A caregiver might be reluctant to disclose information related to FI risk but willing to indicate a need for resources. Moreover, because of the dynamic nature of FI, a family that screens negative for FI on a child's admission may develop a need for support by the time of discharge or may anticipate a need because of expected time away from work during the child's recovery.

To characterize community-based food resource knowledge, need, and use as modifiable factors associated with FI[38–40] in the context of pediatric hospitalization, we use baseline data from a randomized controlled trial (RCT) to describe these factors among families with a hospitalized child and examine their relationship to household food security status.

METHODS
Study Setting and Sample

As previously described, data for this study were obtained from an RCT evaluating a universal social care intervention delivered to parents and other primary caregivers ("caregivers") of hospitalized children as part of the hospital discharge process.[41] The full RCT protocol has been described previously.[42] Participants ($N = 637$) were recruited following their child's admission to the hospital between November 2020 and June 2022 (Fig 1). All participants provided documentation of informed consent. The RCT protocol was approved by the university's institutional review board and registered at clinicaltrials.gov.

This study was performed at a tertiary care children's hospital in a large midwestern urban area that admits ~5300 unique patients annually. The hospital's service area is a densely populated 110-mi^2 geography. Eligible participants included English- and Spanish-speaking individuals (95% of the clinical population at the study site spoke English or Spanish) who identified as the primary caregiver of a child <18 years old hospitalized in the general, intensive care, or transplant units and lived in 1 of 42 study ZIP codes in the hospital's service area. Eligible participants consented to receive text messages, which were used for survey scheduling and appointment reminders and as a component of the intervention[41] (<0.4% of screened caregivers were ineligible on this basis). Caregivers of healthy newborns and children expected to be hospitalized for <24 hours or >30 days (~25% and 7% of admissions, respectively) were ineligible, as were those whose child had a diagnosed eating disorder (per the medical record) or who recalled participating in a previous RCT conducted by our group.

Measures

Eligible participants completed a baseline survey administered during the child's hospital stay by a research interviewer. Items from the 2018 Behavioral Risk Factor Surveillance System[43] survey were used to assess demographic characteristics, including self-reported race and Hispanic/Latino/a ethnicity (known to be associated with FI),[1,44–46] partnership status, education, employment, insurance status and income. Annual household income was dichotomized as < or ≥$25 000 to maximize statistical power based on the distribution of responses in the sample. Household characteristics were assessed by using items from the 2018 American Community Survey.[47] The number of children <18 years in the household was assessed with an item from the 2018 Behavioral Risk Factor Surveillance System questionnaire.[43] Household receipt of Supplemental Nutrition Assistance Program (SNAP) or Special Supplemental Nutrition Program for Women, Infants, and Children (WIC) benefits was determined with items from the 2014 Hunger in America Survey.[48] Gender identity was measured by

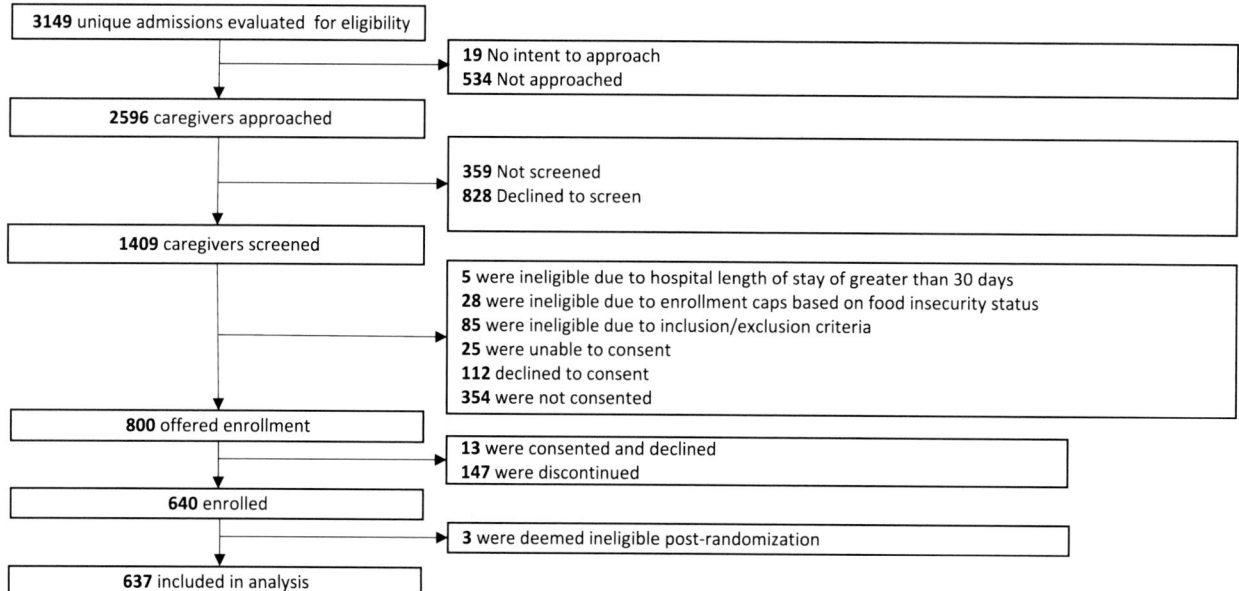

FIGURE 1 Recruitment and enrollment Consolidated Standards of Reporting Trials diagram for the RCT from which the data for the current study were obtained. Not approached: research assistant was unable to make contact with the caregiver to assess interest in screening for inclusion. Includes caregiver not in room when recruiting in-person, no answer to the bedside or cell phone, and no response to recruitment text message. This designation was also chosen if the patient was discharged before contact could be made. No intent to approach: child patient was identified from the electronic medical record database and added to patient list, but caregiver was not approached because of (1) enrollment cap reached, (2) full enrollment completed, (3) physician opted out for this patient, or (4) conflict of interest. Not screened: caregiver expressed interest in study participation but was not screened either due to our inability to reach the caregiver for eligibility screening or the patient was discharged before we could screen them for eligibility. Declined to screen: caregiver was approached for inclusion in the study but declined to be screened for eligibility. Ineligible because of enrollment caps based on FI status: for a 2-week period during enrollment, research team enrolled only caregivers from households classified as FI. During this time, caregivers from FS households were deemed ineligible. Unable to consent: caregiver was unable to provide consent because of technical difficulties with the e-consent process. Declined to consent: caregiver completed eligibility screening but declined to proceed through the informed consent process. Not consented: caregiver did not complete the consent process because of our inability to reach the caregiver for consent, the patient was discharged before we could proceed through the informed consent process, or we reached our target enrollment during the screening process. Consented and declined: caregiver proceeded through the informed consent process but declined to participate. Discontinued: caregiver provided informed consent to participate in the study but did not complete enrollment before the patient was discharged.

using best practices from the Gender Identity in US Surveillance group.[49]

Self-reported food resource knowledge, need, and use were assessed through a series of cascading items developed by our research group and pretested in English and Spanish. These items queried 3 types of food support, including places to obtain free or low-cost food (eg, food banks and pantries), places to obtain free meals (eg, community meal programs), and places to arrange for free or low-cost food delivery (eg, Meals on Wheels). As detailed in Fig 2, responses to these items were used to assign participants to the following dichotomous categories: "Any (Resource) Knowledge" or "No (Resource) Knowledge," "Current Need" or "No Current Need," and "Ever Use" or "Never Use." Assuming that one could not use a resource without previous knowledge of it, participants reporting no resource knowledge were classified as "never use." Participants reporting use who indicated that the resources they used met their food needs were categorized as "no current need," whereas those who indicated that any resources either did

not meet or only somewhat met their needs were categorized as "current need." Participants who responded "don't know" or refused to answer certain items were not assigned to the corresponding categories and were excluded from relevant analyses ("resource knowledge" $n = 20$; "ever use" $n = 21$; "current need" $n = 12$).

Household food security status in the 12 months before hospitalization was measured by using the United States Department of Agriculture 18-item Household Food Security Survey Module (0 = food secure [FS], 1–2 = marginally food secure [MFS], 3–18 = FI).[50] The authors of food security research studies commonly dichotomize scores from this measure as FI and FS.[2] Although some study authors classify the MFS group as FS,[13] several other authors find that MFS households experience adversity at levels intermediate between FS and FI households.[13,51–53] In addition, health and sociodemographic characteristics of MFS households tend to be more similar to those of FI than to those of FS households.[9,10,13,54] Consequently, some have advocated for recognizing

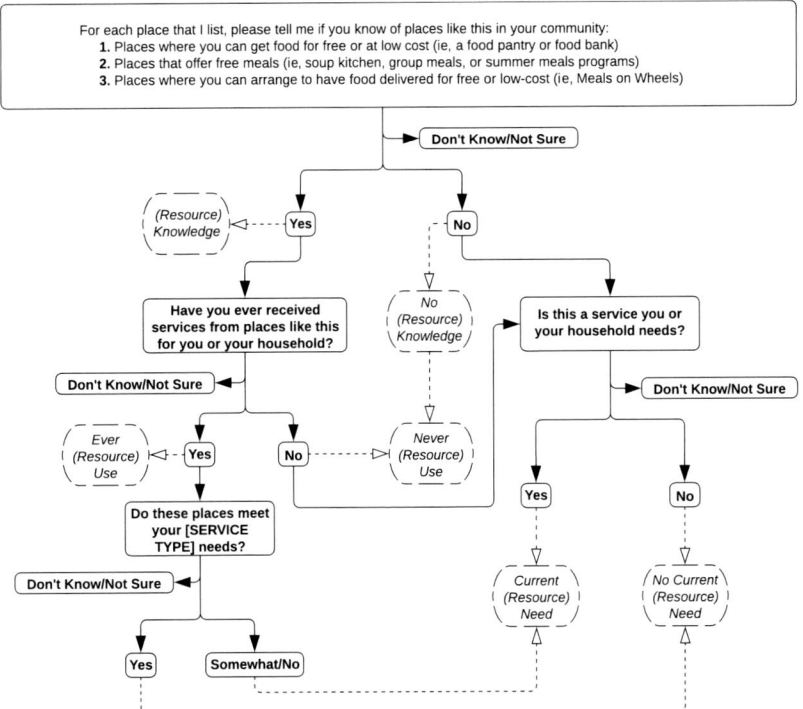

FIGURE 2 Assessment of knowledge, need, and use regarding community-based food resources in the CommunityRx-Hunger baseline survey. Solid lines with filled arrows outline the flow of question and response items. Dotted lines with open arrows indicate the categories to which participants were assigned on the basis of their responses. Participants who responded "Don't Know/Not Sure" to any of the above question items were not assigned to the corresponding categories.

and evaluating MFS as a category distinct from FS and FI,[13,55] as has been done in this study. Authors also frequently dichotomize "low food security" and "very low food security" groups as "food insecure," as has been done here.[2] The decision to aggregate these latter 2 groups was informed by sample size limitations and comparatively limited evidence of differences between these groups.[56–59]

Community-based food resource data were obtained from Unite Us database (Unite USA, Inc, New York, NY),[60] a community resource referral platform. Resources listed as "food pantry" or "fresh fruits and vegetables" within the database were classified as "free/low-cost food" resources (ie, locations where people can obtain food items for off-site meal preparation). Resources listed as "group meals" or "soup kitchen or free meals" were classified as "free meal" resources (ie, locations where people can obtain fully prepared meals for consumption on-or off-site), whereas those listed as "meal delivery" were classified as "free/low-cost food delivery" resources (ie, services that offer delivery of food items or prepared meals to off-site locations).

Statistical Analysis

Sociodemographic and household characteristics were described by food security status and examined for bivariate associations by using χ^2 (categorical variables), Fisher's exact (categorical variables with frequencies <5), and Kruskal–Wallis tests (nonnormal numerical variables). For each sociodemographic and household characteristic, pairwise bivariate comparisons between individual food security status groups (FS vs MFS, FS vs FI, MFS vs FI) were performed by using χ^2, Fisher's exact, and Kruskal–Wallis tests. The Cochran-Armitage test for trend was used to examine for linear trends in the proportion of participants reporting knowledge about, current need for, and ever use of free or low-cost food, free meal, and free or low-cost food delivery resources by food security status. Resources were tabulated and mapped by type and total per ZIP code by using Datawrapper.[61] All other analyses were performed by using Stata software, version 16.1 (StataCorp, College Station, TX). A statistical significance threshold of $P < .05$ was used for all analyses.

RESULTS
Sample Characteristics

Reflecting the study geography, participants ($N = 637$) were predominantly non-Hispanic Black (79.7%). Nearly all were women (94.3%) and identified as the mother of the hospitalized child (88.5%). Median age was 34 years (Table 1). More than half of participant households experienced either FI (35.0%) or MFS (17.6%) in the previous year. Compared with participants from FS

TABLE 1 Caregiver Sociodemographic and Household Characteristics, Stratified by Food Security Status

	Total (*N* = 637)	FS (*n* = 302)	MFS (*n* = 112)	FI (*n* = 223)	*P*[a]
	n (%)	*n* (%)	*n* (%)	*n* (%)	
Median age, y (IQR)	34.0 (11)	33.0 (11)	33.5 (12)	36.0 (13)	.02
Gender					.17
Women	600 (94.3)	279 (92.7)	109 (97.3)	212 (95.1)	
Men	36 (5.7)	22 (7.3)	3 (2.7)	11 (4.9)	
Partnership status					.03
Single	278 (43.8)	116 (38.5)	50 (44.6)	112 (50.5)	
Married/partnered	357 (56.2)	185 (61.5)	62 (55.4)	110 (49.6)	
Caregiver relationship to child					.71
Parent	212 (95.1)	285 (94.7)	103 (92.0)	212 (95.1)	
Grandparent	18 (2.8)	9 (3.0)	4 (3.6)	5 (2.2)	
Other	18 (2.8)	7 (2.3)	5 (4.5)	6 (2.7)	
Caregiver race					.03
Black or African American	505 (79.7)	232 (76.8)	93 (84.6)	180 (81.1)	
White	63 (9.9)	42 (13.9)	6 (5.5)	15 (6.8)	
Other	66 (10.4)	28 (9.3)	11 (10.0)	27 (12.2)	
Caregiver ethnicity					.34
Hispanic, Latino/a, or Spanish origin	91 (14.3)	47 (15.6)	11 (9.9)	33 (14.8)	
Non-Hispanic, Latino/a, Spanish origin	545 (85.7)	255 (84.4)	100 (90.1)	190 (85.2)	
Language preference					.46
Spanish	23 (3.6)	11 (3.6)	3 (2.7)	9 (4.1)	
English	611 (96.4)	291 (96.4)	108 (97.3)	212 (95.9)	
Education					.06
<High school	68 (10.7)	24 (8.0)	12 (10.7)	32 (14.4)	
High school or more	569 (89.3)	278 (92.1)	100 (89.3)	191 (85.7)	
Employed	293 (56.0)	155 (61.5)	45 (50.0)	93 (51.4)	.05
Insurance status					.002
Private insurance	132 (20.9)	80 (26.9)	22 (19.6)	30 (13.5)	
Medicare	30 (4.8)	10 (3.4)	5 (4.5)	15 (6.8)	
Medicaid	447 (70.7)	202 (67.8)	80 (71.4)	165 (74.3)	
Other	3 (0.5)	2 (0.7)	0 (0.0)	1 (0.5)	
Uninsured	20 (3.2)	4 (1.3)	5 (4.5)	11 (5.0)	
Annual household income, USD					<.005
<$25 000	265 (43.0)	105 (36.2)	52 (47.7)	108 (49.8)	
≥$25 000	351 (57.0)	185 (63.8)	57 (52.3)	109 (50.2)	
Household size, median (IQR)	4 (2)	4 (2)	4 (2)	4 (2)	.35
Number of children <18 y old, median (IQR)	2 (2)	2 (1)	2 (2)	2 (3)	.63
SNAP receipt	450 (71.0)	204 (67.8)	79 (71.2)	167 (75.2)	.18
WIC receipt[b]	149 (36.1)	74 (35.8)	25 (33.8)	50 (37.9)	.83

IQR, interquartile range; USD, US dollars.

"Other" category for participant relationship to child included the following responses: "Other relative or legal guardian;" "Someone else." "Other" category for insurance status included the following responses: "TRICARE," "Alaska Native, Indian Health Service, or Tribal Health Services," "Some other source." "Other" category for race includes the following responses: "Asian," "American Indian or Alaska Native," "Native Hawaiian or Pacific Islander," "Other." "Hispanic, Latino/a, or Spanish Origin" category for ethnicity includes the following responses: "Mexican, Mexican American, Chicano/a," "Puerto Rican," "Cuban," "Another Hispanic, Latino/a, or Spanish Origin."

Instances where percentages add up to >100% are a result of rounding.

[a] Values reflect comparisons among all 3 food security status groups. Pairwise comparisons between groups are displayed in Supplemental Table 2.
[b] Includes only caregivers with children meeting WIC age requirements (<5 y of age; *n* = 413).

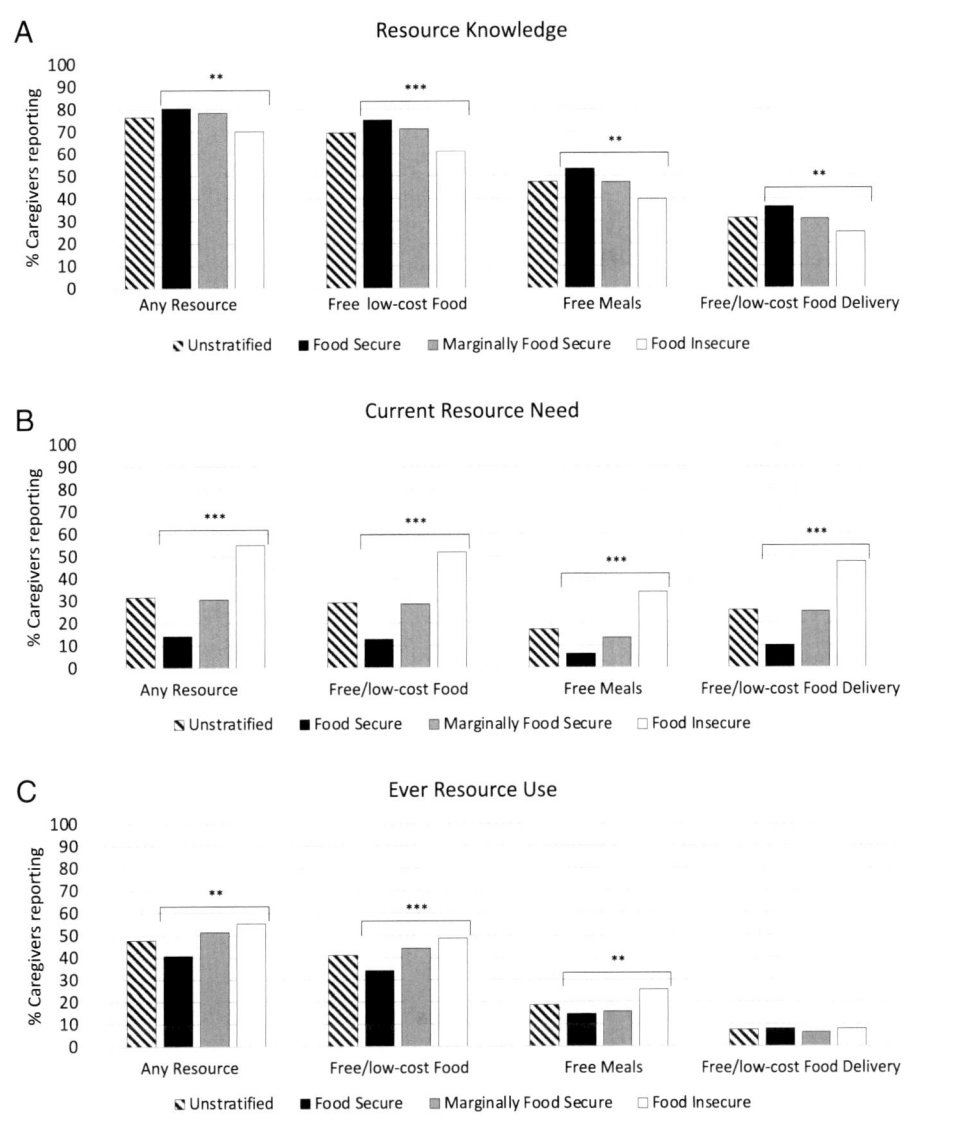

A Resource Knowledge

% Caregivers reporting

☐ Unstratified ■ Food Secure ▨ Marginally Food Secure ☐ Food Insecure

B Current Resource Need

% Caregivers reporting

☐ Unstratified ■ Food Secure ▨ Marginally Food Secure ☐ Food Insecure

C Ever Resource Use

% Caregivers reporting

☐ Unstratified ■ Food Secure ▨ Marginally Food Secure ☐ Food Insecure

FIGURE 3 Caregivers' self-reported food resource knowledge, need and use, stratified by food security status. * $P_{trend} < .05$, ** $P_{trend} < .01$, *** $P_{trend} < .001$.

households, those with FI were older ($P = .004$) and less likely to identify as white ($P = .03$) and more likely to be unpartnered ($P = .007$), have less than a high school education ($P = .02$), be unemployed ($P = .04$), be publicly insured or uninsured ($P < .001$), and report an annual income $<$25 000 ($P < .002$; Supplemental Table 2). Rates of income $<$25 000 were highest among participants from FI households (49.8%), intermediate among MFS household participants (47.7%), and lowest among FS household participants (36.2%).

Food Resource Knowledge, Need, and Use by Food Security Status

One or more participants lived in each of 36 of 42 target ZIP codes in the hospital's service area. In this geography, the resource referral database listed 311 free or low-cost food, free meal, and free or low-cost food delivery resources. The number of resources per ZIP code ranged from 0 to 20 (median = 8). Three-quarters of caregivers (76.5%) knew of ≥1 types of food resources (Fig 3A). The proportion of participants reporting resource knowledge increased linearly with increasing food security (FI to MFS to FS; $P = .008$). Rates of knowledge were highest for free or low-cost food resources and lowest for free or low-cost food delivery resources, consistent with the resource distribution in the study geography (Fig 4).

One-third of caregivers endorsed a current need for ≥1 resource types, including 14.2% of caregivers from FS households (Fig 3B). More than half (55.1%) of caregivers from FI households indicated ≥1 resource needs. The proportion of caregivers

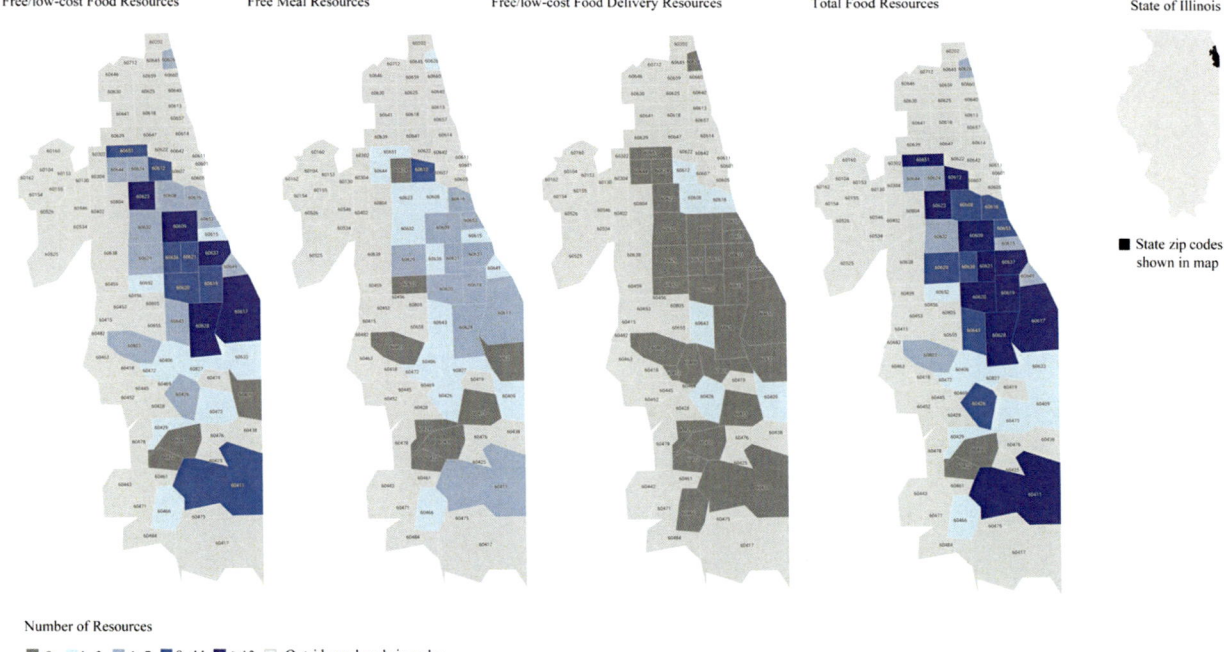

Free/low-cost Food Resources   Free Meal Resources   Free/low-cost Food Delivery Resources   Total Food Resources   State of Illinois

■ State zip codes
shown in map

Number of Resources

■ 0   ■ 1–3   ■ 4–7   ■ 8–11   ■ ≥12   □ Outside analyzed zip codes

FIGURE 4 Community-based food resources in the study region by ZIP code. The distribution of free or low-cost food, free meal, and free or low-cost food delivery resources in ZIP codes having ≥1 study participant was obtained from an online resource referral database and mapped by ZIP code. The lightest grey-shaded ZIP codes include ZIP codes outside the study geography and other ZIP codes that were included in the study geography but in which no participants were enrolled (ZIP codes 60805, 60130, 60153, 60162, 60202, and 60302). The black area in the state legend indicates the region being shown in the 4 maps to the left.

---

endorsing resource need decreased linearly with increasing food security ($P < .001$). The rates of need for free or low-cost food and free or low-cost food delivery resources were higher than those for free meal resources.

Nearly half (47.7%) of caregivers reported having used a community-based food resource, including 40.8% of those from FS households (Fig 3C). The proportion of caregivers reporting resource use decreased linearly with increasing food security ($P = .001$). Usage rates were highest for free or low-cost food resources and lowest for free or low-cost food delivery resources. Among caregivers who used free or low-cost food, free meal, and free or low-cost food delivery resources, 32.5%, 14.8%, and 8.5%, respectively, reported that the resources they used either did not meet or only somewhat met their needs.

DISCUSSION

In a predominantly African American and Black urban community, more than half of families with a child hospitalized at an academic medical center experienced household FI (35%) or MFS (17.6%). Although likely influenced by pandemic conditions, the FI rate in this study cohort (35%) was still more than double contemporaneous population estimates for all US households with

children (12.5% to 14.8%).[1,62] The rate in the current study also exceeded US population and local estimates for African American and Black households with children (22.7% to 27.3% and 32%, respectively).[1,62–65] These findings corroborate previous evidence that FI, which is a modifiable condition, is associated with and may be on the causal pathway to racial and ethnic inequities in illness, injury, and chronic disease among minoritized children.[2,8,20,21,23]

This study fills a gap in evidence about food resource knowledge among caregivers with a hospitalized child. Knowledge of the local community resource landscape influences health-promoting resource utilization and downstream resolution of social needs.[38,40,66] Most caregivers in this study had some knowledge of food resources, and resource knowledge was positively associated with food security. This association is likely bidirectional; knowledge of food resources promotes food security for people in need of resources and FS people likely have better access to resource information.

In a recent national survey, 60.5% of adults from FI households were unaware of any community-based food resources.[39] This rate was approximately twice that of our hospital-based cohort, a finding that may be explained by exposure to resource information and support (eg, Feed1st, our institution's hospital-based food pantry system)[67] during the child's hospitalization. Still, nearly one-third of caregivers experiencing FI in our study indicated no resource knowledge in a region with hundreds of resources. Lack of knowledge may reflect unequal geographic resource distribution, as evidenced by the wide variance in number of resources across caregivers' ZIP codes. Because child hospitalization is a known risk factor for FI,[20] hospital-based interventions to promote local resource knowledge may help mitigate this risk by raising awareness about FI and narrowing resource knowledge gaps.

Importantly, we note that although the presence of food support resources in a community and knowledge of these resources are necessary for access, they are not sufficient. Impediments to food support utilization are well-documented and include geographic- and transportation-related barriers,[68,69] inconsistent quality and quantity of food provided,[70] unavailability of culturally acceptable items,[71,72] stigma associated with obtaining food assistance,[71,73] mismatch between offerings and perceived needs,[74] and logistical barriers like days and hours of operation that do not align with personal obligations.[71–74] Moreover, a substantial number of caregivers in this study who indicated having used community-based food resources reported that the resource they used did not fully meet their needs. Therefore, although information-based FI interventions are likely to assist some families in receiving adequate food support, resource information alone may be insufficient for others.

Nearly one-third of caregivers endorsed ≥1 food resource needs, and resource need was negatively associated with higher food security. Notably, 1 in 7 FS participants indicated current resource need. We also found high rates of economic hardship among FS caregivers, with more than one-third reporting an annual income <$25 000. In addition, among FS household caregivers, more than two-thirds were receiving SNAP benefits and more than one-third of eligible families were receiving WIC benefits. In a previous study performed by our group, we found that 21% of families that screened positive for FI during a child's hospitalization had become FI during that hospitalization.[20] These families' needs would likely go unrecognized in settings where FI screening happens only at the time of admission. Taken together, these findings reflect that FI is a state, not a trait,[24] and food security status is limited as a proxy for identifying people with need for support. As asserted by others, assessing caregiver-prioritized needs in addition to food security status during screening may be important for both identifying FI risk and effectively addressing needs.[75–77]

Nearly half of caregivers in our study, including >40% of those from FS households, had some experience using food resources. Rates of resource use in this cohort were higher than previously reported in this and similar populations.[20,21,78] This difference may be due in part to pandemic-driven resource awareness and use,[79] the relative number of resources in the geography, or exposure to resource information at the time of hospitalization. For example, during the pandemic, all hospital clinicians and staff were provided log-in information to access a community resource referral platform used for a previous RCT.[80]

Consistent with previous studies, we found evidence that MFS participants differ meaningfully from FS and FI participants in several respects. MFS participants were significantly more likely than FS participants, but no more likely than FI participants, to report an annual income <$25 000, confirming previous findings that MFS households are socio-demographically more similar to FI households.[9,10,13,55] Interestingly, we found no such significant relationships for other sociodemographic characteristics commonly associated with food security status (race, ethnicity, employment, education), which may be due in part to the homogeneity of the sample. In our trend analyses of resource knowledge, need, and use across food security status groups, we observed graded relationships, with the MFS group being intermediate between FI and FS on these measures. These findings align with calls for recognition and analysis of MFS households as a distinct group with unique characteristics and outcomes.[13,56]

Limitations

We acknowledge the limitations of this work. First, the cross-sectional design precludes causal inferences. Second, participants' resource knowledge, need, and use were self-reported and, therefore, subject to recall bias. Relatedly, the food resource use questions elicited lifetime recall, limiting our ability to assess the recency and frequency of resource use and its temporal relationship to current resource needs and food security status. Lastly, this study was conducted during a worldwide pandemic, in an urban geography with a predominantly African American and Black population that was disproportionately affected by the pandemic, and in a hospital with an on-site food pantry. Given the high prevalence of FI in our patient population, the presence of the on-site food pantry to address food needs was an important element in the ethical treatment of human subjects in the study. Still, this and other factors may limit the generalizability of study findings.

CONCLUSIONS

Half of families with a hospitalized child experienced FI or MFS in the previous year. Although families exhibited high rates of food resource knowledge and use, nearly half of families with FI had unmet food needs or had never used community-based resources in an area with available support. Hospital-based FI screening and intervention strategies could benefit from considering caregiver-prioritized needs in addition to food security status. Information-based FI interventions may help close community resource knowledge gaps, but resource information alone may not be sufficient for all families.

Acknowledgments

The authors would like to thank Veera Anand and Charlie Fuller for their contributions in verifying the accuracy of the literature citations in this work. The authors also gratefully acknowledge the Feed1st Community Advisory Board for their ongoing guidance, commitment, and collaboration on this work. The authors would like to thank Mellissa Grana for her assistance in editing and proofreading the manuscript.

FUNDING: The efforts of EMA, JSJ, VW, JAM, and STL were supported in part by funding from the National Institutes of Health (R01MD012630, R01AG064949, R01DK127961, R01HL150909, UG3HL154297, P30CA014599). The efforts of SA were supported by funding from the University of Chicago Bucksbaum Institute for Clinical Excellence. The content of this manuscript is solely the responsibility of the authors and does not necessarily represent the official views of the funding organizations. The funding organizations had no role in the design, preparation, review, or approval of this paper.

CONFLICT OF INTEREST DISCLOSURES: Under the terms of grant 1C1CMS330997-01-00 (STL, PI) from the US Department of Health and Human Services, Centers for Medicare & Medicaid Services, awardees were expected to develop a sustainable business model to continue and support the model that was tested after award funding ended. STL was the founder and owner of a social impact company, NowPow, LLC, which was acquired by Unite Us, LLC in 2021. Dr Lindau is an unpaid advisor to, and holds stock in, Unite Us, LLC. STL is an editor on Female Sexual Dysfunction for UpToDate and received royalties <$100/year in 2019 and 2020 for this work. Subsequent royalties have been paid to the University of Chicago. STL and her spouse own equity in Glenbervie Health, LLC. Neither the University of Chicago nor UChicago Medicine is endorsing or promoting Unite Us or its business, products, or services. The remaining authors have indicated they have no potential conflicts of interest relevant to this article to disclose.

COMPANION PAPER: A companion to this article can be found online at www.hosppeds.org/cgi/doi/10.1542/hpeds.2024-007807.

REFERENCES

1. Coleman-Jensen A, Rabbitt MP, Gregory C, Singh A. Household food security in the United States in 2021. Available at: https://www.ers.usda.gov/webdocs/publications/104656/err-309.pdf. Accessed February 21, 2023

2. Gundersen C, Ziliak JP. Food insecurity and health outcomes. *Health Aff (Millwood).* 2015;34(11):1830–1839

3. Coleman-Jensen A, Rabbitt MP, Gregory CA, Singh A. USDA ERS - household food security in the United States in 2019. Available at: https://www.ers.usda.gov/publications/pub-details/?pubid=99281. Accessed February 21, 2023

4. Parekh N, Ali SH, O'Connor J, et al. Food insecurity among households with children during the COVID-19 pandemic: results from a study among social media users across the United States. *Nutr J.* 2021;20(1):73

5. Schanzenbach D, Pitts A. Food insecurity during COVID-19 in households with children: results by racial and ethnic groups. Available at: https://www.ipr.northwestern.edu/documents/reports/ipr-rapid-research-reports-pulse-hh-data-9-july-2020-by-race-ethnicity.pdf. Accessed March 4, 2023

6. Wolfson JA, Leung CW. Food insecurity during COVID-19: an acute crisis with long-term health implications. *Am J Public Health.* 2020;110(12):1763–1765

7. Caspi C, Seligman HK, Berge J, et al; Health Affairs. COVID-19 pandemic-era nutrition assistance: impact and sustainability. Available at: https://www.healthaffairs.org/do/10.1377/hpb20220330.534478/full/. Accessed May 18, 2023

8. Thomas MMC, Miller DP, Morrissey TW. Food insecurity and child health. *Pediatrics.* 2019;144(4):e20190397

9. Shankar P, Chung R, Frank DA. Association of food insecurity with children's behavioral, emotional, and academic outcomes: a systematic review. *J Dev Behav Pediatr.* 2017;38(2):135–150

10. Whitaker RC, Phillips SM, Orzol SM. Food insecurity and the risks of depression and anxiety in mothers and behavior problems in their preschool-aged children. *Pediatrics.* 2006;118(3):e859–e868

11. Abraham S, Breeze P, Sutton A, Lambie-Mumford H. Household food insecurity and child health outcomes: a rapid review of mechanisms and associations. *Lancet.* 2023;402(Suppl 1):S16

12. Schmeer KK, Piperata BA. Household food insecurity and child health. *Matern Child Nutr.* 2017;13(2):e12301 10.1111/mcn.12301

13. Cook JT, Black M, Chilton M, et al. Are food insecurity's health impacts underestimated in the U.S. population? Marginal food security also predicts adverse health outcomes in young U.S. children and mothers. *Adv Nutr.* 2013;4(1):51–61

14. Berkowitz SA, Seligman HK, Meigs JB, Basu S. Food insecurity, healthcare utilization, and high cost: a longitudinal cohort study. *Am J Manag Care.* 2018;24(9):399–404

15. Vessey JA, DiFazio RL, Strout TD, Snyder BD. Impact of non-medical out-of-pocket expenses on families of children with cerebral palsy following orthopaedic surgery. *J Pediatr Nurs.* 2017;37:101–107

16. Shields L, Tanner A. Costs of meals and parking for parents of hospitalised children in Australia. *Paediatr Nurs.* 2004;16(6):14–18

17. Callery P. Paying to participate: financial, social and personal costs to parents of involvement in their children's care in hospital. *J Adv Nurs.* 1997;25(4):746–752

18. Mumford V, Baysari MT, Kalinin D, et al. Measuring the financial and productivity burden of paediatric hospitalisation on the wider family network. *J Paediatr Child Health.* 2018;54(9):987–996

19. Chang LV, Shah AN, Hoefgen ER, et al; H2O Study Group. Lost earnings and nonmedical expenses of pediatric hospitalizations. *Pediatrics.* 2018;142(3):e20180195

20. Makelarski JA, Thorngren D, Lindau ST. Feed first, ask questions later: alleviating and understanding caregiver food insecurity in an urban children's hospital. *Am J Public Health.* 2015;105(8):e98–e104

21. Lee AM, Lopez MA, Haq H, et al. Inpatient food insecurity in caregivers of hospitalized pediatric patients: a mixed methods study. *Acad Pediatr.* 2021;21(8):1404–1413

22. Fortin K, Vasan A, Wilson-Hall CL, et al. Using quality improvement and technology to improve social supports for hospitalized children. *Hosp Pediatr.* 2021;11(10):1120–1129

23. Banach LP. Hospitalization: are we missing an opportunity to identify food insecurity in children? *Acad Pediatr.* 2016;16(5): 438–445

24. US Department of Agriculture. Frequency of food insecurity. Available at: https://www.ers.usda.gov/topics/food-nutrition-assistance/food-security-in-the-u-s/frequency-of-food-insecurity/. Accessed August 30, 2023

25. Gitterman BA, Chilton LA, Cotton WH, et al; Council on Community Pediatrics; Committee on Nutrition. Promoting food security for all children. *Pediatrics.* 2015;136(5):e1431–e1438

26. Seligman HK, Laraia BA, Kushel MB. Food insecurity is associated with chronic disease among low-income NHANES participants. *J Nutr.* 2010;140(2):304–310

27. Hanna SL, Wu CL, Smola C, et al. Food insecurity screening of hospitalized patients: a descriptive analysis. *Hosp Pediatr.* 2022;12(6): e196–e200

28. Beck AF, Solan LG, Brunswick SA, et al; H2O Study Group. Socioeconomic status influences the toll paediatric hospitalisations take on families: a qualitative study. *BMJ Qual Saf.* 2017;26(4):304–311

29. Centers for Medicare & Medicaid Services. CMS issues new roadmap for states to address the social determinants of health to improve outcomes, lower costs, support state value-based care strategies. Available at: https://www.cms.gov/newsroom/press-releases/cms-issues-new-roadmap-states-address-social-determinants-health-improve-outcomes-lower-costs. Accessed February 16, 2023

30. The Joint Commission. New requirements to reduce health disparities. R3 Rep. Available at: https://www.jointcommission.org/-/media/tjc/documents/standards/r3-reports/r3_disparities_july2022-6-20-2022.pdf. Accessed February 16, 2023

31. National Quality Forum. Developing and testing risk adjustment models for social and functional status-related risk within healthcare performance measurement. Available at: https://www.qualityforum.org/Publications/2021/08/Developing_and_Testing_Risk_Adjustment_Models_for_Social_and_Functional_Status-Related_Risk_Within_Healthcare_Performance_Measurement_-_Final_Technical_Guidance.aspx. Accessed February 16, 2023

32. Binger T, Corgel R, Adams Z, et al. Methodology U.S. News & World Report 2021-2022 best hospitals health equity measures. Available at: https://health.usnews.com/media/best-hospitals/Best-Hospitals-Health-Equity-2022-23. Accessed February 17, 2023

33. Markowitz MA, Tiyyagura G, Quallen K, Rosenberg J. Food insecurity screening and intervention in United States children's hospitals. *Hosp Pediatr.* 2022;12(10):849–857

34. Ashbrook A, Essel K, Montez K, Bennett-Tejes D. Screen and intervene: a toolkit for pediatricians to address food insecurity. Available at: https://frac.org/wp-content/uploads/FRAC_AAP_Toolkit_2021.pdf. Accessed December 10, 2022

35. Cullen D, Attridge M, Fein JA. Food for thought: a qualitative evaluation of caregiver preferences for food insecurity screening and resource referral. *Acad Pediatr.* 2020;20(8):1157–1162

36. Fritz CQ, Thomas J, Brittan MS, et al. Referral and resource utilization among food insecure families identified in a pediatric medical setting. *Acad Pediatr.* 2021;21(3):446–454

37. Garg A, Boynton-Jarrett R, Dworkin PH. Avoiding the unintended consequences of screening for social determinants of health. *JAMA.* 2016;316(8):813–814

38. Sharareh N, Wallace AS. Applying a health access framework to understand and address food insecurity. *Healthcare (Basel).* 2022;10(2):380

39. Salas J, Gupta P, Waxman E. How many food-insecure adults need help but don't know where to get it? Findings from the Well-Being and Basic Needs Survey, December 2022. Available at: https://www.urban.org/sites/default/files/2023-08/How Many Food-Insecure Adults Need Help but Don't Know Where to Get It.pdf. Accessed January 15, 2023

40. Tung EL, Abramsohn EM, Boyd K, et al. Impact of a low-intensity resource referral intervention on patients' knowledge, beliefs, and use of community resources: results from the CommunityRx trial. *J Gen Intern Med.* 2020;35(3):815–823

41. Abramsohn EM, De Ornelas M, Borson S, et al. CommunityRx, a social care assistance intervention for family and friend caregivers delivered at the point of care: two concurrent blinded randomized controlled trials. *Trials.* 2023;24(1):681

42. Glasser NJ, Lindau ST, Wroblewski K, et al; CommunityRx-Hunger Collaborators. Effect of a social care intervention on health care experiences of caregivers of hospitalized children: a randomized clinical trial. *JAMA Pediatr.* 2023;177(12):1266–1275

43. Centers for Disease Control and Prevention. 2018 behavioral risk factor surveillance system questionnaire. Available at: https://www.cdc.gov/brfss/questionnaires/index.htm. Accessed August 19, 2023

44. Hunt BR, Benjamins MR, Khan S, Hirschtick JL. Predictors of food insecurity in selected Chicago community areas. *J Nutr Educ Behav.* 2019;51(3):287–299

45. Bartfeld J, Dunifon R. State-level predictors of food insecurity among households with children. *J Policy Anal Manage.* 2006;25(4): 921–942

46. Goldberg SL, Mawn BE. Predictors of food insecurity among older adults in the United States. *Public Health Nurs.* 2015;32(5): 397–407

47. U.S. Census Bureau. The American community survey. Available at: https://www2.census.gov/programs-surveys/acs/methodology/questionnaires/2018/quest18GQ.pdf. Accessed January 5, 2024

48. Feeding America. Hunger in America 2014 executive summary. Available at: https://www.feedingamerica.org/sites/default/files/research/hunger-in-america/hia-2014-executive-summary.pdf. Accessed August 9, 2023

49. Gender Identity in U.S. Surveillance (GenIUSS) Group. Best practices for asking questions to identify transgender and other gender minority respondents on population-based surveys. Available

at: http://williamsinstitute.law.ucla.edu/wp-content/uploads/geniuss-report-sep-2014.pdf. Accessed August 8, 2023

50. U.S. Household Food Security Survey Module; Economics Research Service, USDA. Three-stage design, with screeners. Available at: https:www.ers.usda.gov/datafiles/Food_Security_in_the_United_States/Food_Security_Survey_Modules/hh2012.pdf. Accessed October 5, 2022

51. Herman DR, Westfall M, Bashir M, Afulani P. Food insecurity and mental distress among WIC-eligible women in the United States: a cross-sectional study. *J Acad Nutr Diet.* 2024;124(1):65–79

52. Parker ED, Widome R, Nettleton JA, Pereira MA. Food security and metabolic syndrome in U.S. adults and adolescents: findings from the National Health and Nutrition Examination Survey, 1999–2006. *Ann Epidemiol.* 2010;20(5):364–370

53. Ford ES. Food security and cardiovascular disease risk among adults in the United States: findings from the National Health and Nutrition Examination Survey, 2003–2008. *Prev Chronic Dis.* 2013;10:E202

54. Dean EB, French MT, Mortensen K. Food insecurity, health care utilization, and health care expenditures. *Health Serv Res.* 2020;55(Suppl 2 Suppl 2):883–893

55. Men F, Tarasuk V. Classification differences in food insecurity measures between the United States and Canada: practical implications for trend monitoring and health research. *J Nutr.* 2022;152(4):1082–1090

56. Soldavini J, Berner M. The importance of precision: differences in characteristics associated with levels of food security among college students. *Public Health Nutr.* 2020;23(9):1473–1483

57. Soldavini J, Ammerman AS. Marginal, low, and very-low food security among children are associated with intake of select dietary factors during summer. *J Acad Nutr Diet.* 2021;121(4):728–737

58. Bhandari S, Campbell JA, Walker RJ, et al. Dose response relationship between food insecurity and quality of life in United States adults: 2016-2017. *Health Qual Life Outcomes.* 2023;21(1):21

59. Johnson AD, Markowitz AJ. Associations between household food insecurity in early childhood and children's kindergarten skills. *Child Dev.* 2018;89(2):e1–e17

60. Unite Us. Your partner for social care. Available at: https://uniteus.com/?utm_term=&utm_campaign=&utm_source=adwords&utm_medium=ppc&hsa_acc=1725281010&hsa_cam=20151014834&hsa_grp=150858131204&hsa_ad=658809854040&hsa_src=g&hsa_tgt=dsa-437115340933&hsa_kw=&hsa_mt=&hsa_net=adwords&hsa_ver=3&gclid=CjOKCQjwsp6pB. Accessed October 12, 2023

61. Datawrapper. Datawrapper. Available at: https://www.datawrapper.de/. Accessed January 10, 2023

62. Coleman-Jensen A, Rabbitt MP, Gregory C, Singh A. Household food security in the United States in 2020. Available at: https://www.ers.usda.gov/webdocs/publications/102076/err-298.pdf. Accessed February 21, 2023

63. Chicago's Food Bank. Hunger in our community: a 2020 status report. Available at: https://www.chicagosfoodbank.org/wp-content/uploads/2020/12/Food-Depository-Hunger-Report-Dec-2020.pdf. Accessed January 14, 2024

64. Chicago's Food Bank. Hunger in our community: summer 2021. Available at: https://www.chicagosfoodbank.org/wp-content/uploads/2021/08/Food-Depository-Hunger-Report-Summer-2021.pdf. Accessed January 14, 2024

65. Chicago's Food Bank. Hunger in our community: a spring 2022 status report. Available at: https://www.chicagosfoodbank.org/news/hunger-in-our-community-spring-2022/. Accessed January 17, 2024

66. Levasseur M, Gauvin L, Richard L, et al; NuAge Study Group. Associations between perceived proximity to neighborhood resources, disability, and social participation among community-dwelling older adults: results from the VoisiNuAge study. *Arch Phys Med Rehabil.* 2011;92(12):1979–1986

67. Frazier CRM, Pinkerton EA, Grana M, et al. Feed1st, no questions asked: how a hospital-based food pantry program grew its impact during the COVID-19 pandemic. *Am J Public Health.* 2022;112(10):1394–1398

68. Ginsburg ZA, Bryan AD, Rubinstein EB, et al. Unreliable and difficult-to-access food for those in need: a qualitative and quantitative study of urban food pantries. *J Community Health.* 2019;44(1):16–31

69. Rajasooriar D, Soma T. Food access, mobility, and transportation: a survey and key informant interviews of users of non-profit food hubs in the City of Vancouver before and during the COVID-19 crisis. *BMC Public Health.* 2022;22(1):6

70. Loopstra R. Interventions to address household food insecurity in high-income countries. *Proc Nutr Soc.* 2018;77(3):270–281

71. Marriott JP, Fiechtner L, Birk NW, et al. Racial/ethnic disparities in food pantry use and barriers in Massachusetts during the first year of the COVID-19 pandemic. *Nutrients.* 2022;14(12):2531

72. Gany F, Bari S, Crist M, et al. Food insecurity: limitations of emergency food resources for our patients. *J Urban Health.* 2013;90(3):552–558

73. Fong K, Wright R, Wimer C. The cost of free assistance: why low-income individuals do not access food pantries. *J Sociol Soc Welf.* 2016;43(1):71–93

74. Loopstra R, Tarasuk V. The relationship between food banks and household food insecurity among low-income Toronto families. *Can Public Policy.* 2012;38(4):497–514

75. Luke MJ, Fernandes DM, Leon Rodriguez F, et al. Caregiver perspectives on social needs screening and interventions in an urban children's hospital. *Hosp Pediatr.* 2023;13(8):670–681

76. Gottlieb LM, Hessler D, Long D, et al. Effects of social needs screening and in-person service navigation on child health: a randomized clinical trial. *JAMA Pediatr.* 2016;170(11):e162521

77. Tuzzio L, Wellman RD, De Marchis EH, et al. Social risk factors and desire for assistance among patients receiving subsidized health care insurance in a US-based integrated delivery system. *Ann Fam Med.* 2022;20(2):137–144

78. Hendrickson MA, O'Riordan MA, Arpilleda JC, Heneghan AM. Effects of food insecurity on asthma outcomes in the pediatric emergency department. *Pediatr Emerg Care.* 2010;26(11):823–829

79. Gupta P, Salas J, Waxman E. Two years into the pandemic, charitable food remains a key resource for one in six adults: findings from the December 2021 well-being and basic needs survey. Available at: https://www.urban.org/research/publication/two-years-pandemic-charitable-food-remains-key-resource-one-six-adults#:~:text=Adults %7C Urban Institute-,Two Years into the Pandemic%2C Charitable Food Remains a Key,for One in Six Adults&text=Despite federal s. Accessed September 10, 2023

80. Shumacher ME, Markman S, Scales K, et al. Use of an innovation center to foster high-value COVID-19 care at an academic healthcare system. *J Hosp Med.* 2022;17(5):384–388

Addressing Food Insecurity Among Hospitalized Children: Upstream and Downstream Approaches

Michael J. Luke, MD, Aditi Vasan, MD, MSHP

Hospitalization can be a traumatic experience for patients and their caregivers. Recognizing the emotional toll that acute illness can have on families, children's hospitals often provide a range of services focused on easing the adjustment to life in the hospital, from toothbrushes and laundry rooms for personal hygiene, to chaplaincy services for spiritual counsel. However, health systems do not always recognize or address the significant financial impacts of hospitalization on their patients and families. Hospitalization can lead to or exacerbate financial strain resulting from lost wages; travel, food, and parking expenses; medication copays; and other costs incurred during a child's hospital stay.[1] Hospitalization can also lead to the development of new social needs, such as the need for child care or elder care for family members at home, or new housing instability if families are evicted from a shelter or lose temporary housing during their hospital stay.

Recent research has highlighted the risk of food insecurity (FI) among families admitted to the hospital.[2,3] Many hospitals provide free meals for admitted children, but caregivers accompanying these children often have to purchase meals from a limited selection of expensive local vendors.[4] Time spent at their child's bedside may also mean that caregivers are unable to prepare food at home, instead relying on more expensive take-out or delivery options to feed other family members. And for caregivers without flexible schedules or paid family medical leave, compounded financial strain from lost wages may limit expendable income.[5,6]

To address these concerns, many children's hospitals have implemented universal FI screening. Although workflows vary across institutions, hospitals typically respond to positive screens with some combination of (1) referral to local community-based resources (eg, food banks, community meal programs, food delivery services), (2) direct provision of hospital-based food resources (eg, meal vouchers, in-hospital food pantry access), (3) information about government nutrition benefit programs, including the Supplemental Nutrition Assistance Program (SNAP) and the Special Supplemental Nutrition Program for Women, Infants, and Children (WIC), and (4) connection to a social worker for more tailored guidance and support.[7,8]

In this issue of *Hospital Pediatrics*, Asay et al present findings from a cross-sectional survey of caregivers of children admitted to an urban children's hospital investigating their awareness and use of local food resources.[9] In

www.hospitalpediatrics.org

DOI:https://doi.org/10.1542/hpeds.2024-007807

Copyright © 2024 by the American Academy of Pediatrics

Address correspondence to Michael J. Luke, MD, 3500 Civic Center Blvd, Philadelphia, PA 19104. E-mail: lukem1@chop.edu

HOSPITAL PEDIATRICS (ISSN Numbers: Print, 2154-1663; Online, 2154-1671).

Dr Luke conceptualized, wrote, and revised the commentary; and Dr Vasan reviewed and revised the commentary.

FUNDING: Dr Luke's effort contributing to this manuscript was in part funded by the NICHD (grant T32HD060550). Dr Vasan's effort contributing to this manuscript was in part funded by the Agency for Healthcare Research and Quality (grant K08HS029396). The funders had no role in the conceptualization or creation of this manuscript.

CONFLICT OF INTEREST DISCLOSURES: The authors have indicated they have no potential conflicts of interest relevant to this article to disclose.

COMPANION PAPER: A companion to this article can be found online at www.hosppeds.org/cgi/doi/10.1542/hpeds.2023-007597.

Clinical Futures, and PolicyLab, Children's Hospital of Philadelphia, Philadelphia, Pennsylvania; Department of Pediatrics, and Leonard David Institute of Economics, Perelman School of Medicine, University of Pennsylvania, Philadelphia, Pennsylvania

this hospitalized population, the authors found that rates of FI were more than double the national average among households with children. Although rates of food resource knowledge in their population were relatively high, almost half of their food-insecure cohort had never used available food resources. Their findings suggest that hospital-based FI screening and provision of resource information may increase awareness of local food resources among families of hospitalized children.

As the authors note, there are some limitations to the generalizability of their findings. This study was conducted during the SARS-CoV-2 pandemic, a period when national FI rates more than tripled and many emergency food systems rapidly mobilized and increased outreach to meet these escalating demands.[10] Additionally, this study population included mostly caregivers living in urban communities, where residents might have greater awareness of and closer geographic proximity to available food resources compared with families in suburban or rural areas.[11,12] Finally, this study was conducted in a health system with a hospital-based food pantry, which may have led to greater awareness of local food resources among their participants.[13]

Despite these limitations, their findings offer several insights to help guide implementation of FI screening and resource provision in the pediatric inpatient setting. The authors found that rates of FI in their hospitalized population were substantially higher than national and local estimates of FI among households with comparable social demographics. They use these findings to reinforce the idea that food security is a dynamic state, rather than a static trait. As such, even families who were previously food secure could acutely develop FI from the socioeconomic burdens of hospitalization. Therefore, in addition to screening questions assessing FI over a 12-month period, such as those in the validated Hunger Vital Sign, hospitals should consider incorporating screening questions that specifically assess for acute FI during a child's hospital stay.[3,14] Similarly, there is no consensus on the appropriate frequency for implementing social needs screening to optimize family support while minimizing screening burden. Although quarterly or semiannual screening may be the ideal cadence in an outpatient setting, the authors' findings suggest that the potential for new FI resulting from a child's admission may warrant screening families at every hospitalization.

The authors conclude that hospital-based FI screening and provision of resource information can increase awareness of local food resources among families of hospitalized children. It is important to consider these findings in the context of known limitations of health care–based social interventions. Although hospital-based food resources, such as the Feed1st Program referenced in this study, and paper or electronic referrals to local community-based resources, can help meet the needs of marginalized communities living near the hospital, there are several reasons why these interventions might not be the best way to reach all families in need.

First, health system–provided referrals to local food resources may overwhelm these programs, limiting their capacity to serve other families in need. These interventions could have the unintended consequence of decreasing availability of food resources for children and families without adequate access to health care, if limited community-based resources are preferentially channeled toward individuals who received referrals in health care settings. Second, as a growing number of state governments devote funding to addressing health-related social needs through their Medicaid programs,[15] they may have less funding available to improve outreach for and boost participation in government nutrition benefit programs like WIC and SNAP, which are available to all state residents regardless of health status. Last, food resources that are located at the hospital or in the surrounding communities may not be feasible long-term resources for families living farther away, particularly families in rural communities. These families may face greater socioeconomic strains in the event of hospitalization because of longer travel times, prolonged absences from work, and limited access to resources at home.[16] As many smaller children's hospitals and pediatric units within safety-net hospitals close, and the geographic catchment area for children's hospitals continues to broaden, hospital social workers are challenged with maintaining up-to-date lists of relevant resources for an expanding population.[17]

To address these challenges, health systems should ideally invest in both health system–based and community-based approaches to identifying social needs and connecting families to resources, prioritize connecting families with both local food resources and key government nutrition benefit programs, including WIC and SNAP, and consider leveraging geocoded resource technology, such as the online resource map used in this study, to ensure they are able to locate available and appropriate food resources for all families.

Health systems should also recognize that they might not always be equipped to effectively address social adversity. Proper investment in social care is costly, and much of the health care workforce may not have the time, experience, or expertise needed to adequately address social needs.[18] Health system investment in key personnel including social workers (who have the knowledge and experience required to manage these needs), community health workers (who can build a trusted connection with patients they serve through shared lived experiences), and community advisory boards (which can gather direct input from community members on healthcare-based social care initiatives) may help bridge this gap. Nonprofit hospitals should also use their community benefit spending to invest directly in community-based organizations focused on reducing FI and promoting food justice. These organizations have often built trust with the communities they serve and may have more specialized expertise in addressing nuanced issues related to FI within marginalized communities.

In addition, although health system–based interventions to address FI can meaningfully impact individual patients and families, these interventions are less likely to move the needle on FI at the population level. Health systems should therefore also intervene upstream, using their role as anchor institutions to advocate for a stronger social safety net and more equitable social policies. Addressing FI at the population level requires influencing the political structures leading to inequities in access to affordable, nutritious food.[19] For example, federal nutrition programs such as SNAP, WIC, and the National School Lunch Program typically undergo congressional reauthorization every 5 years. This period serves as an opportune window to advocate for critical policy changes like increasing the value of monthly SNAP benefits, protecting WIC and SNAP eligibility among low-income households regardless of employment or immigration status, and modernizing the WIC and SNAP programs to boost participation, particularly in underresourced and non–English-speaking communities.[20]

Addressing food insecurity requires a multipronged approach that ideally includes both health system–based social care interventions and upstream policy changes. To mitigate the adverse effects of food insecurity on child health, children's hospitals should not only invest in social care programs and conduct rigorous evaluations of these programs, like the work done by Asay et al, but also advocate for policy changes that mitigate inequities in food access and promote a more just and equitable food system.

REFERENCES

1. Callery P. Paying to participate: financial, social and personal costs to parents of involvement in their children's care in hospital. *J Adv Nurs.* 1997;25(4):746–752

2. Makelarski JA, Thorngren D, Lindau ST. Feed first, ask questions later: alleviating and understanding caregiver food insecurity in an urban children's hospital. *Am J Public Health.* 2015;105(8):e98–e104

3. Lee AM, Lopez MA, Haq H, et al. Inpatient food insecurity in caregivers of hospitalized pediatric patients: a mixed methods study. *Acad Pediatr.* 2021;21(8):1404–1413

4. Shields L, Tanner A. Costs of meals and parking for parents of hospitalised children in Australia. *Paediatr Nurs.* 2004;16(6):14–18

5. Mumford V, Baysari MT, Kalinin D, et al. Measuring the financial and productivity burden of paediatric hospitalisation on the wider family network. *J Paediatr Child Health.* 2018;54(9):987–996

6. Chang LV, Shah AN, Hoefgen ER, et al; H2O Study Group. Lost earnings and nonmedical expenses of pediatric hospitalizations. *Pediatrics.* 2018;142(3):e20180195

7. Banach LP. Hospitalization: are we missing an opportunity to identify food insecurity in children? *Acad Pediatr.* 2016;16(5):438–445

8. COUNCIL ON COMMUNITY PEDIATRICS; COMMITTEE ON NUTRITION. Promoting food security for all children. *Pediatrics.* 2015;136(5):e1431–e1438

9. Asay S, Abramsohn EM, Winslow V, et al. Food insecurity and community-based food resources among caregivers of hospitalized children. *Hosp Pediatr.* 2024;14(7):e2023007597

10. Wolfson JA, Leung CW. Food insecurity during COVID-19: an acute crisis with long-term health implications. *Am J Public Health.* 2020;110(12):1763–1765

11. Rabbitt MP, Hales LJ, Burke MP, Coleman-Jensen A. *Household food security in the United States in 2022*

12. Byker Shanks C, Andress L, Hardison-Moody A, et al. Food insecurity in the rural united states: an examination of struggles and coping mechanisms to feed a family among households with a low-income. *Nutrients.* 2022;14(24):5250

13. Salas J, Gupta P, Waxman E. *How Many Food-Insecure Adults Need Help but Don't Know Where to Get It?* Fact Sheet; 2023

14. Hager ER, Quigg AM, Black MM, et al. Development and validity of a 2-item screen to identify families at risk for food insecurity. *Pediatrics.* 2010;126(1):e26–e32

15. Hanson E, Albert-Rozenberg D, Garfield KM, et al. The evolution and scope of Medicaid Section 1115 demonstrations to address nutrition: a US survey. *Health Affairs Scholar.* 2024;2(2):qxae013

16. Baumgaertner E. As hospitals close children's units, where does that leave Lachlan. *The New York Times.* Oct 12, 2022

17. Joseph AM, Davis BS, Kahn JM. Association between hospital consolidation and loss of pediatric inpatient services. *JAMA Pediatr.* 2023;177(8):859–860

18. Glied S, D'Aunno T. Health systems and social services-a bridge too far? *JAMA Health Forum.* 2023;4(8):e233445

19. Berkowitz SA. Multisector collaboration vs. social democracy for addressing social determinants of health (published online ahead of print). *Milbank Q.* 2023. DOI:10.1111/1468-0009.12685

20. Hartline-Grafton H, Hassink SG. Food insecurity and health: practices and policies to address food insecurity among children. *Acad Pediatr.* 2021;21(2):205–210

Identifying Food Insecurity in Cardiology Clinic and Connecting Families to Resources

Allison K. Black, MD,[a] Julia Pantalone, BA,[b] Anna-Claire Marrone, MD,[c] Evonne Morell, DO,[b,d] Robin Telles, MSW,[d] Mark DeBrunner, MD[b,d]

BACKGROUND: Food insecurity (FI) increases children's risk for illness and developmental and behavioral problems, which are ongoing concerns for congenital heart disease (CHD) patients. In 2020, 14.8% of households with children suffered from FI. The Hunger Vital Signs (HVS) asks 2 questions to assess FI. The global aim of the project is to implement HVS and connect FI families to resources.

METHODS: Stakeholders identified 6 critical drivers in implementing FI screening at an outpatient cardiology clinic and conducted plan-do-study-act (PDSA) cycles to implement HVS. Over the 13-month study period, time series analyses were performed to assess our process measure (FI screening) and outcome measure (connection of FI families to resources). Demographics and severity of CHD were analyzed for FI families.

RESULTS: Screening rates increased from 0% to >85%, screening 5064 families. Process evaluations revealed roadblocks including screening discomfort. FI families were more likely to identify as Black or multiple or other ethnicity. Severe CHD patients were at higher risk for FI ($n = 106$, odds ratio [OR] 1.67 [1.21–2.29], $P = .002$). Face-to-face meetings with social work and community partnerships reduced loss to follow-up and our ability to offer all FI families individualized FI resources.

CONCLUSION: HVS screening can be implemented in a cardiology clinic to improve identification of FI families. A written tool can combat screening discomfort and improve identification of FI families. Children with severe CHD may be at increased risk for FI. A multidisciplinary team and community partnerships can improve individualized resource distribution.

[a]*Norton Children's Hospital and School of Medicine, University of Louisville, Louisville, Kentucky;* [b]*University of Pittsburgh School of Medicine, Pittsburgh, Pennsylvania;* [c]*Children's Healthcare of Atlanta, Atlanta, Georgia; and* [d]*Children's Hospital of Pittsburgh, Pittsburgh, Pennsylvania*

Dr Black conceptualized and designed the study, drafted the initial manuscript, and reviewed and revised the manuscript; Dr DeBrunner supervised the project from its conceptualization and study design and reviewed and revised the manuscript; Ms Pantalone and Dr Marrone designed the data collection instruments, collected data, carried out the initial analyses, and reviewed and revised the manuscript; Dr Morell provided quality improvement expertise for the study design and reviewed and revised the manuscript; Ms Telles is a clinical social worker and helped design the project implementation and resource utilization for the project in addition to revising the manuscript; and all authors approved the final manuscript as submitted and agree to be accountable for all aspects of the work.

DOI: https://doi.org/10.1542/peds.2020-011718

Accepted for publication Nov 29, 2021

Address correspondence to Allison K. Black, MD, University of Louisville, 571 S. Floyd St., Suite 113, Louisville, KY 40202. E-mail: Allison.Black@Louisville.edu

PEDIATRICS (ISSN Numbers: Print, 0031-4005; Online, 1098-4275).

FUNDING: No external funding.

CONFLICT OF INTEREST DISCLOSURES: The authors have indicated they have no conflicts of interest relevant to this article to disclose.

Food insecurity (FI), defined as limited or uncertain access to adequate food, is detrimental to the growth and development of children.[1] In 2020, approximately 14.8% of households with children were FI.[2] The association between household FI and adverse health outcomes in children includes risk of neurodevelopmental disabilities, asthma, depressive symptoms, and poor academic performance.[3–10]

The American Academy of Pediatrics (AAP) recognizes the importance of screening for FI, specifically at health maintenance visits.[11] Formal screening is preferred as associations between anthropometric data and FI have been unreliable to identify food insecure children.[12] The validated 2-question "Hunger Vital Signs" (HVS) asks: (1) "within the past 12 months we worried whether our food would run out before we got money to buy more" and (2) "within the past 12 months the food we bought just didn't last and we didn't have money to get more." Thirteen HVS have

To cite: Black AK, Pantalone J, Marrone A-C, et al. Identifying Food Insecurity in Cardiology Clinic and Connecting Families to Resources. *Pediatrics.* 2022;149(5):e2020011718

QUALITY REPORT

been instrumental in identifying FI families because of its accuracy (97% sensitivity and 83% specificity) and ease of administration.[13] This screening tool does not impose additional time or workflow barriers, facilitating incorporation into clinic flow.[14,15] FI is recurrent or episodic in nature, and scheduled screenings limited to annual well-child visits may delay intervention during vulnerable times.[2]

The AAP's 2015 policy statement on "Promoting food security for all children" recommends screening at health maintenance visits or sooner as indicated. Children with chronic medical conditions may be at increased risk for FI because of high resource burden on the family.[16] FI is associated with decreased access to health care services, resulting in poor adherence to prescription medication, decreased use of preventative services, and increased hospitalizations.[17-19] According to the Hunger in America 2014 National Report, 66% of FI families Feeding America client households reported deciding between paying for medical care and paying for food each year, and 31% did so every month.[20] Consequently, children in FI families are more likely to delay medical care.[21] Thus, expanding FI screening to pediatric subspecialty care is likely to increase timely identification of an at-risk household.

Children with congenital heart disease (CHD) are at risk for problems associated with FI, including altered growth and neurodevelopmental disabilities.[22] In CHD children, socioeconomic status is a predictor of neurodevelopmental outcomes and academic achievement, and children with more severe defects have worse outcomes.[23] A recent study by Newberger et al highlights the increased risk of financial hardship among families of children with CHD, which was associated with high rates of FI and delays in care.[24] Yet, FI screening and the potential impact of FI in children with CHD remains underinvestigated. Our specific, measurable, achievable, realistic and timely (SMART) aim was to screen 80% of pediatric cardiology clinic patients for FI from a baseline of 0% and to connect 100% of FI families to resources in 1 year.

METHODS

Setting and Context

This study was part of a larger quality improvement (QI) initiative to improve FI screening at Children's Hospital of Pittsburgh (CHP) in conjunction with a FI task force. CHP is a large, urban academic medical center in Allegheny County. Of 1.2 million people living in Allegheny County, nearly 1 in 7 are FI, constituting 42 000 children.[25] The hospital-based outpatient cardiology office primarily serves patients living in Pennsylvania (>90%), with a small percentage from other referral locations. The payor mix is 42% publicly insured, 56% private insurance, and 2% self-pay.

QI Team and Model

A pediatric cardiology fellow served as team leader and attended departmental meetings for QI support and CHP FI task force meetings for resource expansion. Clinic stakeholders were identified and included clinic intake providers, frontline physicians and advanced practice providers, and our social worker (SW). Data was monitored and collected by our QI team.

Interventions: Planning

Critical key drivers were identified to achieve our aim to screen CHD patients for FI and to connect families to resources. Given the human nature of our intake process, we anticipated a maximum level of reliability (LOR) of 1 to 2. A LOR of 1 allows 2 failures out of 10 opportunities. We set our SMART aim to screen 80% of patients from a baseline of 0% in 1 year and connect all FI families to resources. Six primary drivers were identified: (1) increase FI awareness, (2) identify FI families via a defined protocol, (3) stakeholder buy-in, (4) connect FI families to resources, (5) follow-up with FI families, and (6) assess risk of FI based on CHD severity (Fig 1).

Interventions: Education, Training, and the Screening Process

The intake team received training on FI and the HVS via a verbal presentation supplemented by information sheets. The FI task force and nursing leaders trained new staff and updated staff on electronic medical record (EMR) changes and new resources. Frontline providers (FLP) were educated about FI and informed of the screening processes and resources via E-mail training. Clinic hand-outs included basic needs support information, emergency food resources, national program resources, and programs specific to Western Pennsylvania and other counties (Supplemental Fig 6).

The HVS were implemented utilizing a verbal screening protocol during clinic intake. Early insights revealed discomfort by medical intake staff and low response rate from families. A standardized verbal screening script was trialed with limited success for positive screens.[26] On the basis of stakeholder input, the process was transitioned to a written screen with verbal screen back-up. The initial HVS were collected on paper and recorded in a temporary location in the EMR, which later became standardized.

SW was notified of positive screens via EMR messages and followed up

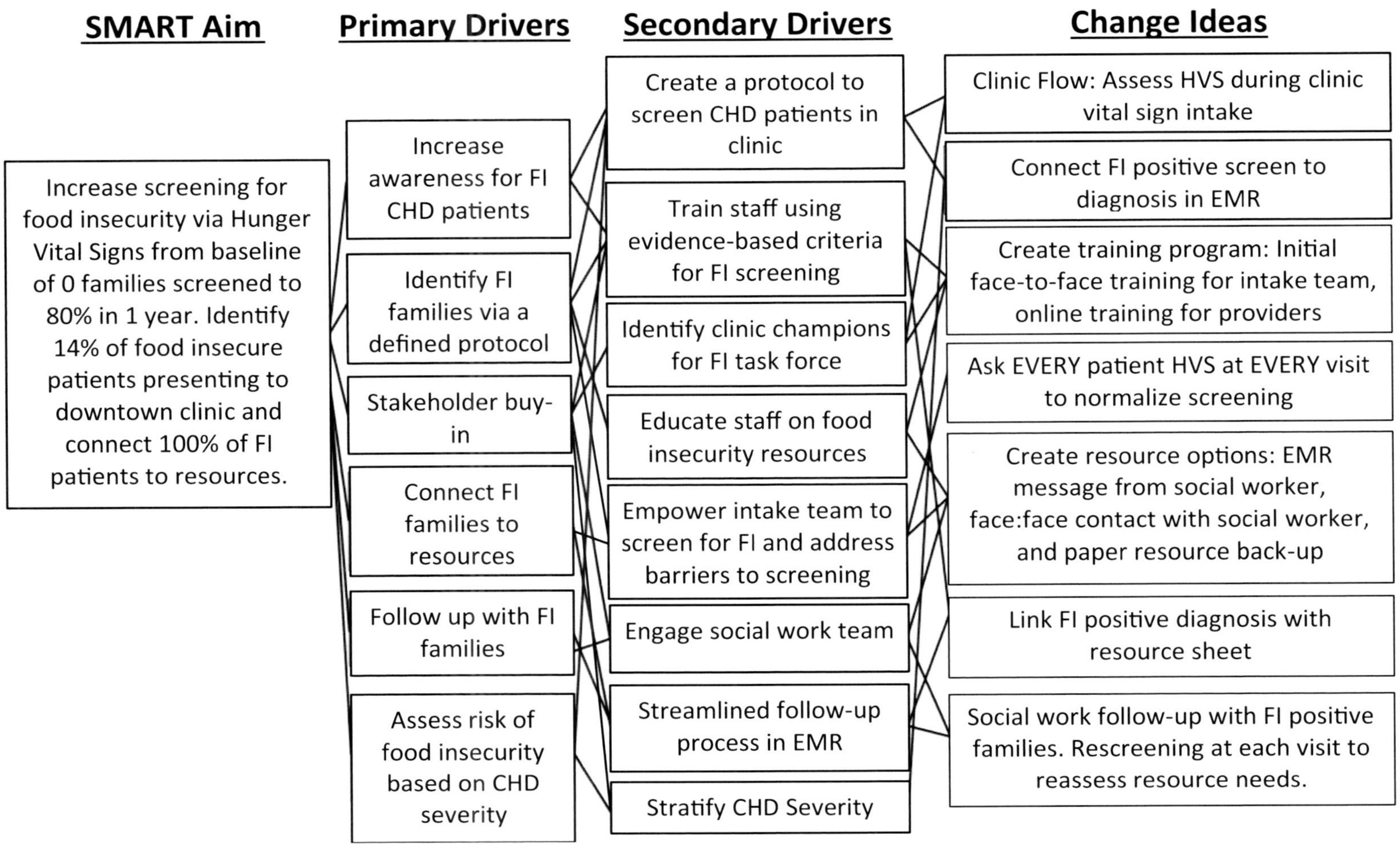

SMART Aim

Increase screening for food insecurity via Hunger Vital Signs from baseline of 0 families screened to 80% in 1 year. Identify 14% of food insecure patients presenting to downtown clinic and connect 100% of FI patients to resources.

Primary Drivers

Increase awareness for FI CHD patients

Identify FI families via a defined protocol

Stakeholder buy-in

Connect FI families to resources

Follow up with FI families

Assess risk of food insecurity based on CHD severity

Secondary Drivers

Create a protocol to screen CHD patients in clinic

Train staff using evidence-based criteria for FI screening

Identify clinic champions for FI task force

Educate staff on food insecurity resources

Empower intake team to screen for FI and address barriers to screening

Engage social work team

Streamlined follow-up process in EMR

Stratify CHD Severity

Change Ideas

Clinic Flow: Assess HVS during clinic vital sign intake

Connect FI positive screen to diagnosis in EMR

Create training program: Initial face-to-face training for intake team, online training for providers

Ask EVERY patient HVS at EVERY visit to normalize screening

Create resource options: EMR message from social worker, face:face contact with social worker, and paper resource back-up

Link FI positive diagnosis with resource sheet

Social work follow-up with FI positive families. Rescreening at each visit to reassess resource needs.

FIGURE 1
Key driver diagram. FI, food insecure; CHD, congenital heart disease; EMR, electronic medical record.

with FI families by phone. This transitioned to paging SW during the clinic visit for an in-person meeting or introduction. If a meeting was not possible, the family was offered a resource sheet with the SW's introductory note. The SW attempted to call FI families; those families who could not be reached were mailed any additional resources on the basis of their address on file. Eventually, we also offered an assessment by our community partner, Just Harvest. With consent, even in the absence of a SW, Just Harvest could perform a needs assessment of FI families.

Demographic data including age, gender, and race and ethnicity in addition to anthropometric body mass index (BMI) data and disease severity were collected to assess FI risk in our cohort. This data were included in our heart institute meetings to promote provider buy-in through data sharing.

Study of the Intervention

We executed tests of change by conducting rapid cycle plan-do-study-act (PDSA) ramps with change concepts focused on staff education, screening process, documentation, and resource distribution (Table 1). Each ramp was composed of 6 PDSA cycles on the basis of hypothesis-driven interventions to implement HVS. We adopted, adapted, or abandoned changes after data review and stakeholder insights at each stage of interventions. We evaluated cardiology visits at our CHP downtown prospectively from January 29, 2018 to February 8, 2019. Baseline data were established from January 29 to March 5, 2018, and testing started thereafter. We tracked EMR data and paper back-up copies for FI screening and extracted EMR data for demographic information and CHD security.

Measures

The primary process measure was proportion of patients screened for FI to total number of patients seen at each visit.

Our outcome measure was the proportion of all FI families connected to resources. Initially, all FI families were offered a general resource handout that met this definition. Our clinic process was refined to offer more individualized resources to FI families. As such, our outcome measure was redefined reflecting proportion of FI families offered individualized resources. All data presented reflects this new definition. As a measure of screening success our secondary outcome measure was the proportion of FI patients identified per patients screened.

This project was implemented in a busy cardiology clinic. For our balancing measure, we assessed acceptance of FI screening and perception of clinic workflow impact via an anonymous survey.

Analysis

A time series analysis was performed for our process and outcome measures. Measures were plotted on statistical process control (SPC) charts. Because these measures were yes or no responses, the chart selected was a p-chart.

For our process measure (patients screened for FI), each point on the respective SPC chart represents a combination of 5 clinic days. SPC methods were used to identify significant changes in system performance. The process was initially assessed biweekly. Centerline (mean) was shifted, and control limits were recalculated when persistent special cause variation was seen, defined as at least 8 consecutive points above the mean. Control limits were set at

±3 σ and, when recalculated, the original centerline was continued as a dotted line to visualize system change. Control limits were recalculated when stable process change was achieved with each PDSA cycle. Our goal line was set at 80% patients screened and 14% positive screening rate to match Allegheny County's FI rate.

For our primary outcome measure (FI families connected to resources), each plot on the corresponding annotated p-chart represents a total of 7 clinic days with positive FI screens. Our goal was set at 100% families connected to individualized resources. Our secondary outcome measure (FI families identified) was tracked on the respective SPC chart points, which represent a combination of 5 clinic days. SPC methods were used to identify significant changes in system performance.

Addressing our balancing measure, we assessed acceptance of FI screening and perception of workflow after implementation. Via an anonymous survey tool, we assessed staff acceptance by (1) if providers felt clinic workflow was negatively impacted as a result of screening, (2) if providers felt that their patients have benefited from screening, and (3) additional comments on the process.

To promote buy-in and to better understanding our patient population's FI resource needs, we analyzed FI risk on the basis of patient demographics and CHD disease severity. We modified the stratification scheme used by Hoffman et al to include all structural and acquired CHD (Supplemental Table 3).[27] Those patients without CHD were labeled as "none." Mild CHD included processes requiring cardiology follow-up without intervention. Moderate disease required intervention or more frequent

TABLE 1 Multiple Change, Rapid-Cycle PDSA Ramp with 4 Change Concepts and 6 PDSA Cycles

Multiple Change, Rapid-Cycle PDSA Ramp

	Change 1: Staff Education	Change 2: Screening Process	Change 3: Documentation	Change 4: Resource Distribution
Cycle 1: 3/5–3/23/18	Intake team: In-person HVS training[a] FLP: E-mail training[a] Insights: Discomfort with verbal HVS screening tool	Implementation of verbal HVS screening tool Insights: Increase in screening, below goal	Temporary EMR location for HVS documentation with paper back-up Insights: Need location in EMR	Paper resources, EMR message to SW Insights: High rate of loss to follow-up for FI+ families
Cycle 2: 3/24–5/11/18	Review standardized script and clinic process Insights: Discomfort with verbal HVS screening tool	Standardized script Insights: Increase in screening, below goal. Early increase in FI+ screen	Temporary EMR location with paper back-up Insights: Paper back-up identified FI+ screens not documented in EMR	Paper resources, EMR SW note, and mailed resources Insights: High rate of loss to follow-up for FI+ families
Cycle 3: 5/12–7/2/18	Review HVS written tool Insights: Written HVS screening tool alleviates discomfort with screening	Implement written HVS Insights: Centerline shift. Screening for FI and identification of FI+ families	Trial standardized location of EMR Insights: All FI+ screens in EMR	Paper resources with SW introductory note to family, EMR SW note, mailed resources Insights: High rate of loss to follow-up for FI+ families
Cycle 4: 7/3–8/21/18	Review screening process and findings with Heart Center Insights: Data sharing promotes buy-in	Stable screening process, unchanged Insights: The team meets screening goal of 80%	Standardized EMR location Insights: FLP knows location of FI+ screens	Meaningful assessment by SW when available in clinic[b] Insights: Inconsistent resource distribution, face-to-face meeting improves follow-up
Cycle 5: 8/22–11/14/18	Educate FLP: FI screening can impact care Insights: Data sharing promotes buy-in	Stable screening process, unchanged Goal met: The team maintains screening goal of 80%	Goal met: Standardized EMR location for HVS	Previous resources with paging SW Insights: Centerline shift: Paging SW during clinic visit improves individualized resource distribution
Cycle 6: 11/15–12/28/18	Reeducation at times of staff turn-over Insights: High staff turnover impacts screening (Outlier). New staff educated on process and maintained HVS screening goal	Stable screening process, but outlier during high staff turnover Goal met: Screening goal of 80%, focus on education during staff turnover to maintain goal	Goal met: Standardized EMR location for HVS	Previous resources and consent for community partner, Just Harvest Insights/Goal met Centerline shift: Addition of community partners improves individualized resources

[a] Frontline provider resources: FI definition, clinic flow review, AAP FI policy statement, HVS facts, and sample resource sheet.

[b] FI families endorse issues with medical assistance loophole insurance enrollment, health care costs, obtaining medication, high cost of healthy and nutritious food.

Table of multiple change, rapid-cycle PDSA ramp. Each circle on subsequent run charts represents a PDSA cycle described in the table.

TABLE 2 Characteristics of Patients by Food Security Status

	Food Secure, n = 4802	Food Insecure, n = 262	P
Age, months	120 (24–204)	96 (20–192)	.07
Sex, female	2196 (45.7)	114 (43.5)	.65
Race/Ethnicity			<.0001
Asian	86 (1.8)	6 (2.3)	
Black	619 (12.8)	76 (29.0)	
Hispanic	86 (1.8)	7 (2.7)	
White, non-Hispanic	3779 (78.7)	154 (58.8)	
Other or multiple	67 (1.4)	12 (4.6)	
Not specified	165 (3.5)	7 (2.7)	
BMI, kg/m^2	18 (16–24)	18 (16–24)	.37
BMI classification			.21
Underweight	364 (7.6)	15 (5.7)	
Normal BMI	2839 (59.1)	142 (54.2)	
Overweight	750 (15.6)	50 (19.1)	
Obese	847 (17.6)	55 (21.0)	

Values are reported as median (IQR) or n (%).

cardiology follow-up. Severe disease included those anticipated to have intervention in the newborn period and frequent cardiology follow-up.

Ethical Considerations

Approval was given on the basis of the hospital QI project submission guidelines, which did not require institutional review board (IRB) submission.

RESULTS

Study Population

Of 6885 cardiology patients seen, 5064 were screened for FI. Of the families screened, children in FI households were similar in age to children in food secure families. There was no association between FI and gender (43.5% vs 45.7% female, P = .65) or BMI classification (54.2% vs 59.1% normal BMI). Most families (3933 of 5064, 77.7%) seen in clinic identified as White, non-Hispanic. FI families were more likely to be Black (29.0% vs 12.8%) or identify as multiple or other racial and ethnic groups (4.6% vs 1.4%) and were less likely to be White (58.8% vs 78.7%) (Table 2).

Measures

Baseline screening was 0%. On implementation with verbal screening, there was a rapid, initial shift of FI screening rate to 60% within 2 months. When transitioned to a written screening tool, the process improved to 87% screened (Fig 2). At baseline, our clinic did not identify any patients experiencing FI. At the conclusion of our testing period, identification of FI rose to an average of 6%. After 3 months, we identified at least 1 family struggling with FI every week (Fig 3).

Initially, all FI families were offered a general paper resource, and a note was sent to SW for follow-up allowing us to meet our goal. In the

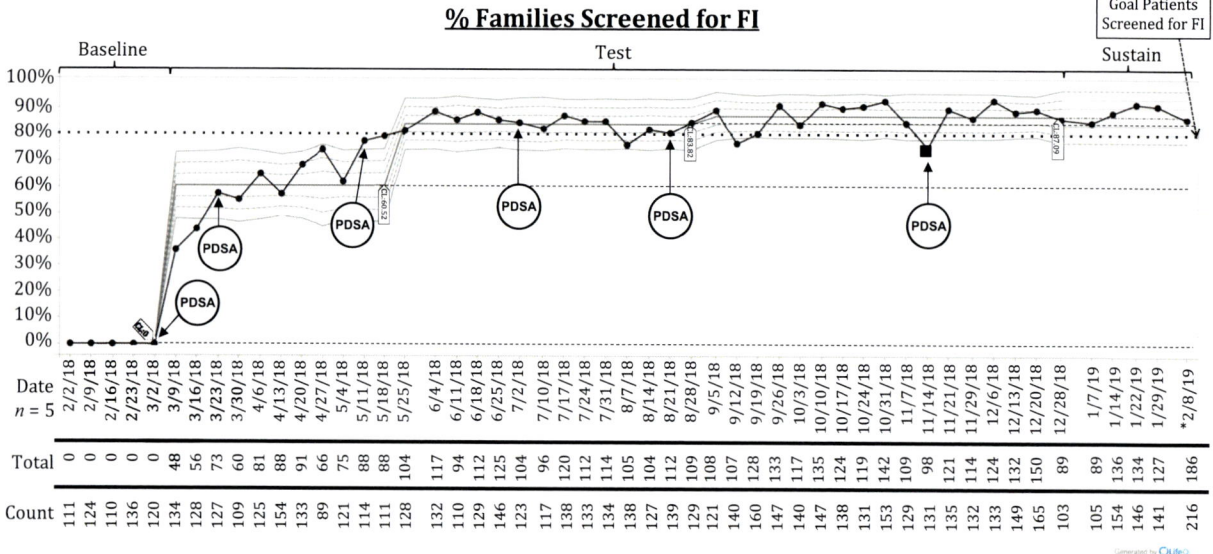

FIGURE 2

P-Chart of families screened in cardiology clinic for food insecurity. *n = 5 clinic days, except February 8, 2019 includes 8 combined clinic days. Black circles indicate outliers due to high turnover of intake staff. Retrained staff and assessed education process. See details on each PDSA cycle in Table 1.

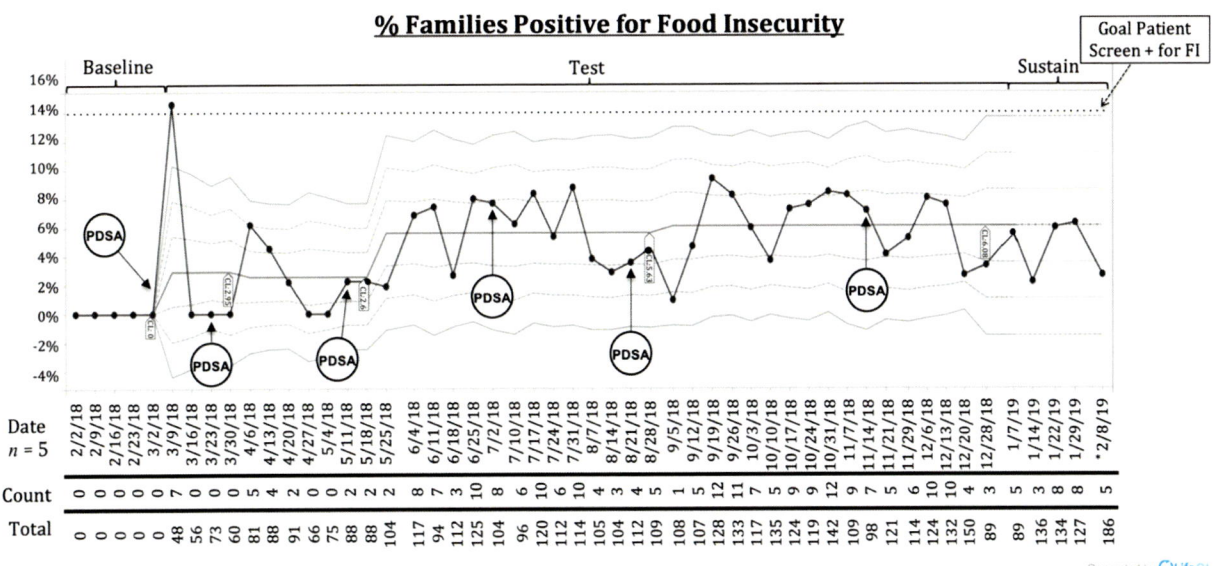

FIGURE 3
P-Chart of families screened positive for food insecurity. *n = 5 clinic days, except February 8, 2019 includes 8 clinic days. Refer to Fig 2 for details on each PDSA cycle.

early stages, many families were lost to follow-up. Insights from early outliers with highly successful resource distribution and input from the SW team revealed that face-to-face introduction on the day of the clinic greatly reduced loss to follow-up as compared to phone call follow-up alone. After the incorporation of paging the SW during the clinic visit for an in-person assessment or, if unavailable, after an introduction to the SW follow-up phone call, our centerline shifted to 84% individualized resource distribution. After the addition of Just Harvest consent, all families were offered what were considered appropriate, individualized resources by our team (Fig 4).

Individualized assessments revealed potential areas of intervention. For example, lack of Medicaid enrollment in children with special health care needs or lack of knowledge about resources (Women, Infant, and Children [WIC],

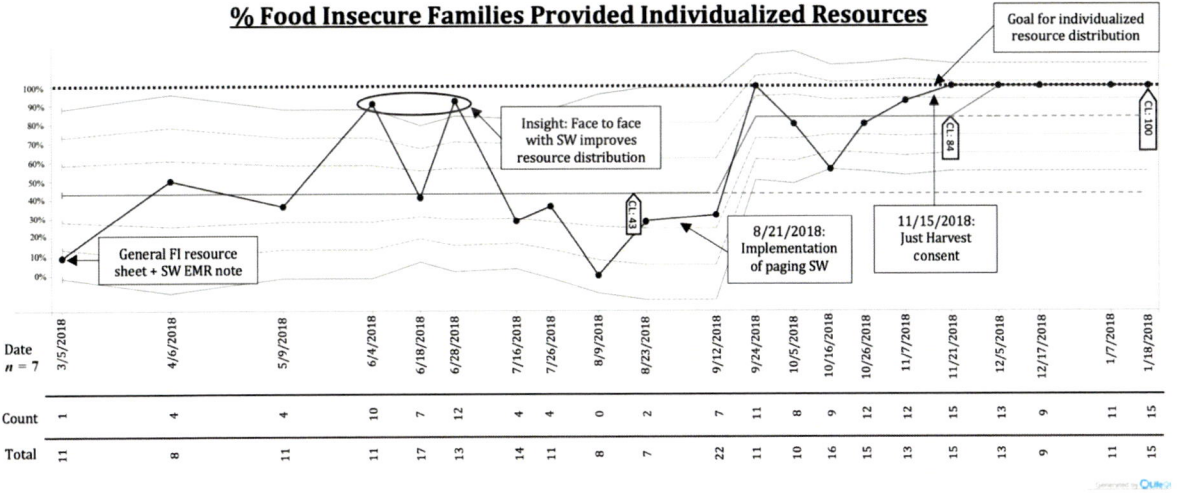

FIGURE 4
P-Chart of individualized resource distribution to FI families n = 7 combined clinic days with + FI screens. Abbreviated annotated insights included on p-chart, refer to Fig 2 for details on each PDSA cycle.

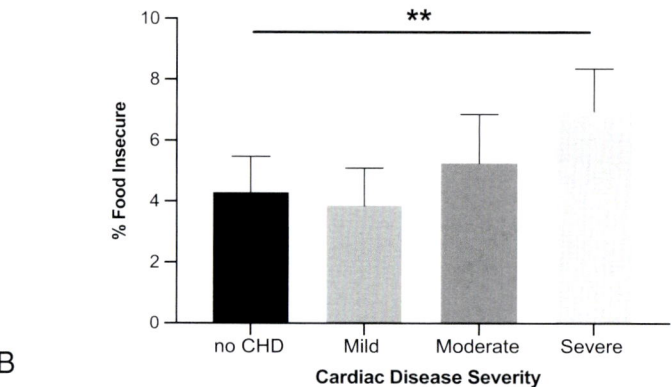

A

B

	Total n = 5064	Food Secure n = 4802	Food Insecure n = 262	OR [95% CI]	p-value
No CHD	1399	1339 (95.7%)	60 (4.3%)	Reference	Reference
Mild CHD	1193	1147 (96.1%)	46 (3.9%)	0.90 (0.60, 1.33)	.62
Moderate CHD	951	901 (94.7%)	50 (5.3%)	1.24 (0.85, 1.81)	.28
Severe CHD	1521	1415 (93.0%)	106 (7.0%)	1.67 (1.21, 2.29)	.002

FIGURE 5

A, Graph of food insecurity by congenital heart disease severity. B, table of food insecurity by congenital heart disease severity. **, statistically significant.

Supplemental Nutrition Assistance Program benefits, or food pantries) and immediate food support needs, including food pantry locations, were targeted areas of support. Families also endorsed difficulty obtaining healthy food recommended by the provider (Produce to People), job instability surrounding hospital stays, or shifts in income as family members stayed home to take care of their child. This helped create our finalized resource sheet (Supplemental Fig 6) and ability to offer all FI families individualized resources.

As a balancing measure, we evaluated staff acceptance of screening. Our clinic had 26 cardiologists and 9 cardiology fellows at screening initiation. Four attending physicians had moved at the time of survey, and 4 did not have clinic at our main hospital. Twenty-three individuals completed the survey (completion

rate of 85%). One hundred percent of respondents felt that implementation of FI screening never negatively impacted workflow. Seventy percent strongly agreed that FI screening is of great benefit to all patients, 30% agreed that FI screening benefited some patients, and no respondents responded neutral, disagreed, or strongly disagreed that FI screening was beneficial. All comments shared by physician respondents were positive (Supplemental Table 4).

Congenital Heart Disease and Food Insecurity

FI was more frequent in patients with moderate CHD, although the difference was not statistically significant (OR 1.24 [0.85–1.81], $P = .28$). FI was most frequent in patients with severe CHD compared to any other group, and 7% of families ($n = 106$) screened positive for FI (OR 1.67 [1.21–2.29], $P = .002$) (Fig 5 A and B). This

association held true regardless of race and/or ethnicity; however, minority patients with severe CHD may be particularly vulnerable (Supplemental Table 5).

DISCUSSION

To our knowledge, this report is the first describing implementation of FI screening in a pediatric cardiology clinic. We demonstrated the ability to reliably assess FI in a busy outpatient cardiology office. Our screening rate and FI identification improved using a written version of HVS, which mitigated provider-reported and subjective parental discomfort. There was overwhelming support of FI screening by our clinic physicians, and they did not feel their clinic workflow was negatively impacted by screening.

We reached our screening goal during our study period, but there were limitations in FI screening and risk assessment. Our study relied on human screeners. Implementation of an automated intake form directly imported into the EMR may further increase screening rates through improved LOR. A specified EMR location for screening helped improve our screening rate, but hard stops in the EMR may improve completion rates. Whereas we identified multiple families struggling with FI, our positivity rate did not reach that of Allegheny County (14%).[25] Although our clinic is located in Allegheny County, our referral basis is from surrounding areas and even outside states. Additionally, although we screened every patient to create normalization, there continues to be stigmatization surrounding FI.

Our primary outcome was to connect all FI families to resources. Early distribution of a generalized FI form resulted in limited success for follow-up and revealed that FI is not a 1-size-fits-all solution. Needs assessments uncovered underused resources, which exacerbated risk for FI. Collaboration with SW and community partners allowed our families to connect with local, individualized food resources and greatly improved our success in resource connection. Partnership with community programs may be a way to address FI issues in the absence of a SW. A meeting with our SW near the time of screening was integral to connecting families with appropriate resources and prevented loss to follow-up. An established FI team and SW allowed our clinic to have refined, individualized resources for families impacted by FI. As a result, our clinic served as a standard for screening and resource distribution for expansion to other clinics.

The results of our study reveal that patients with severe CHD may be at particular risk for FI. This held true across race and ethnicity groups, except those who did not specify race, and it highlighted that minority patients with severe CHD may be particularly vulnerable. This information was used to promote provider buy-in highlighting the risk to our most vulnerable clinic population. In addition, it helped focus individualized resource connection for moderate and severe CHD patients, including SW assessment for Medicaid enrollment and assessment surrounding hospitalizations, which were cited by families as a particular source of resource strain. A limitation to this analysis was that it did not address possible confounding factors, such as household income for FI families. Further studies are needed to assess FI in our patient population to expand on opportunities for intervention.

The impact of CHD severity on FI is not unexpected. Changes in financial stability may limit families' ability to gain access to adequate food.[2,28] Families of children with cancer lost >40% of their annual household income 6 months after their child's diagnosis.[29] Severe CHD patients undergo multiple procedures requiring hospitalizations with homebound recovery for varying lengths of time. As we continue to search for ways to reduce morbidity in our patient population, addressing the impact of complex CHD on social influencers of health (including FI) by creating individualized resources is integral. This can be done through community partnerships and social work support.

Whereas the majority of our patient population identified as White, our study highlights racial disparities in FI families in our clinic population. As a medical community, targeting racial inequities that may impact medical outcomes is essential. In CHD, low neighborhood socioeconomic status is associated with worse outcomes after the Norwood procedure, suggesting that socioeconomic factors are important, potentially modifiable determinants of outcome.[30] Further, FI families are more likely to delay medical care because of cost.[20,21] Thus, addressing FI in CHD patients by using the HVS may improve access to timely care in these high-risk patients.

CONCLUSION

FI screening is feasible in an outpatient cardiology office. Severe CHD patients may be at higher risk for FI, and more focused studies are needed for this population. As FI is a modifiable risk factor, identifying and addressing FI may improve outcomes for CHD patients. Community partnerships and SW support improves individualized, targeted FI interventions.

ACKNOWLEDGMENTS

We thank the Heart Institute at CHP, including our social work team and our FI Task Force.

ABBREVIATIONS

AAP: American Academy of Pediatrics
BMI: body mass index
CHD: congenital heart disease
CHP: UPMC Children's Hospital of Pittsburgh
EMR: electronic medical record
FI: food insecurity
FLP: frontline providers
HVS: Hunger Vital Signs
LOR: level of reliability
PDSA: plan-do-study-act
QI: quality improvement
SPC: statistical process control

REFERENCES

1. Shankar P, Chung R, Frank DA. Association of food insecurity with children's behavioral, emotional, and academic outcomes: a systematic review. *J Dev Behav Pediatr.* 2017;38(2): 135–150

2. Coleman-Jensen A, Rabbitt MP, Gregory CA, Singh A; Economic Research Service, US Department of Agriculture. Household food security in the United States in

2020. Economic research report. 2021. Available at: https://www.ers.usda.gov/publications/pub-details/?pubid=102075 Accessed March 31, 2022

3. Laraia BA. Food insecurity and chronic disease. *Adv Nutr.* 2013;4(2):203–212

4. Cook JT, Frank DA, Berkowitz C, et al. Food insecurity is associated with adverse health outcomes among human infants and toddlers. *J Nutr.* 2004; 134(6):1432–1438

5. Zaslow M, Bronte-Tinkew J, Capps R, Horowitz A, Moore KA, Weinstein D. Food security during infancy: implications for attachment and mental proficiency in toddlerhood. *Matern Child Health J.* 2009;13(1):66–80

6. Hernandez DC, Jacknowitz A. Transient, but not persistent, adult food insecurity influences toddler development. *J Nutr.* 2009;139(8):1517–1524

7. Whitaker RC, Phillips SM, Orzol SM. Food insecurity and the risks of depression and anxiety in mothers and behavior problems in their preschool-aged children. *Pediatrics.* 2006;118(3):e859–e868

8. Weinreb L, Wehler C, Perloff J, et al. Hunger: its impact on children's health and mental health. *Pediatrics.* 2002;110(4):e41

9. McLaughlin KA, Green JG, Alegría M, et al. Food insecurity and mental disorders in a national sample of U.S. adolescents. *J Am Acad Child Adolesc Psychiatry.* 2012;51(12):1293–1303

10. Eisenmann JC, Gundersen C, Lohman BJ, Garasky S, Stewart SD. Is food insecurity related to overweight and obesity in children and adolescents? A summary of studies, 1995–2009. *Obes Rev.* 2011;12(5): e73–e83

11. Council on Community Pediatrics; Committee on Nutrition. Promoting food security for all children. *Pediatrics.* 2015; 136(5):e1431–e1438

12. Drennen CR, Coleman SM, Ettinger de Cuba S, et al. Food insecurity, health, and development in children under age four years. *Pediatrics.* 2019;144(4):e20190824

13. Hager ER, Quigg AM, Black MM, et al. Development and validity of a 2-item screen to identify families at risk for food insecurity. *Pediatrics.* 2010;126(1): e26–e32

14. De Marchis EH, Torres JM, Fichtenberg C, Gottlieb LM. Identifying food insecurity in health care settings: A systematic scoping review of the evidence. *Fam Community Health.* 2019;42(1):20–29

15. Adams E, Hargunani D, Hoffmann L, Blaschke G, Helm J, Koehler A. Screening for food insecurity in pediatric primary care: A clinic's positive implementation experiences. *J Health Care Poor Underserved.* 2017;28(1):24–29

16. O'Malley JA, Klett BM, Klein MD, Inman N, Beck AF. Revealing the prevalence and consequences of food insecurity in children with epilepsy. *J Community Health.* 2017;42(6):1213–1219

17. Kushel MB, Gupta R, Gee L, Haas JS. Housing instability and food insecurity as barriers to health care among low-income Americans. *J Gen Intern Med.* 2006;21(1):71–77

18. Ma CT, Gee L, Kushel MB. Associations between housing instability and food insecurity with health care access in low-income children. *Ambul Pediatr.* 2008;8(1):50–57

19. Peltz A, Garg A. Food insecurity and health care use. *Pediatrics.* 2019;144(4):e20190347

20. Weinfield NS, Mills G, Borger C, et al. Hunger in America 2014. Available at: http://help.feedingamerica.org/HungerInAmerica/hunger-in-america-2014-full-report.pdf. Accessed March 31, 2018

21. Thomas MMC, Miller DP, Morrissey TW. Food insecurity and child health. *Pediatrics.* 2019;144(4):e20190397

22. Marino BS, Lipkin PH, Newburger JW, et al; American Heart Association Congenital Heart Defects Committee, Council on Cardiovascular Disease in the Young, Council on Cardiovascular Nursing, and Stroke Council. Neurodevelopmental outcomes in children with congenital heart disease: evaluation and management: a scientific statement from the American Heart Association. *Circulation.* 2012;126(9):1143–1172

23. Moons P, Van Deyk K, De Geest S, Gewillig M, Budts W. Is the severity of congenital heart disease associated with the quality of life and perceived health of adult patients? *Heart.* 2005;91(9):1193–1198

24. Ludomirsky AB, Bucholz EM, Newburger JW. Association of financial hardship because of medical bills with adverse outcomes among families of children with congenital heart disease. *JAMA Cardiol.* 2021;6(6):713–717

25. Just Harvest. Hunger in Allegheny County. Available at: https://www.justharvest.org/wp-content/uploads/2015/06/Just-Harvest-Fact-Sheet-on-Hunger-in-Allegheny-County-2017.pdf. Accessed March 31, 2018

26. Stenmark SH, Steiner JF, Marpadga S, Debor M, Underhill K, Seligman H. Lessons learned from implementation of the food insecurity screening and referral program at Kaiser Permanente Colorado. *Perm J.* 2018;22:18–093

27. Hoffman JI, Kaplan S. The incidence of congenital heart disease. *J Am Coll Cardiol.* 2002;39(12):1890–1900

28. Coleman-Jensen William McFall Mark Nord A, McFall W, Nord M. Food insecurity in households with children: prevalence, severity, and household characteristics 2010–11. *Econ Res Serv.* 2013;113: 2010–2011

29. Bona K, London WB, Guo D, Frank DA, Wolfe J. Trajectory of material hardship and income poverty in families of children undergoing chemotherapy: A prospective cohort study. *Pediatr Blood Cancer.* 2016;63(1): 105–111

30. Bucholz EM, Sleeper LA, Newburger JW. Neighborhood socioeconomic status and outcomes following the Norwood procedure: An analysis of the pediatric heart network single ventricle reconstruction trial public data aet. *J Am Heart Assoc.* 2018;7(3):e007065

Establishing a Permanent Food Pantry in a Pediatric Emergency Department

Brit Anderson, MD,[a] Elizabeth Lehto, DO, MS, MSc,[a] Frances Hardin-Fanning, PhD, RN,[b] Joelle Hirst, BSN, RN, SANE, SANE-A,[c] Joy Storm, MPH, RN, SANE,[c] Elizabeth Montgomery, APRN,[c] Amber Hussain, MD,[d] Kerry Caperell, MD, MS, MBA[a]

Childhood food insecurity is associated with adverse health outcomes. Food pantries housed within healthcare facilities have the potential to reduce childhood food insecurity. An interdisciplinary team established a permanent food pantry in the pediatric emergency department of a metropolitan children's hospital. Members of the team included attending and resident physicians, nurse practitioners, nurses, patient care technicians, a volunteer coordinator, Prevention and Wellness staff, and environmental services staff. The development process, formative evaluation, and impact of the pantry during the first 15 months of use is described. Families presenting to the emergency department were notified of the food pantry and offered a bag of groceries. Data collected included number of adult and children in the household, age ranges of family members, and whether food was accepted. The food pantry provided aid to 2199 households from January 2021 to April 2022. Recipients of food assistance included 4698 children, 3565 adults, and 140 seniors. In addition, the interdisciplinary approach to the development process elucidated barriers to and facilitators of the project's success, thereby maximizing the food assistance outcome.

[a]Norton Children's Medical Group affiliated with the University of Louisville School of Medicine Division of Pediatric Emergency Medicine, Louisville, Kentucky; [b]University of Louisville School of Nursing, Louisville, Kentucky; [c]Norton Children's Hospital, Louisville, Kentucky; and [d]Department of Pediatrics, University of Louisville, Louisville, Kentucky

Dr Anderson conceptualized the design, collected and analyzed data, and drafted the initial manuscript; Drs Lehto and Hussain conceptualized the design, trained student volunteers, and collected data; Ms Hirst and Ms Montgomery conceptualized the design and collected data; Dr Hardin-Fanning contributed to project design, analyzed data, and drafted the initial manuscript; Ms Storm conceptualized the design and collected data; Dr Caperell conceptualized the design and analyzed the data; and all authors critically reviewed and revised the manuscript, approved the final manuscript, and agreed to be accountable for all aspects of the work.

DOI: https://doi.org/10.1542/peds.2023-061757

Accepted for publication Jun 28, 2023

Address correspondence to Brit Anderson, MD, 571 S Floyd St, Louisville, KY 40202. E-mail: brit.anderson@louisville.edu

PEDIATRICS (ISSN Numbers: Print, 0031-4005; Online, 1098-4275).

FUNDING: Funding for the food pantry described was primarily provided by The Norton Children's Hospital Foundation. An additional donation was received from individuals and a local nonprofit, Recipe to End Hunger. Dare to Care, a regional Feeding America food bank, is a key collaborator providing food for the pantry. This project was designed in a multi-disciplinary fashion which included input from funders.

CONFLICT OF INTEREST DISCLOSURES: The authors have indicated they have no conflicts of interest relevant to this article to disclose.

To cite: Anderson B, Lehto E, Hardin-Fanning F, et al. Establishing a Permanent Food Pantry in a Pediatric Emergency Department. *Pediatrics.* 2023; 152(4):e2023061757

Food insecurity, defined as inconsistent access to safe and nutritious foods that meet dietary needs and preferences for a healthy life, is associated with lifelong health consequences in children.[1-4] Despite decades of public health interventions, food insecurity remains prevalent in the United States.[5] Food insecurity is a social determinant of health categorized in the Healthy People 2030 Economic Stability domain.[6] Healthy People 2030 objectives include eliminating very low food security among children and reducing household food insecurity and subsequently, hunger.[6]

In 2019, food insecurity rates in the United States were significantly lower (10.5%) for the first time since the 2007 prerecession level (11.1%).[5] However, the 2020 and 2021 food insecurity rates (10.5% and 10.2%, respectively) were not significantly different from the 2019 prevalence.[5] In 2020, more than 38 million Americans, including 12 million children, were unable to meet their dietary needs.[7] Despite this critical need, community food banks and food assistance programs are often underused because of the stigma associated with needing assistance.[7,8] However, food assistance affiliated with health care facilities may not be associated with the same stigma as it can be viewed as an integral component of health care if approached empathetically.[9,10] Hospital-based food pantry usage allows individuals to feel more comfortable receiving food assistance, trust the food provided, have high satisfaction with food quality, and experience less stigma than when accessing other food assistance programs.[9] In addition, previous hospital-based food pantry programs have reported significant improvements in fruit and vegetable consumption in patrons.[11]

Food assistance partnerships with clinical providers have the potential to reduce food insecurity and serve as primary prevention strategies aimed at reducing chronic illness.[12-15] Despite the existence of multiple community food banks and pantries, food insecurity is still a significant issue in Jefferson County, Kentucky, where this initiative took place. A recent Louisville Community Health Assessment found that 22% of Jefferson County families had experienced food insecurity at some point in the last 12 months.[16] More than a third of the nearly 90 000 Jefferson County residents experiencing food insecurity in 2019 were above the 200% poverty rate of food assistance eligibility.[17] At this range of income, the families are limited in how they can resolve food insecurity and are most likely to benefit from community food resources.

OBJECTIVES

A pediatric emergency department (ED)-based food pantry was established to prioritize the distribution of food and resource information to families who needed it, address concerns related to food assistance stigma, and maintain respect for frontline provider time. The objectives of this analysis are to report the number of households, children, adults, and seniors who received aid from the pantry and to describe potential improvements to the development and implementation of the food assistance process. Cost of food per recipient family was also analyzed.

METHODS AND PROCESS

Setting

In January 2021, a permanent food pantry was opened in the emergency department at Norton Children's Hospital, Louisville, Kentucky. Norton Children's is an urban, tertiary care, free-standing children's hospital providing care to approximately 50 000 ED patients annually. The food pantry is in an office just outside the ED. Each month, food is ordered and delivered by a local food bank based upon usage during the previous month. A 90-day pilot began on January 25, 2021 to provide data for a formative evaluation. During this time, incremental infrastructure was added with the goal of making all caregivers in the ED aware of food resources. Results are reported for January 25, 2021 through April 30, 2022, unless otherwise noted. The fast-track area of the ED was selected as the initial area of focus because the higher acuity of the main ED limited interaction time with families.

Stakeholders and Funding

This project was implemented in collaboration with Norton Children's Prevention and Wellness, which had previously opened more than 20 food pantries in primary care clinics around the city. Established in 1991, Norton's Prevention and Wellness focuses on childhood injury prevention and healthy lifestyle promotion. This project greatly benefited from the expertise of this organization and their previous work. For this project, a local food bank, Dare to Care,

supplied nonperishable foods to the pantry during monthly deliveries. Funding was primarily provided by the Norton Children's Hospital Foundation, the philanthropic arm of the Norton Healthcare Systems. The Foundation's Board of Trustees and members include healthcare providers and community stakeholders from multiple disciplines. Ongoing communication with stakeholders throughout programmatic development and implementation has contributed toward sustainability.

Ethical Considerations

The interdisciplinary team discussed the ethics of interacting with families in the ED who may need food assistance. A core tenet of our project was the distribution of food to ED families in a respectful manner. Consideration was given to the use of validated food insecurity or hunger screeners.[18,19] However, given established high rates of food insecurity in pediatric EDs,[20,21] concerns about increased nursing burden with screening[22,23] and potential caregiver discomfort with formal screening in an environment where families do not have an established relationship with the care team,[24] the decision was made to simply notify families of the food pantry and offer a bag of groceries.

Resource allocation equity was also considered. Food insecurity screening procedures were discussed by the team and consensus was reached that screening could potentially contribute to hesitancy to accept food and would also add additional workload to our healthcare personnel. Although offering food resources to all is equality, rather than equity, dignity and comfort were central values. Caregivers in one ED-based study reported fear of negative consequences, including judgement if they disclosed food insecurity to ED personnel but were more comfortable reporting food insecurity to their established primary care provider.[24]

Based on the current evidence of stigma and concerns of negative consequences, resources were offered in the absence of food insecurity screening. It is certainly possible that families who would not have screened positive for food insecurity may have accepted resources. However, food distribution occurred during a time when the economic effects of the coronavirus disease 2019 (COVID-19) pandemic were still prevalent and in a location known to provide services for families with low economic resources. Therefore, the greater community need not justify the provision of food resources without screening procedures.

This evaluation was considered nonhuman subjects research by the University of Louisville Institutional Review Board.

Variables

Pantry usage data for the first 15 months were analyzed. Data included the number of people in the household, age of household members, number of children, and whether food was accepted. Age was categorized as preschool (ie,

<6 years), school age (ie, 6 to <18 years), adults (ie, 18 to <60 years), and seniors (ie, 60+ years). These categories were selected at the request of the regional food bank that supplied the food items and are reflective of aggregate data reported by the US Department of Agriculture (USDA) Food and Nutrition Services.[5] These data also provided insight into how much food should be distributed to each household. Because of concern that patients may be hesitant to discuss food insecurity if their acceptance of food became part of the medical record, responses were recorded on paper forms. No identifying information was collected. Food allergies were queried before distribution.

Implementation

Initially, when families accepted food, they were given a checklist of foods to choose from, and a staff member packed a bag with the foods selected. However, because this was time-consuming and most families checked all options, personnel began prepackaging bags and storing several near the nurses' station. All food was shelf-stable and included canned fruits and vegetables, soups, beans, rice, whole wheat pasta, milk, and cereal. Opaque, reusable grocery bags were used for ease of carrying. In addition to food, each bag contained a handout with Quick Response codes for more information about resources, including the Supplemental Nutrition Assistance Program, Women Infants and Children, school meal programs, and local community-based organizations. Recipes using food from the pantry were included, along with other donated items when available.

The pilot phase was implemented on weekends and evenings in the fast-track area of the ED, an 8-bed unit within the main ED, where, in 2021, approximately 10 000 lower acuity patients received care. We later expanded to round-the-clock assistance with the goal of offering food to every family seen in fast-track. Signage in English and Spanish was placed in all ED rooms to encourage families to ask providers about the pantry service if it was not formally offered to them. Interpreters were used if needed.

Challenges

An interdisciplinary food pantry council was formed in April 2021 to address challenges in our process. The 20 members of the council include attending and resident physicians, nurse practitioners, nurses, patient care technicians, a volunteer coordinator, Prevention and Wellness staff, and environmental services staff. This council identified frontline staff (nurses and physicians) burden as a barrier to the food pantry's success. The pilot phase took place early in the COVID-19 pandemic, a time of lower patient volumes, and it became clear as ED volumes returned to prepandemic levels that additional support was necessary. Initially, ED clinical staff were responsible for all operations of the pantry, including ordering food,

unloading the truck, stocking shelves, packing bags, offering food, and collecting data. Council members aimed to improve frontline provider acceptance of the project by asking interested staff to join the council, providing educational opportunities and identifying opportunities to ease the daily burden of the operation of the pantry.

Although there were challenges in adapting the program to an emergency department environment, a formative evaluation with the first 10 families was conducted in the first 90 days and procedures were revised to provide services more efficiently. Early in the program, bags were filled with large quantities of food and more money was spent on the contents in each bag. However, families were leaving bags behind because they were too heavy. Flexibility and the input from the interdisciplinary teams was critical to the financial sustainability of the program.

OUTCOMES

From January 25, 2021 through April 30, 2022, total ED volume was 54 775; of these, 12 705 (23.2%) were seen in the fast-track. A total of 3981 families (31.3% of fast-track patients) were offered food from the ED pantry. Of these, 2199 (55%) families accepted food. These families were comprised of 8811 people: 2253 children <6 years old, 2445 children aged 6 to <18 years, 3565 adults aged 18 to <60 years, and 140 seniors (60+). Family size was documented beginning March 1, 2021 through April 30, 2022. Average family size was 4.1 members and family size ranged 1 to 13 members. The pantry distributed 35 600 pounds of food at a cost of $25 208 when purchased through the food bank. The cost per family served was approximately $11.

LESSONS LEARNED

Childhood Food Insecurity

Pediatric ED food pantries have a significant potential benefit given patrons' high rates of food insecurity, the unique ability to provide services to those who do not have an established primary care physician, and the inherent accessibility at times when other resources are unavailable. These services also help develop a strong emotional connection and increased trust with the care center.[14,24] Previous studies have shown that around 20% of ED patients screen positive for food insecurity.[18] In our program, 55% of families accepted food when offered. Inconsistent data collection may have contributed to this discrepancy, with possibly fewer staff completing a form if a family declined food assistance. Despite these potential missing data, the ED-based food pantry was generally well-received and highly used. There are several factors in the process that may have contributed to this level of usage. Support was offered by asking patients and families if they wanted a bag of food instead of asking screening questions. Food was immediately available to take home from their ED visit, overcoming resource inaccessibility (limited transportation, wait times at food assistance agencies), which can be challenging to navigate. Food acceptance was not recorded in the medical record and therefore, families may have been more willing to accept resources. Additionally, food pantries in clinical settings transition the perception of food assistance from charity to "food as medicine" and part of health care.[9,10]

Rates of food insecurity increased during the COVID-19 pandemic.[24] This program took place during the initial phases of the COVID-19 pandemic and this may also partially explain why there were higher acceptance rates than reported in previous studies. The USDA forecasts continued food price increases in 2023.[5] This anticipated increase in food costs will likely exacerbate food insecurity in low and middle-income households, particularly those with children. Food insecurity will continue to be an essential health issue, and innovative strategies to increase food assistance options are vital to meet nutritional needs.

Continuity of care in partnership with primary care providers poses a challenge. Future considerations for documentation of food security status in the electronic health record would provide a way to track food security outcomes over time. A core tenet of this project was to provide patient anonymity to enhance comfort in accepting food. Although a list of food resources was provided in each bag, future discussions will address how to notify primary care providers of the need for continued food assistance.

Interprofessional Collaboration Opportunities

The interdisciplinary leadership team for the ED food pantry is unique compared with other projects in the healthcare setting. Monthly meetings of the food pantry council are well-attended. The council has engaged in other projects, such as the development of a novel medical student curriculum, nursing training, and the development of a hospital-wide food insecurity screening and resource referral. This continued process illustrates the impact that is possible when working together in healthcare outside of traditional silos. Further work to evaluate care provider perspectives and to complete development of the medical education program is underway. The education program with preclinical medical students, started in October 2021, includes educational modules, simulated conversations with families about food insecurity, and experiential volunteering in the pantry. Students can receive elective credit for participation. In addition, a series of Norton Children's Nursing Grand Rounds are currently being conducted. These include presentations related to identification of food insecure children, reduction of stigma and fear of consequences, and enhanced awareness of food resources from food insecurity researchers, ED physicians, and Prevention and Wellness leaders.

Workflow

The pediatric ED food pantry process is iterative. Although key emergency department personnel have responsibilities in the food pantry (delivery supervision, data collection, ordering of food items), volunteers now complete many tasks (packing bags, stocking shelves, and offering food) during times of high ED volume. Volunteers include preclinical medical students who have been integral in providing feedback to the team. Other ancillary staff (social workers, patient care techs, patient liaisons) now notify families of available resources. Although the pantry services are still centered upon the fast-track areas given the more complex flow of the main ED, there are signs in main ED rooms that notify families of the services. Many of the interventions were beneficial, but the team continues formative and summative evaluations to address challenges as they arise. Personnel who expressed interest in the project now hold key positions and have work time allocated to support the pantry.

LIMITATIONS

Because there was no documentation in the medical record, there was no communication of need to primary care providers, who could have provided continued support for families. Replication of this type of service should include a communication pathway by which primary care providers are notified of the need for food assistance so that continuity of nutritional care can be established. Additionally, analysis of the program and its potential impact on health equity was limited by lack of granular data collection. Inclusion of demographic variables, such as self-reported race and insurance status, would strengthen future studies.

FUTURE RESEARCH

A qualitative study of recipients' perceptions of the food pantry would inform future processes. Although formal feedback was not elicited, families did spontaneously report positive comments. Qualitative studies are needed to explore the impact on reduced stigma, quality of food and interaction with personnel, and the degree of comfort in seeking future food assistance. In addition, future impact analysis using a validated measure of food security (USDA Household Food Security Survey Module) will strengthen the rationale for continued funding of the pantry and replication in other facilities.[19] In addition, rigorous methodologies should be employed to evaluate the impact of these resource-based primary prevention projects on frontline provider burnout and on racial and ethnic nutrition-related health disparities.[25,26]

CONCLUSIONS

This project demonstrates that an ED-based food pantry is a potential venue to provide emergency food assistance to the community. Educational and food insecurity impact outcomes will continue to be evaluated.

ACKNOWLEDGMENTS

We thank Nicole Greenwell, Brenda O'Bryan, Tracy Morrison, Angie Garman, Adrienne Griten, Kelly Hibbs, Dr Erin Frazier, Norton Children's Hospital Foundation, and Norton Children's Hospital. This project was implemented in collaboration with Norton Children's Prevention and Wellness, which had previously opened more than 20 food pantries in primary care clinics around the city. Established in 1991, Norton's Prevention and Wellness focuses on childhood injury prevention and healthy lifestyle promotion, and the emergency department staff and volunteers who support this project.

ABBREVIATION

ED: emergency department

REFERENCES

1. Abdurahman AA, Chaka EE, Nedjat S, Dorosty AR, Majdzadeh R. The association of household food insecurity with the risk of type 2 diabetes mellitus in adults: a systematic review and meta-analysis. *Eur J Nutr.* 2019;58(4):1341–1350

2. Bishop NJ, Wang K. Food insecurity, comorbidity, and mobility limitations among older U.S. adults: findings from the Health and Retirement Study and Health Care and Nutrition Study. *Prev Med.* 2018;114:180–187

3. Ford ES. Food security and cardiovascular disease risk among adults in the United States: findings from the National Health and Nutrition Examination Survey, 2003-2008. *Prev Chronic Dis.* 2013;10:E202

4. Thomas MMC, Miller DP, Morrissey TW. Food insecurity and child health. *Pediatrics.* 2019;144(4):e20190397

5. United States Department of Agriculture Economic Research Services. Food insecurity key statistics and graphics. Available at: https://www.ers.usda.gov/topics/food-nutrition-assistance/food-security-in-the-u-s/key-statistics-graphics/#trends. Accessed March 3, 2022

6. United States Office of Disease Prevention and Health Promotion. Healthy people 2020. Available at: https://www.healthypeople.gov/2020/topics-objectives/topic/social-determinants-of-health. Accessed March 3, 2022

7. Coleman-Jensen A, Rabbitt M, Christian AG, Singh A. *Household Food Security in the United States in 2020.* Washington, District of Columbia: U.S. Department of Agriculture, Economic Research Service; 2021

8. Middleton G, Mehta K, McNaughton D, Booth S. The experiences and perceptions of food banks amongst users in high-income countries: an international scoping review. *Appetite.* 2018;120:698–708

9. Greenthal E, Jia J, Poblacion A, James T. Patient experiences and provider perspectives on a hospital-based food pantry: a mixed methods evaluation study. *Public Health Nutr.* 2019;22(17):3261–3269

10. Greenway FL. Food as medicine for chronic disease: a strategy to address non-compliance. *J Med Food.* 2020;23(9):903–904

11. Hu D, Cherian A, Chagin K, et al. Food as medicine clinic: early results and lessons learned. *Cureus.* 2022;14(11):e31912

12. Mirsky JB, Zack RM, Berkowitz SA, Fiechtner L. Massachusetts General Hospital Revere Food Pantry: addressing hunger and health at an academic medical center community clinic. *Healthc (Amst).* 2021;9(4):100589

13. Wetherill MS, White KC, Seligman H. Charitable food as prevention: Food bank leadership perspectives on food banks as agents in population health. *Community Dev (Columb).* 2019;50(1):92–107

14. Cullen D, Blauch A, Mirth M, Fein J. Complete eats: summer meals offered by the emergency department for food insecurity. *Pediatrics.* 2019;144(4):e20190201

15. Council on Community Pediatrics; Committee on Nutrition. Promoting food security for all children. *Pediatrics.* 2015;136(5):e1431–e1438

16. Louisville Metro Department of Public Health and Wellness. Louisville metro community health assessment. Available at: https://louisvilleky.gov/health-wellness/document/2018communityhealthneedsassessmentdetailedfindigspdf. Accessed July 17, 2022

17. Feeding America. Food insecurity among overall (all ages) population in Kentucky. Available at: https://map.feedingamerica.org/county/2017/overall/kentucky?msclkid=bfe91387b1fd11ecaeefeab531698688. Accessed July 17, 2022

18. Gattu RK, Paik G, Wang Y, Ray P, Lichenstein R, Black MM. The hunger vital sign identifies household food insecurity among children in emergency departments and primary care. *Children (Basel).* 2019;6(10):107

19. United States Department of Agriculture Economic Research Serve. Household food security survey module. Available at: https://www.ers.usda.gov/topics/food-nutrition-assistance/food-security-in-the-u-s/survey-tools/. Accessed March 3, 2022

20. Gonzalez JV, Hartford EA, Moore J, Brown JC. Food insecurity in a pediatric emergency department and the feasibility of universal screening. *West J Emerg Med.* 2021;22(6):1295–1300

21. Cullen D, Woodford A, Fein J. Food for thought: a randomized trial of food insecurity screening in the emergency department. *Acad Pediatr.* 2019;19(6):646–651

22. Pabalan L, Dunn R, Gregori K, et al. Assessment of food insecurity in children's hospital of wisconsin's emergency department. *WMJ.* 2015;114(4):148–151

23. Robinson T, Bryan L, Johnson V, McFadden T, Lazarus S, Simon HK. Hunger: a missed opportunity for screening in the pediatric emergency department. *Clin Pediatr (Phila).* 2018;57(11):1318–1325

24. Cullen D, Attridge M, Fein JA. Food for thought: a qualitative evaluation of caregiver preferences for food insecurity screening and resource referral. *Acad Pediatr.* 2020;20(8):1157–1162

25. Hickey E, Phan M, Beck AF, Burkhardt MC, Klein MD. A mixed-methods evaluation of a novel food pantry in a pediatric primary care center. *Clin Pediatr (Phila).* 2020;59(3):278–284

26. Gundersen C, Hake M, Dewey A, Engelhard E. Food insecurity during COVID-19. *Appl Econ Perspect Policy.* 2021;43(1):153–161

SNAP Participation and Emergency Department Use

Rajan Anthony Sonik, PhD, JD, MPH,[a] Alisha Coleman-Jensen, PhD,[b] Timothy B. Creedon, PhD,[c] Xinyu Yang, MPH[c]

OBJECTIVES: To examine whether Supplemental Nutrition Assistance Program (SNAP) participation is associated with emergency department use among low-income children and whether any such association is mediated by household food hardship and child health status and/or moderated by special health care needs (SHCN) status. We hypothesized SNAP to be associated with reduced likelihoods of emergency department use, with greater effect sizes for children with SHCN and mediation by food hardship and health status.

METHODS: In this secondary analysis, we estimated a bivariate probit model (with state-level SNAP administrative policies as instruments) within a structural equation modeling framework using pooled cross-sectional samples of children in low-income households from the 2016 to 2019 iterations of the National Survey of Children's Health ($n = 24\,990$).

RESULTS: Among children with and without SHCN, respectively, SNAP was associated with: 22.0 percentage points (pp) (95% confidence interval [CI] 12.2–31.8pp) and 17.1pp (95% CI 7.2–27.0pp) reductions in the likelihood of household food hardship exposure (4.8pp difference-in-differences, 95% CI 2.3–7.4pp), 9.7pp (95% CI 3.9–15.5pp) and 7.9pp (95% CI 2.2–13.6) increases in the likelihood of excellent health status (1.9pp difference-in-differences, 95% CI 0.7–3.0pp), and 7.7pp (95% CI 2.9–12.5pp) and 4.3pp (95% CI 1.0–7.6pp) reductions in the likelihood of emergency department use (3.4pp difference-in-differences, 95% CI 1.8–5.1pp).

CONCLUSIONS: We found SNAP participation was associated with lower likelihoods of emergency department use, that better food hardship and health statuses mediated this association, and that effect sizes were larger among children with SHCN. Food hardship relief may improve outcomes for vulnerable children and the health systems serving them.

[a]*AltaMed Institute for Health Equity, AltaMed Health Services, Los Angeles, California,* [b]*Economic Research Service, United States Department of Agriculture, Washington, District of Columbia; and* [c]*Health Equity Research Lab, Cambridge Health Alliance, Cambridge, Massachusetts*

Dr Sonik conceptualized and designed the study, coordinated and supervised the data analysis, interpreted the findings, drafted the initial manuscript, and reviewed and revised the manuscript; Dr Coleman-Jensen conceptualized and designed the study, reviewed the data analysis, interpreted the findings, and reviewed and revised the manuscript; Dr Creedon supervised and reviewed the data analysis, interpreted the findings, and reviewed and revised the manuscript; Ms Yang led the data analysis, interpreted the findings, and reviewed and revised the manuscript; and all authors approved the final manuscript as submitted and agree to be accountable for all aspects of the work.

DOI: https://doi.org/10.1542/peds.2022-058247

Accepted for publication Oct 26, 2022

Address correspondence to Rajan Anthony Sonik, AltaMed Institute for Health Equity, AltaMed Health Services Corporation, 2035 Camfield Ave, 3rd Floor, Los Angeles, CA 90040. E-mail: rsonik@altamed.org

PEDIATRICS (ISSN Numbers: Print, 0031-4005; Online, 1098-4275).

WHAT'S KNOWN ON THIS SUBJECT: The Supplemental Nutrition Assistance Program reduces food hardship, but associations with health and healthcare outcomes among children have received limited study. Potential relationships may differ for children with special health care needs, who have heightened social and health care complexity.

WHAT THIS STUDY ADDS: Supplemental Nutrition Assistance Program participation was associated with lower likelihoods of emergency department use. Moderation of this relationship by special health care needs status and mediation by food hardship and health status were also found.

To cite: Sonik RA, Coleman-Jensen A, Creedon TB, et al. SNAP Participation and Emergency Department Use. *Pediatrics.* 2023;151(2):e2022058247

ARTICLE

The Supplemental Nutrition Assistance Program (SNAP), formerly the Food Stamp Program, is the largest food hardship relief program in the United States, serving >25 million adults and nearly 15 million children.[1,2] SNAP has been found to reduce but not eliminate exposures to household food hardship. Broadly, food hardship is inadequate access to affordable, appropriate food, with 2 common measures being food insecurity and food insufficiency.[3] Among SNAP-eligible households, exposure to food hardship rises disproportionately for eventual participants before their initial participation (compared with eligible households never seeking benefits),[4,5] typically because of family, health, or employment shocks.[6,7] Exposure then falls disproportionately for participants after benefits begin,[4,5,8,9] albeit not fully to preshock levels.[10–14]

Even this partial relief, however, may yield discernible health and health care benefits. Associations of food hardship with poor health outcomes (from impaired development[15] and depression[16,17] to obesity,[18,19] poor sleep,[20] and iron deficiency[21]) and poor health care outcomes (from postponed preventive care and medication access[22–24] to increased emergency visits, inpatient care, and expenditures,[24–26] including worse health status and increased emergency visits among children[27]) have led to examinations into whether SNAP may address or prevent these harms. Among adults, several studies have associated SNAP with reduced inpatient use and expenditures,[28–31] particularly for people with chronic illnesses and disabilities.[28–30] Food hardship and health outcomes are hypothesized to mediate relationships between SNAP and health care outcomes,[32] but this has not been examined directly.

Among children, some studies have associated SNAP participation with better health status.[33–35] The relationship between SNAP and health care utilization among children has received less study, however, apart from an association between SNAP and reduced emergency visits for childhood asthma[36] and another between emergency visits and the ends of monthly benefit cycles.[37] The potential for different levels of sensitivity to SNAP benefits among different populations of children has also remained unexplored. In this regard, children with special health care needs (SHCN), identified as those with heightened medical, educational, or therapeutic service needs due to any chronic condition expected to last for at least 1 year[38] (a service-need-based definition distinct from the more socially complex concept of disability) warrant attention given their prevalence (18.5% of US children),[39] medical complexity, and high exposures to material hardships generally[40] and food hardship specifically.[27,41]

To address these gaps, we aimed to examine whether (1) food hardship and health status mediated relationships between SNAP and emergency health care use among children and (2) whether SHCN status moderated any such relationships. We hypothesized that SNAP participation would be negatively associated with emergency health care use, that this relationship would be mediated through lower exposure to food hardship and an increased likelihood of having a positive health status, and that SHCN status would increase the magnitude of these associations.

METHODS

Among those eligible to participate, households with greater levels of food hardship disproportionately self-select into SNAP.[4,5] To attend to this bias, we estimated a bivariate probit model with instrumental variables.[5,9] To simultaneously estimate the hypothesized mediation and moderation relationships, we embedded this model within a structural equation modeling framework. We detail our data, measures, and approach in the sections below.

Data and Sample

We analyzed data from the 2016 to 2019 iterations of the National Survey of Children's Health (NSCH), a nationally representative sample of noninstitutionalized children in the United States aged 0 to 17.[42] These were the first iterations to include a food hardship measure. Children with SHCN and children aged 0 to 5 are oversampled in the survey, and weights are provided to allow for nationally representative estimates.[42] After previous studies assessing the associations between SNAP and food hardship, we limited our analytic sample to children living in households with income <150% of the federal poverty level to focus on families most likely to be eligible for SNAP benefits.[5,9] This resulted in a final unweighted sample of 24 990 children, 6644 with and 18 346 without SHCN.

Measures

The exposure of interest was a bivariate indicator of whether a household had any SNAP participation in the previous year. The mediators were household food hardship and parent-reported child health status. Exposure to household food hardship over the previous year was measured through a single-item food insufficiency question ("Which of these statements best describes your household's ability to afford the food you need during the past 12 months?") with 4 possible responses: (1) "We could always afford to eat good nutritious meals," (2) "We could always afford enough to eat but not always the kind of food we should eat," (3) "Sometimes we could not afford enough to eat"; or (4) "Often we could not afford enough to eat." Household food hardship was flagged as present if any of the latter 3 responses were chosen, given the associations between these responses and worse health and health care outcomes among children.[27] This definition incorporates marginal food sufficiency and food insufficiency,[3] and it is roughly equivalent to a measure incorporating both low and very low food security.[3]

The 5 potential parent-reported child health statuses were dichotomized as excellent versus very good, good, fair, or poor; this dichotomization has been found to be a more relevant predictor of unfavorable health care outcomes among children than adult groupings of excellent with very good and good.[27] SHCN status was the moderator of interest, defined in the validated NSCH instrument as having heightened health care needs in at least 1 of 5 areas due to an underlying condition expected to last for at least 1 year.[43] The ultimate outcome was any emergency health care utilization. This was indicated by either 1 or "2 or more" visits to a "hospital emergency room" in the previous year (vs no visits).

We adjusted for individual, parent/caregiver, household, and state-level covariates. These included the child's age in years, sex (male/female were the only options in the survey), and race/ethnicity (aggregated to non-Hispanic white, non-Hispanic Black, non-Hispanic other, or Hispanic), whether any parent/caregiver was employed and whether any had a high school degree, household income as a

percentage of the federal poverty level and whether there was a smoker in the household, and state-level unemployment, GDP, and income per capita.[9] Adjusting for state, year, and state-by-year variables did not significantly alter model findings (Supplemental Tables 4 and 5), so we did not include them in the final model for parsimony.

For instrumental variables, we follow previous studies[5,9,30] in using state-level SNAP policies tracked in the US Department of Agriculture Economic Research Service SNAP Policy Database.[44] Benefits are federally funded, but states control policies related to ease of benefits access and maintenance. These policies are significantly associated with program enrollment. We, therefore, used as instruments the 2 policies that had the strongest associations with SNAP participation in our sample without being directly associated with the mediators or ultimate outcome: whether a state uses broad-based categorical eligibility for SNAP (through which certain households are deemed eligible on the basis of qualifying for other social programs)[45] and the proportion of nonearning, nonelderly SNAP units that have 1- to 3-month recertification periods (ie, a high administrative burden for participants; a SNAP unit is an individual or group of people living together who participate in SNAP).[9]

Statistical Approach

We conducted bivariate comparisons of child, parent/caregiver, household, and state-level covariates, SNAP participation, household food hardship, excellent health status, and any emergency health care use by SHCN status. For our fully adjusted model, given the binary nature of our exposure and outcome variables and the presence of covariates, we used the instrumental variables discussed

above in the context of a bivariate probit model.[46] To assess the hypothesized mediation relationships, we estimated this model within a structural equation modeling frame in which household food hardship and health status mediated relationships between SNAP participation and emergency health care use. This involved modeling a latent variable for which SNAP participation and household food hardship were the measurement variables and the parameters for the relationships between this latent variable and each measurement variable were constrained to be equal to one another.[47] We modeled SNAP participation (and therefore the interaction of SNAP participation and SHCN status) as operating through household food hardship both on conceptual grounds (ie, SNAP is intended to reduce food hardships, and previous studies have revealed evidence for this effect[4,5,8–14]) and for parsimony. For interpretability, we calculated predicted probabilities (accounting for both direct and indirect relationships when relevant) on the basis of the results of our model.

Because of model complexity, incorporating survey weights proved computationally infeasible. To assess potential bias from excluding weights, we compared weighted and unweighted results from simpler versions of our model (ie, an unadjusted version and versions with varying subsets of our covariates). Parameters from each did not meaningfully differ. At most, parameters in weighted versions had marginally larger magnitudes, indicating a slight bias toward the null from using an unweighted full model. Another potential concern was that computational difficulties in weighted models were caused by significant correlations between instrumental variables and residuals in the bivariate probit portion of the

TABLE 1 Demographics of Sample Children With and Without SHCN

Demographic Variable[a]	Children With SHCN (n = 6644)	Children Without SHCN (n = 18 346)	Mean Difference (95% CI)	P
Age, mean (SD)	10.6 (4.5)	8.7 (5.3)	1.9 (1.8 to 2.0)	<.001
Female, n (%)	2789 (42.0)	9194 (50.1)	8.1 (6.7 to 9.5)	<.001
Race/ethnicity, n (%)				
Non-Hispanic white	3694 (55.6)	9310 (50.8)	4.9 (3.5 to 6.3)	<.001
Non-Hispanic Black	1073 (16.2)	2352 (12.8)	3.3 (2.4 to 4.3)	<.001
Non-Hispanic other	762 (11.5)	2661 (14.5)	−3.0 (−4.0 to −2.1)	<.001
Hispanic	1115 (16.8)	4023 (21.9)	−5.1 (−6.3 to −4.0)	<.001
Household income as % of federal poverty level, mean (SD)	87.9 (33.3)	90.1 (33.7)	−2.3 (−3.2 to −1.3)	<.001
Smoker in household, n (%)	2014 (30.9)	4085 (22.9)	8.0 (6.8 to 9.3)	<.001
≥1 caregiver employed, n (%)	4383 (75.6)	14 109 (81.7)	−11.7 (−12.9 to −10.5)	<.001
≥1 caregiver with high school degree, n (%)	6025 (93.5)	16 357 (92.2)	1.2 (0.5 to 2.0)	.001

SD, standard deviation.

[a] Sample included children in households with income <150% of the federal poverty level aged 0 to 17 in the National Survey of Children's Health.

model because weights could theoretically magnify these correlations and cause the model to not converge. However, we assessed this possibility and found no significant correlations that could lead to such an issue. Relying on these checks, our data conformed with scenarios in which previous analyses have suggested that unweighted models can be used without a significant risk of bias,[48] and we, thus, proceeded with an unweighted final model. As such, for consistency, we also provide unweighted bivariate comparisons, which also did not qualitatively differ from weighted ones. Stata (Version 16) was used for all estimations.

RESULTS

Child, household, and parent/caregiver characteristics for our analytic sample are provided in Table 1. Compared with children without SHCN, children with SHCN were more likely to live in a household with someone who smokes cigarettes and have no employed parent or caregiver, despite being more likely to have at least 1 parent/caregiver with at least a high school level of education. Children with SHCN were also more likely to be in a household that participated in SNAP, be in a household that experienced food hardship, have less than excellent health status, and have had at least 1 emergency department visit in the past year (Table 2).

We present results from our final model graphically in Figure 1 (full model results provided in Supplemental Table 4). We provide adjusted predicted probabilities of each outcome variable (household food hardship, excellent child health status, and any child visit to a hospital emergency department) based on these results in Table 3. SHCN status was associated with a greater likelihood of experiencing household food hardship, nonexcellent health status, and at least 1 emergency department visit in the past year. Conversely, for all children, SNAP participation was associated with a lower likelihood of experiencing household food hardship, nonexcellent health status, and at least 1 emergency department visit in the past year. The magnitude of the associations between SNAP and each outcome was larger for children with versus without SHCN: 29% larger for household food hardship (−22.0 percentage points [pp] vs −17.1pp), 23% larger for excellent health status (+9.7pp vs +7.9pp), and 79% larger for visits to a hospital emergency department (−7.7pp vs −4.3pp; Table 3).

DISCUSSION

We found that household SNAP participation was associated with a lower likelihood of emergency health care use among children, that this relationship was mediated by a lower likelihood of household food hardship and a higher likelihood of excellent parent-reported child health status, and that the magnitude of these associations was larger among children with SHCN.

TABLE 2 SNAP Participation and Outcome Measures Among Sample Children With and Without SHCN

Variable[a]	Children With SHCN (n = 6644)	Children Without SHCN (n = 18 346)	Mean Difference (95% CI)	P
Household SNAP participation, n (%)	3198 (49.8)	6728 (38.2)	11.5 (10.1 to 12.9)	<.001
Household food hardship, n (%)	4083 (63.2)	8597 (48.6)	14.6 (13.2 to 16.0)	<.001
Excellent child health status, n (%)	1906 (28.8)	12 115 (66.3)	−37.5 (−38.8 to −36.1)	<.001
Any child visit to a hospital emergency department, n (%)	2354 (35.7)	3934 (21.6)	14.1 (12.8 to 15.3)	<.001

[a] Sample included children in households with income <150% of the federal poverty level aged 0 to 17 in the National Survey of Children's Health.

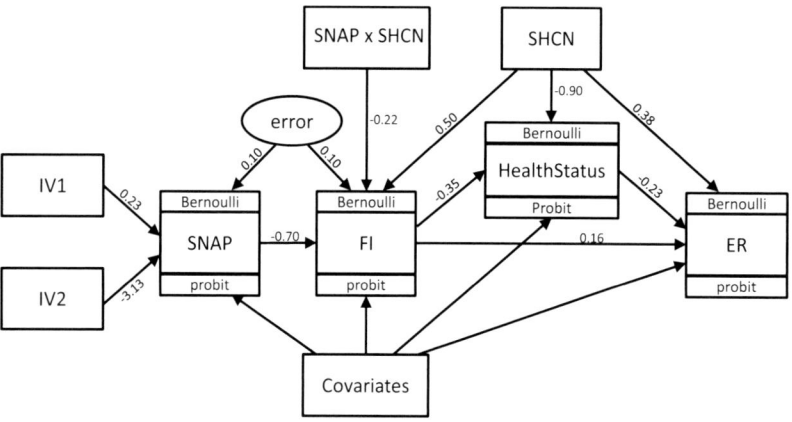

FIGURE 1
Structural equation model with key coefficients.
IV1, instrumental variable 1 (broad-based categorical eligibility); IV2, instrumental variable 2 (1- to 3-month recertification periods); SNAP, Supplemental Nutrition Assistance Program participation; FI, household food hardship (measured using a household food insufficiency question); SHCN, special health care needs status; ER, any child visit to a hospital emergency room.
Covariates included the child's age in years, sex, and race/ethnicity, whether any parent/caregiver was employed and whether any had a high school degree, household income as a percentage of the federal poverty level and whether there was a smoker in the household, and state-level unemployment, GDP, and income per capita; observed variables are represented in rectangles and the latent variable used to model the bivariate probit model within the structural equation modelling frame is represented in an oval.

The association of SNAP with a 31% reduction in the likelihood of experiencing household food hardship in the overall sample (an 18.3pp reduction from 59.7%) was similar to associations of SNAP with 31%[5] and 38%[9] reductions in the likelihood of household food hardship found in previous studies using similar methods (as measured by having either low or very low food security, a measure roughly equivalent to our measure of having either marginal food sufficiency or food insufficiency[3,49]).

This suggests that our use of the single-item food insufficiency measure available in the NSCH, although not offering as much nuance as lengthier food insecurity tools,[3] was unlikely to have altered our main findings. However, exploring the effects of using different food hardship measures may offer additional insights. For example, among all SNAP-participating households (not only those including children), Ratcliffe and colleagues[5] found that SNAP was associated with a smaller reduction in the likelihood of more severe food security compared with food insecurity generally, indicating that more extreme food hardship experiences may be less elastic than milder ones. Future studies with additional food hardship measures may allow even richer assessments of associations between SNAP participation and downstream health and health care outcomes than have been found to date,[50] especially for children.

Still, we find evidence for meaningful associations with these downstream measures within our data. The conceptual model for the relationship between food hardship and negative health care consequences proposes mechanisms through which cycles of hyper and hypoglycemia drive long-term chronic disease development and short-term exacerbations of these conditions,[32] the latter of which are likely applicable to children with chronic conditions even if not developed over long timeframes. If the associations in the present data have a causal component, then it is most likely that the shorter-term pathways dominate what we detected.

However, even if SNAP alleviates harmful cycles of deprivation and sustenance with regard to food, the structural factors driving food hardship disparities in the first place remain intact. For example, the flow from racism to disparities in housing, health care, education, and other facets of life,[51-53] and the resulting long-term patterns of embodied stressors that increase risks for chronic disease development, are unlikely to be unwound by SNAP alone (even if SNAP yields benefits unrelated to food through substitution effects[9]). This is consistent with findings that most SNAP applicants seek benefits after spikes in food hardship experiences, indicating it is sought to prevent additional rather than initial harms.[4-7] In addition, shorter-term pathways are likely especially dominant among children for whom chronic disease onset is typically less related to long-term factors than for adults. Still, the potential benefits of SNAP alleviating shorter-term exacerbations are significant. Each exacerbation or insult to health that is not prevented can contribute to significant long-term harm,[54,55] particularly for children.[56-58]

Our finding of larger effect sizes among children with SHCN is consistent with previous work suggesting that the health status of these children is especially sensitive to food hardship.[27] It also emphasizes the potential importance of the shorter-term pathways through which SNAP benefits may improve health. Given the heightened material

TABLE 3 Adjusted Predicted Probabilities of Outcomes by SNAP Participation and SHCN Status

Group			Household Food Hardship			Excellent Child Health Status			Any Child Visit to a Hospital Emergency Department		
SNAP	SHCN	n	Adjusted[a] Predicted Probability, % (95% CI)	Difference, pp (95% CI)	Difference in Difference, pp (95% CI)	Adjusted[a] Predicted Probability, % (95% CI)	Difference, pp (95% CI)	Difference in Difference, pp (95% CI)	Adjusted[a] Predicted Probability, % (95% CI)	Difference, pp (95% CI)	Difference in Difference, pp (95% CI)
No		14 096	59.7 (56.0 to 63.3)	—		51.7 (49.1 to 54.4)	—		28.9 (26.6 to 31.3)	—5.2[c] (−8.8 to −1.5)	—
Yes		9926	41.3 (35.1 to 47.5)	−18.3[d] (−28.1 to −8.6)		59.9 (56.8 to 62.9)	8.1[c] (2.6 to 13.7)		23.8 (22.3 to 25.3)		
	No	18 346	49.6 (48.9 to 50.4)			64.4 (63.4 to 65.3)			20.7 (19.8 to 21.6)	21.5[d] (19.9 to 23.1)	
	Yes	6644	59.5 (58.0 to 61.0)	9.8[d] (8.3 to 11.4)		29.2 (27.9 to 30.5)	−35.2[d] (−37.0 to −33.4)		42.2 (40.6 to 43.7)		
No	No	10 868	56.6 (52.6 to 60.6)	—		61.0 (57.9 to 64.1)	—		22.7 (20.4 to 24.9)	−4.3[b] (−7.6 to −1.0)	
Yes	No	6728	39.5 (33.5 to 45.5)	−17.1[c] (−27.0 to −7.2)		68.9 (66.1 to 71.6)	7.9[c] (2.2 to 13.6)		18.4 (17.0 to 19.7)		
No	Yes	3228	68.2 (65.1 to 71.4)	—		25.5 (23.5 to 27.5)	—		45.4 (42.4 to 48.5)	−7.7[c] (−12.5 to −2.9)	
Yes	Yes	3198	46.3 (39.3 to 53.2)	−22.0[d] (−31.8 to −12.2)	−4.8[d] (−7.4 to −2.3)	35.2 (30.8 to 39.5)	9.7[c] (3.9 to 15.5)	1.9[c] (0.7, 3.0)	37.7 (35.2 to 40.2)		−3.4[d] (−5.1 to −1.8)

[a] Based on a structural equation model adjusting for the child's age in years, sex, and race/ethnicity, whether any parent/caregiver was employed and whether any had a high school degree, household income as a percentage of the federal poverty level and whether there was a smoker in the household, and state-level unemployment, GDP, and income per capita.

[b] P < .05.

[c] P < .01.

[d] P < .001.

—, cells without a relevant difference or difference-in-difference to present.

hardships experienced by children with SHCN generally,[40] it was conceivable that the benefits of SNAP participation would be muted for this group as the damage done by other concurrent challenges lessoned its potential effects. That this was not observed suggests that the immediate relief provided by SNAP may be strong enough to yield health gains even in the face of other long-term harms.

LIMITATIONS

The current study has limitations. Although our modeling approach was designed to reduce bias caused by self-selection into SNAP and other potential confounding, the cross-sectional nature of our data still limits our ability to make causal inferences and rule out unmeasured sources of variation. Also, it is possible that parent-reported data could be imprecise, particularly for relatively subjective questions such as general health status. However, past research has revealed that parent-reported poor child health is associated with increased health care utilization,[59] a relatively more objective measure. We found the same association here, which serves to validate this child health status measure. The stigma associated with reporting poorly rated health status (as well as SHCN status, food hardship, and emergency health care) could produce bias, but stigma leading to underreporting of these conditions would have tended to bias our results toward the null. Additionally, our dichotomization of health status is generally a more conservative approach, and therefore more likely to lead to null results. However, we identified important relationships with this variable, which strengthens the study.

The simple measure of any SNAP participation over the past year limited the nuance of our analyses as well, although, again, the imprecision here would tend to bias results to the null. Relatedly, SNAP exists within an ecosystem of public benefit programs that are likely correlated. Although the instruments we chose were both significantly correlated with participation in SNAP but not with participation 3 other programs measured in the data (the Special Supplemental Nutrition Program for Women, Infants, and Children, Temporary Assistance for Needy Families, and the National School Lunch Program; Supplemental Table 6), the data did not ask about other programs, like child Supplemental Security Income, which may affect household food hardship as well.[60] Additionally, although food hardship is associated with leading causes[61] of pediatric emergency visits (eg, respiratory disorders,[36,62] injury,[63] mental health[64]), our inability to distinguish reasons for emergency health care visits prevented more nuanced analyses.

Our use of unweighted analyses also raises the specter of sampling error, nonresponse bias, and design effects; however, the fact that estimates did not differ between our weighted and unweighted versions of simpler versions of our model alleviates this concern. Additionally, concerns of overly tight standard errors in our final model were reduced given that the weighted models did not result in larger standard errors. Lastly, although we modeled multiple relationships, we ultimately measure an oversimplified version of reality. For example, the relationship between health status and emergency health care use is likely bidirectional. Future work with longitudinal data will likely be needed to further investigate such complexities.

CONCLUSIONS

We find evidence SNAP is associated with reduced food hardship, improved health status, and reduced emergency health care use among low-income children, with larger effects among children with SHCN. These relationships are important to weigh amid federal policy discussions determining SNAP benefit levels and state policy discussions determining the relative administrative ease or difficulty of SNAP access. They suggest access to SNAP may have additional benefits for children. These findings also suggest SNAP may have benefits beyond food hardship relief, through possible reductions in emergency health care use and associated healthcare spending. In addition, given the larger effects among children with SHCN, efforts to increase their access may be especially beneficial.

ACKNOWLEDGEMENTS

We thank Dr William Crown of Brandeis University for his thoughtful contributions to our approach to sensitivity analyses.

ABBREVIATIONS

CI: confidence interval
NSCH: National Survey of Children's Health
pp: percentage points
SHCN: special health care needs
SNAP: Supplemental Nutrition Assistance Program

FUNDING: This research was supported in part by a Cooperative Agreement with the US Department of Agriculture Economic Research Service, grant number R03HS026317 from the Agency for Healthcare Research and Quality, and grant number R01MD013837 from the National Institute on Minority Health and Health Disparities.

The funders had no role in the design and conduct of the study. The findings and conclusions in this publication are those of the authors and should not be construed to represent any official USDA, HHS, or US Government determination or policy.

CONFLICT OF INTEREST DISCLOSURES: The authors have indicated they have no potential conflicts of interest relevant to this article to disclose.

REFERENCES

1. Food and Nutrition Service. National level annual summary: SNAP tables. Available at: fns.usda.gov/pd/supplemental-nutrition-assistance-program-snap. Accessed November 10, 2022

2. King MD, Giefer KG; United States Census Bureau. Nearly a third of children who receive SNAP participate in two or more additional programs. Available at: https://www.census.gov/library/stories/2021/06/most-children-receiving-snap-get-at-least-one-other-social-safety-net-benefit.html. Accessed November 10, 2022

3. Coleman-Jensen A, Rabbitt MP, Hashad RN, et al; USDA Economic Research Service. Measurement. Available at: https://www.ers.usda.gov/topics/food-nutrition-assistance/food-security-in-the-u-s/measurement/. Accessed November 10, 2022

4. Nord M, Golla AM; US Department of Agriculture. Does SNAP decrease food insecurity: untangling the self-selection effect. Economic research report 85. Available at: https://www.ers.usda.gov/webdocs/publications/46295/10977_err85_1_.pdf?v=42317. Accessed November 10, 2022

5. Ratcliffe C, McKernan S-M, Zhang S. How much does the Supplemental Nutrition Assistance Program reduce food insecurity? *Am J Agric Econ.* 2011;93(4):1082–1098

6. Leete L, Bania N. The effect of income shocks on food insufficiency. *Rev Econ Househ.* 2010;8:505–526

7. Kim J, Shaefer HL. Are household food expenditures responsive to entry into the Supplemental Nutrition Assistance Program? *Soc Sci Q.* 2015;96(4): 1086–1102

8. Mabli J, Ohls J. Supplemental Nutrition Assistance Program participation is associated with an increase in household food security in a national evaluation. *J Nutr.* 2015;145(2):344–351

9. Shaefer HL, Gutierrez IA. The Supplemental Nutrition Assistance Program and material hardships among low-income households with children. *Soc Serv Rev.* 2013;87(4):753–779

10. Alaimo K, Briefel RR, Frongillo EA Jr, Olson CM. Food insufficiency exists in the United States: results from the third National Health and Nutrition Examination Survey (NHANES III). *Am J Public Health.* 1998;88(3):419–426

11. Cohen B, Ohls J, Andrews M, et al; US Food and Nutrition Service. Food stamp participants' food security and nutrient availability: final report. Available at: https://naldc.nal.usda.gov/catalog/46423. Accessed November 10, 2022

12. Jensen HH. Food insecurity and the Food Stamp Program. *Am J Agric Econ.* 2002;84(5):1215–1228

13. Ribar DC, Hamrick KS; USDA Economic Research Service. Dynamics of poverty and food sufficiency. Available at: https://www.ers.usda.gov/publications/pub-details/?pubid=46766. Accessed November 10, 2022

14. Wilde P, Nord M. The effect of Food Stamps on food security: a panel data approach. *Rev Agric Econ.* 2005;27(3): 425–432

15. Alaimo K, Olson CM, Frongillo EA Jr. Food insufficiency and American school-aged children's cognitive, academic, and psychosocial development. *Pediatrics.* 2001;108(1):44–53

16. Leung CW, Epel ES, Willett WC, et al. Household food insecurity is positively associated with depression among low-income supplemental nutrition assistance program participants and income-eligible nonparticipants. *J Nutr.* 2015;145(3):622–627

17. Whitaker RC, Phillips SM, Orzol SM. Food insecurity and the risks of depression and anxiety in mothers and behavior problems in their preschool-aged children. *Pediatrics.* 2006;118(3):e859–e868

18. Caspi CE, Tucker-Seeley RD, Adamkiewicz G, et al. Food hardship and obesity in a sample of low-income immigrants. *J Immigr Minor Health.* 2017;19(1): 130–137

19. Jones SJ, Frongillo EA. Food insecurity and subsequent weight gain in women. *Public Health Nutr.* 2007;10(2):145–151

20. Ding M, Keiley MK, Garza KB, et al. Food insecurity is associated with poor sleep outcomes among US adults. *J Nutr.* 2015;145(3):615–621

21. Park CY, Eicher-Miller HA. Iron deficiency is associated with food insecurity in pregnant females in the United States: National Health and Nutrition Examination Survey 1999-2010. *J Acad Nutr Diet.* 2014;114(12):1967–1973

22. Mayer VL, McDonough K, Seligman H, et al. Food insecurity, coping strategies and glucose control in low-income patients with diabetes. *Public Health Nutr.* 2016;19(6):1103–1111

23. Ma CT, Gee L, Kushel MB. Associations between housing instability and food insecurity with health care access in low-income children. *Ambul Pediatr.* 2008; 8(1):50–57

24. Kushel MB, Gupta R, Gee L, Haas JS. Housing instability and food insecurity as barriers to health care among low-income Americans. *J Gen Intern Med.* 2006;21(1):71–77

25. Tarasuk V, Cheng J, de Oliveira C, et al. Association between household food insecurity and annual health care costs. *CMAJ.* 2015;187(14):E429–E436

26. Berkowitz SA, Seligman HK, Meigs JB, Basu S. Food insecurity, healthcare utilization, and high cost: a longitudinal cohort study. *Am J Manag Care.* 2018; 24(9):399–404

27. Sonik RA, Coleman-Jensen A, Parish SL. Household food insufficiency, health status and emergency healthcare utilisation among children with and without special healthcare needs. *Public Health Nutr.* 2020;23(17):3204–3210

28. Sonik RA. Massachusetts inpatient Medicaid cost response to increased Supplemental Nutrition Assistance Program benefits. *Am J Public Health.* 2016; 106(3):443–448

29. Sonik RA, Parish SL, Mitra M. Inpatient Medicaid usage and expenditure patterns after changes in Supplemental Nutrition Assistance Program benefit levels. *Prev Chronic Dis.* 2018;15(E120): E120

30. Berkowitz SA, Seligman HK, Rigdon J, et al. Supplemental Nutrition Assistance Program (SNAP) participation and health care expenditures among low-income adults. *JAMA Intern Med.* 2017; 177(11):1642–1649

31. Samuel LJ, Szanton SL, Cahill R, et al. Does the Supplemental Nutrition Assistance Program affect hospital utilization among older adults? The case of Maryland. *Popul Health Manag.* 2018; 21(2):88–95

32. Seligman HK, Schillinger D. Hunger and socioeconomic disparities in chronic disease. *N Engl J Med.* 2010;363(1):6–9

33. Ettinger de Cuba SA, Bovell-Ammon AR, Cook JT, et al. SNAP, young children's health, and family food security and healthcare access. *Am J Prev Med.* 2019;57(4):525–532

34. Morrissey TW, Miller DP. Supplemental Nutrition Assistance Program participation improves children's health care use: an analysis of the American Recovery and Reinvestment Act's natural experiment. *Acad Pediatr.* 2020;20(6): 863–870

35. Bitler MP, Seifoddini A. Health impacts of food assistance: evidence from the United States. *Annu Rev Resour Econ.* 2019;11:261–287

36. Heflin C, Arteaga I, Hodges L, et al. SNAP benefits and childhood asthma. *Soc Sci Med.* 2019;220:203–211

37. Cotti CD, Gordanier JM, Ozturk OD. Hunger pains? SNAP timing and emergency room visits. *J Health Econ.* 2020;71: 102313

38. McPherson M, Arango P, Fox H, et al. A new definition of children with special health care needs. *Pediatrics.* 1998; 102(1 Pt 1):137–140

39. Maternal and Child Health Bureau, Health Resources and Services Administration. Children with special health care needs: NSCH data brief. Available at: https://mchb.hrsa.gov/sites/default/files/mchb/Data/NSCH/nsch-cshcn-data-brief.pdf. Accessed November 10, 2022

40. Parish SL, Rose RA, Grinstein-Weiss M, et al. Material hardship in U.S. families raising children with disabilities. *Except Child.* 2008;75(1):71–92

41. Rose-Jacobs R, Fiore JG, Ettinger de Cuba S, et al. Children with special health care needs, supplemental security income, and food insecurity. *J Dev Behav Pediatr.* 2016;37(2):140–147

42. United States Census Bureau, United States Department of Commerce. 2019 national survey of children's health. Available at: https://www2.census.gov/programs-surveys/nsch/technical-documentation/methodology/2019-NSCH-Methodology-Report.pdf. Accessed November 10, 2022

43. Bethell CD, Read D, Stein REK, et al. Identifying children with special health care needs: development and evaluation of a short screening instrument. *Ambul Pediatr.* 2002;2(1):38–48

44. Economic Research Service (ERS), U.S. Department of Agriculture (USDA). SNAP policy database, SNAP policy data sets. Available at: https://www.ers.usda.gov/data-products/snap-policy-data-sets/. Accessed November 10, 2022

45. Food and Nutrition Service, United States Department of Agriculture. Broad-based categorical eligibility (BBCE). Available at: https://www.fns.usda.gov/snap/broad-based-categorical-eligibility. Accessed November 10, 2022

46. Chiburis RC, Das J, Lokshin M. A practical comparison of the bivariate probit and linear IV estimators: World Bank policy research working paper no. WPS 5601. Available at: https://openknowledge.worldbank.org/bitstream/handle/10986/3368/WPS5601.pdf?sequence=1&isAllowed=y. Accessed November 10, 2022

47. Canette I; Stata. Using generalized structural equation models to fit customized models without programming, and taking advantage of new features of –margins–. Available at: https://www.stata.com/meeting/portugal15/abstracts/materials/portugal15_canette.pdf. Accessed November 10, 2022

48. Solon G, Haider SJ, Wooldridge JM. What are we weighting for? *J Hum Resour.* 2015;50(2):301–316

49. Scott RI, Wehler CA; University of Wisconsin Institute for Research on Poverty. Food insecurity/food insufficiency: an empirical examination of alternative measures of food problems in impoverished U.S. households: Institute for Research on Poverty discussion papers 1176–98. Available at: https://ideas.repec.org/p/wop/wispod/1176-98.html. Accessed November 10, 2022

50. Gregory CA, Deb P. Does SNAP improve your health? *Food Policy.* 2015;50:11–19

51. Bailey ZD, Feldman JM, Bassett MT. How structural racism works - racist policies as a root cause of U.S. racial health inequities. *N Engl J Med.* 2021;384(8):768–773

52. Egede LE, Walker RJ. Structural racism, social risk factors, and Covid-19 - a dangerous convergence for Black Americans. *N Engl J Med.* 2020;383(12):e77

53. Odoms-Young A, Bruce MA. Examining the impact of structural racism on food insecurity: implications for addressing racial/ethnic disparities. *Fam Community Health.* 2018;41(Suppl 2 Food Insecurity and Obesity):S3–S6

54. Margüello MS, Garrastazu R, Ruiz-Nuñez M, et al. Independent effect of prior exacerbation frequency and disease severity on the risk of future exacerbations of COPD: a retrospective cohort study. *NPJ Prim Care Respir Med.* 2016;26:16046

55. Sadatsafavi M, Xie H, Etminan M, Johnson K, FitzGerald JM; Canadian Respiratory Research Network. The association between previous and future severe exacerbations of chronic obstructive pulmonary disease: updating the literature using robust statistical methodology. *PLoS One.* 2018;13(1):e0191243

56. Forrest CB, Riley AW. Childhood origins of adult health: a basis for life-course health policy. *Health Aff (Millwood).* 2004;23(5):155–164

57. Halfon N, Hochstein M. Life course health development: an integrated framework for developing health, policy, and research. *Milbank Q.* 2002;80(3):433–479, iii

58. Halfon N, Larson K, Lu M, Tullis E, Russ S. Lifecourse health development: past, present and future. *Matern Child Health J.* 2014;18(2):344–365

59. O'Hara B, Caswell K; US Census Bureau. Health status, health insurance, and medical services utilization: 2010, current population reports P70-133. Available at: https://www2.census.gov/library/publications/2013/demo/p70-133.pdf. Accessed November 10, 2022

60. Sonik RA, Parish SL, Mitra M. Food insecurity patterns before and after initial receipt of Supplemental Security Income. *Public Health Nutr.* 2019;22(10):1909–1913

61. McDermott KW, Stocks C, Freeman WJ. *Overview of Pediatric Emergency Department Visits, 2015: Statistical Brief #242.* Rockville, MD: Healthcare Cost and Utilization Project, Agency for Healthcare Research and Quality; 2018

62. Mangini LD, Hayward MD, Dong YQ, Forman MR. Household food insecurity is associated with childhood asthma. *J Nutr.* 2015;145(12):2756–2764

63. Men F, Urquia ML, Tarasuk V. Examining the relationship between food insecurity and causes of injury in Canadian adults and adolescents. *BMC Public Health.* 2021;21(1):1557

64. Spencer AE, Baul TD, Sikov J, et al. The relationship between social risks and the mental health of school-age children in primary care. *Acad Pediatr.* 2020;20(2):208–215

Perspectives From Urban WIC-Eligible Caregivers to Improve Produce Access

Priyanka Joshi, MD,[a],* Brittany J. Van Remortel, MD, MPH,[b],* Danielle L. Cullen, MD, MPH, MSHP[a]

OBJECTIVES: The Farmer's Market Nutrition Program (FMNP) provides fresh, locally grown fruits and vegetables (FV) to eligible participants in the Special Supplemental Nutrition Program for Women, Infants, and Children (WIC). However, redemption of FMNP benefits remains low. This qualitative study explores facilitators and barriers to produce access and FMNP redemption for caregivers of WIC-eligible children in Philadelphia during the COVID-19 pandemic.

METHODS: We conducted semistructured phone interviews with caregivers between August and December 2020 to understand experiences with produce access and programming preferences to increase benefit redemption and produce consumption. We used content analysis with constant comparison with code interviews inductively and identified emerging themes through an iterative process.

RESULTS: Participants ($n = 30$) wanted their children to eat more produce but described barriers to produce access, including limited availability, higher cost, and limited time. The Supplemental Nutrition Assistance Program and WIC benefits improved the ability to purchase produce, but difficulties with electronic benefit transfer and pandemic-related office closures limited use of WIC benefits. Similarly, lack of convenient market locations and hours prohibited use of FMNP benefits. Caregivers described that an ideal food program would be delivery based, low cost, offer a variety of FV, and provide recipes and educational activities.

CONCLUSIONS: WIC-eligible caregivers want their children to eat more produce; however, they face multiple barriers in redeeming their benefits to access fresh produce. Delivery-based, low-cost produce programs may lead to increased produce access as well as benefit use. Future study is needed on feasibility and acceptability of produce delivery options among WIC-eligible families.

Divisions of *a*Emergency Medicine and *b*Oncology, The Children's Hospital of Philadelphia, Philadelphia, Pennsylvania

*Contributed equally as co-first authors

Dr Joshi conceptualized and designed the study, drafted the initial manuscript, designed the data collection instruments, collected data, carried out the initial analyses, and reviewed and revised the manuscript. Dr Van Remortel conceptualized and designed the study, designed the data collection instruments, collected data, carried out the initial analyses, and reviewed and revised the manuscript. Dr Cullen conceptualized and designed the study, supervised the design of the data collection instruments and data analysis, and reviewed and revised the manuscript. All authors approved the final manuscript as submitted and agree to be accountable for all aspects of the work.

DOI: https://doi.org/10.1542/peds.2022-058536

Accepted for publication Nov 8, 2022

Address correspondence to Priyanka Joshi, Division of Emergency Medicine, 3401 Civic Center Blvd, Philadelphia, PA 19104. E-mail: joship@chop.edu.

PEDIATRICS (ISSN Numbers: Print, 0031-4005; Online, 1098-4275).

WHAT'S KNOWN ON THIS SUBJECT: Rates of fruit and vegetable consumption are particularly poor among children from low-income families. Public assistance programs help improve produce access and increase food security among low-income populations. However, many of these programs go underused, including the Special Supplemental Nutrition Program for Women, Infants, and Children's Farmer's Market Nutrition Program.

WHAT THIS STUDY ADDS: Little is known about contributors to low Farmer's Market Nutrition Program redemption and experiences with produce access among Special Supplemental Nutrition Program for Women, Infants, and Children participants. Our study provides actionable feedback from caregivers on barriers to use of benefits and how to optimize benefit use and increase produce access.

To cite: Joshi P, Van Remortel BJ, Cullen DL. Perspectives From Urban WIC-Eligible Caregivers to Improve Produce Access. *Pediatrics.* 2023;151(2):e2022058536

ARTICLE

The majority of children in the United States have insufficient intake of fruits and vegetables (FV), contributing to lifelong dietary patterns and poorer health outcomes.[1-5] From 2007 to 2010, only 40% of children aged 1 to 18 years met US Department of Agriculture recommendations for daily fruit intake and a mere 7% met recommendations for daily vegetable intake.[1] Eating patterns developed in childhood carry into adulthood and impact long-term health, underscoring the importance of early development of healthy eating behaviors.[6-10]

Low intake of FV can be a sequela of food insecurity (FI)—the disruption of food intake or eating patterns because of lack of money and other resources—disproportionally affecting African American and Hispanic populations and contributing to the increasing incidence of obesity and chronic disease among children in these populations.[10-17] FI affected nearly 22% of children in Philadelphia in 2019, and rates worsened during the COVID-19 pandemic, with more than 40% of mothers with children younger than age 12 years reporting FI in April 2020.[15,18]

Public assistance programs, such as the Special Supplemental Nutrition Program for Women, Infants, and Children (WIC), improve produce access and increase food security among low-income populations.[19] African Americans and Hispanics account for more than one-half of all WIC participants, so programmatic changes in WIC have the potential to improve racial/ethnic disparities in both diet and obesity.[16,17] However, these programs are often underused, with only 51% of those eligible in the United States participating in WIC in 2017.[20] Further, only one-half of those who participate in WIC redeem Farmer's Market Nutrition Program

(FMNP) vouchers, which provide additional funds to purchase produce from farmer's markets.[21-23] Redemption of FMNP vouchers is associated with higher FV intake; however, participation varies across states.[24-26] In Philadelphia, FMNP voucher redemption has been far below the national average of 55%; redemption rates were 26% in 2018 and plummeted to 17.5% in 2020 during the COVID-19 pandemic (Bureau of Food Assistance, Pennsylvania Department of Agriculture, unpublished data; 2018).[23]

Little is known about contributors to low FMNP redemption and experiences with produce access among WIC participants, particularly during the COVID-19 pandemic. This qualitative study, conducted in partnership with the Philadelphia WIC program (N.O.R.T.H. Inc.), sought to explore facilitators and barriers to (1) intake of FV among WIC-eligible families, (2) use of available food benefits, specifically the FMNP, and (3) understand caregiver preferences for programs aimed at increasing produce consumption. Through direct community feedback, we aimed to elucidate actionable steps to improve produce access and food benefit use among WIC-eligible families as well as inform future programming and policies.

METHODS

Study Design and Participant Recruitment

Recruitment occurred at an urban primary care clinic located in West Philadelphia serving about 14 000 children annually, of which 75% are publicly insured and approximately 27% are WIC eligible (P.J., T.G., personal communication, 2022). Among clinic patients, 88% of patients identify as African American, 4% as Latino, and 3% as

non–English speaking (P.J., T.G., personal communication, 2022). Eligible caregivers were recruited by 2 study team members (P.J. and B.J.V.) via 2 methods. Between December 2019 and February 2020, participants were recruited via telephone from a list of families who initially completed surveys in the clinic waiting room to gauge interest in a mobile WIC office and who consented to future contact. Subsequently, because of pandemic-related changes in office practices, electronic medical records were queried to identify families that received a WIC letter between January 2020 and July 2020, and eligible caregivers were recruited via phone. Participants were assessed for study eligibility at the time of the initial recruitment call. To participate in the study, caregivers had to be >18 years, live in Philadelphia, speak English, and have a WIC-eligible child younger than age 5 years who received care at the previously mentioned clinic. Although all participants were asked about FMNP use, redemption of FMNP benefits was not a requirement for study participation.

Data Collection

A semistructured interview guide was developed from literature review and expert opinion.[27] Interview questions were grouped into general categories including family's current and ideal produce intake, facilitators and barriers to produce access, use of food benefits and local food programs, and perceived characteristics of an ideal program to increase produce access. The interview guide was reviewed and modified through an iterative process after the first 2 interviews were conducted. Interviews were performed via telephone by 2 study team members (P.J. and B.J.V.) between August and December 2020 after verbal consent was obtained; the study team members received training in interview techniques and qualitative analysis from a researcher (D.L.C.) with expertise in qualitative research methods. P.J. is a South Asian American female, native English and Hindi and proficient Spanish speaker, and childless. B.J.V. is a white American female, native English speaker, and childless. Both P.J. and B.J.V. were providers at the previously mentioned clinic. Each interview lasted 30 minutes on average. Participants were provided a $25 gift card as compensation for their time. Demographics including sex, race, ethnicity, insurance coverage, and body mass index were abstracted from the electronic medical record for the WIC-eligible child. Caregivers were asked to identify the total number of children and the number of WIC-eligible children in their household and were screened for FI using the 2-question validated Hunger Vital screening tool.[28] All study procedures were deemed exempt from ongoing review by the Children's Hospital of Philadelphia institutional review board.

Analysis

Interviews were digitally recorded and deidentified as transcribed verbatim. Transcripts were entered into NVivo 12 Software (QRS International) for organization, coding, and data analysis. The initial coding dictionary was established based on questions in the interview guide. We used content analysis with constant comparison with code interviews inductively and deductively to identify emerging themes.

Two study team members (P.J. and B.J.V.) coded the first 2 transcribed interviews and met to examine interrater reliability, resolve coding disagreements by consensus, and revise code definitions. The revised coding dictionary was then used for the next 3 interviews, after which team members again resolved coding disagreements and finalized code definitions. The remaining 25 interviews were coded separately, with 8 additional interviews double coded at set intervals to ensure that interrater reliability remained stable over time with $\kappa > 0.8$ at each assessment. Coded transcript sections were reviewed to uncover emerging subthemes and direct quotations were chosen to exemplify these themes. Interviews were conducted until thematic saturation was reached (Table 1).

RESULTS

Caregiver Demographics

Of the 200 eligible caregivers, 89 were contacted up to 3 times by phone for recruitment on a rolling basis. Of those contacted, 4 (5%) declined to participate, 50 (56%) were unable to be reached, and 5 (6%) phone numbers were disconnected or invalid. Our sample of 30 caregivers was primarily female ($n = 29$) and had an average of 3 children per household (Table 2). Fifty-seven percent of participants screened positive for FI.

Facilitators and Barriers to Intake of Fruits and Vegetables

Major Barriers to Produce Access Include Limited Availability, Higher Cost, and Lack of Childcare

Many caregivers described limited produce options in their neighborhood and shared that available produce is of lower quality than that offered in more affluent areas. Because of this, many reported the need to travel to other neighborhoods to purchase FV. Additionally, time constraints and higher cost of produce relative to other foods in the setting of competing financial priorities were significant factors affecting access for many caregivers. Some expressed that junk food and fast food were more affordable and convenient than fresh produce. One caregiver described, "…the burger is 99 cents. The salad is like $5.49. Which are you going to choose if you're low income? You're going to choose the burger for your kids. And then they wonder why kids are so obese. They're obese because they can't afford to give them the right FV that they need" [Participant 8].

Difficulty finding childcare was reported as a barrier to being able to go to the store or market by many caregivers. Caregivers also noted that traveling and shopping with young children created challenges to obtaining produce. Many caregivers reported worsening of barriers to produce access during the COVID-19 pandemic given produce shortages, increased food prices, childcare center closures, and decreased income sources.

Reliable Transportation and Federal Benefit Programs are Facilitators to Produce Access

Some caregivers shared that having a car makes it easier to obtain produce because it provides reliable transportation and allows them to travel to stores with their preferred produce. One caregiver reported, "I drive so it's not like me getting there or getting back was a problem…If I didn't have transportation, then it would be a different story for me to be able to go get produce" [Participant 2]. Caregivers expressed that enrollment in both WIC and Supplemental Nutrition Assistance Program (SNAP) increased produce access by allowing them to use limited funds toward other essential purchases such as diapers and medical bills. Some caregivers felt that SNAP benefits were overall more helpful than WIC benefits given the amount of funds provided, reliability of the system, and increased options for use of benefits.

TABLE 1 Interview Themes With Representative Quotes From Participating WIC-Eligible Caregivers

Topic	Themes	Illustrative Quotes [Participant No.]
Facilitators and barriers to intake of fruits and vegetables	Major barriers to produce access include limited availability, higher cost, and lack of childcare	"When you want good produce sometimes you got to travel a little bit and I don't think that should be the case." [9] ".. it's either gone or they don't look too good so you've got to drive far out and I'm a person that doesn't drive on the highway. So the only thing is that you have to drive out farther than what's in your community." [21] "I wish I could buy more. It seems like it's the same amount of money for less." [30] "When you have little kids, it's hard especially if you're not driving." [26] "I don't have anybody nearby to watch them for me, so it was hard for me to get to the store." [28] "I don't have that much time. That's a big problem, the fact that I can only go to one [store]. That might be the one that's the closest." [181] "I'm more so time, I need time. Everything is just so constant moving with me in my life right now." [2]
	Reliable transportation and federal benefit programs are facilitators to produce access	" ... It's a big issue because sometimes SEPTA get broken down and stuff like that. It's really irritating ... " [19] "It's very helpful, especially when you're basically the only provider for your baby. It's very helpful because it's like, even though you work, that money still has to go towards other things like bills or clothing, diapers, things like that. SNAP and WIC definitely helps out a lot."[14] "I've been relying on the food stamps to get fruits and vegetables... I don't have to worry about them cutting it off...They're always there every month... It's been a very, a very big impact. Like, it was like, we needed it. We eat more because we got food stamps." [15]
Barriers to use of WIC and the FMNP	The transition to electronic benefit transfer in the setting of pandemic-driven WIC office closures has made accessing benefits challenging	"One thing I would say, the access to WIC. Now, they switched their whole system. You can't just get your card reloaded in person. You have to drop it off in a dropbox, wait for them to mail it back. One time I waited 3 weeks for the card to come and I had to go out of my pocket and get the milk. That access has been a little weird now because of COVID." [11] "...they've been closed and they've been canceling appointments. And we haven't got any emails or any calls or anything about them reopening or anything." [10]
	Caregivers are aware of the FMNP but are unable to regularly access farmer's markets	"Well, I had gotten it, but I haven't had a chance to go to the farmer's market. I know that it's basically fresher, I should say, foods that they have there. I just have not had a chance to go to it." [26] "I use[d] it before, but a lot of times those checks don't fit, to be honest. I'm just being honest because the same thing with the time, with the time and the location." [20]

TABLE 1 Continued

Topic	Themes	Illustrative Quotes [Participant No.]
Family level preferences for programs aimed at increasing produce consumption	Caregivers want their children to eat more fruits and vegetables	"I feel like she could eat more, but she's very picky in general. It's hard to pretty much try to get her to eat a lot more vegetables." [25] "I wish they'd do better on the fruit than snacks but I wish it was a little more. Every time they want a snack, I wish they'd grab a fruit instead of a bag of chips." [21] "I would like for him to eat more of a variety of fruits and vegetables." [10]
	An ideal food program would be delivery-based, low or no cost, and provide supplemental resources about produce	"It would be like a care package, including a variety of different fruits and vegetables and it would be like delivered to the home to make it more accessible...more easy to obtain." [26] "I would try like different things. There would be days that I would offer them normal fruits and vegetables, but I also would have like different things that I would offer like exotic fruits and vegetables. Things that are from like different countries and things that they would like to try, maybe they would maybe be interested in or trying different things to cook with..." [3] "What I think is really great to have inside of a box is the fresh string beans and the fresh broccoli and introduce some things the kids that like... Introduce some fruits to families that they don't know about..." [8] "I think it should completely be covered by WIC or SNAP." [3] "I would want to pick it out myself with your family. It could be a learning experience. A lot of kids don't know the different fruits and vegetables. They don't know what's a fruit, what's a vegetable ... Get to know your fruits and vegetables that you're going to eat." [22] "Recipes would probably be good for people so they could broaden their horizons and have other different ways of making foods and stuff. That might be helpful because when I see stuff like that, I actually read it." [20] "A list or something like that, or a booklet to show you how to make it and different ways you could put fruits and vegetables and the kids' who said they won't know it or have fun food maybe for the kids that try to eat." [6]

Barriers to Use of WIC and the FMNP

The Transition to Electronic Benefit Transfer in the Setting of Pandemic-Driven WIC Office Closures Made Accessing Benefits Challenging

At the time when interviews were conducted (August–December 2020), WIC benefits were available on electronic benefit transfer (EBT) cards but had to be manually reloaded by WIC staff in person or by mail every 3 to 4 months. Many caregivers described challenges with the overall transition to EBT, including fear of misplacing their card, with subsequent loss of benefits while awaiting replacement, as well as unfamiliarity with the process.

Most caregivers commented that WIC office closures during the pandemic created significant barriers to accessing benefits, given difficulty communicating with WIC staff and reliance on postal mail for reloading. One caregiver shared her experience: "I just stopped going ... because they want me to drop off the card, come pick up the card ... I don't have the time with the

TABLE 2 Sociodemographic Characteristics of Study Participants and Their Primary WIC-Eligible Child

	Participants/Caregivers n = 30
Caregiver sex, n (%)	
Female	29 (97)
Male	1 (3)
Household characteristics	
Median number of children (IQR)	3 (1–4)
Median number of WIC-eligible children (IQR)	1 (1–2)
Mean age of children, y (SD)	5.3 (3.6)
Mean age of WIC-eligible children, y (SD)	1.8 (1.1)
Characteristics of WIC-eligible child	
Sex	
Female	13 (43)
Male	17 (57)
Race	
Black or African American	24 (80)
White	1 (3)
Asian	1 (3)
Other	2 (7)
Multiracial	2 (7)
Ethnicity	
Not Hispanic or Latinx	29 (97)
Hispanic or Latinx	1 (3)
Insurance coverage	
Public	28 (93)
Private	2 (7)
Weight for length/BMI percentile, mean (SD)	50.4 (40)
Caregiver-reported food insecurity	
Yes	17 (57)
No	11 (37)
Not reported	2 (7)

BMI, body mass index; IQR, interquartile range; SD, standard deviation.

hours that they give me … Then they want to mail it back to me instead of me just being [able] to …load the benefits" [Participant 20].

Caregivers Are Aware of the FMNP but are Unable to Regularly Access Farmer's Markets

FMNP voucher amounts and eligibility vary by state.[22] In Pennsylvania, pregnant, breastfeeding, and postpartum women, and children ages 6 months to 5 years who participate in WIC are eligible to receive $24 (4 checks of $6 each).[29,30] Vouchers are provided during WIC appointments in the spring and summer for redemption between June 1 and November 30.[29,30] During the COVID-19 pandemic, vouchers were mailed to participants' homes because of office closures. Most caregivers described that they were aware of FMNP, but it was challenging to access the markets. Caregivers described that the markets were located far from them and required access to a car. Furthermore, parking costs and limited market hours were prohibitive to using them regularly. One caregiver commented, "At least having one in the city instead of so far away where people have to pay more money to get to …and then we got to end up paying for parking. There's a lot that goes with it" [Participant 29]. Several caregivers described that they would like to use their FMNP benefits to purchase produce in grocery stores rather than at farmer's markets alone. Finally, some felt that the amount provided by the vouchers was too low.

Family Level Preferences for Programs Aimed at Increasing Produce Consumption

Caregivers Want Their Children to Eat More FV

Most caregivers expressed a desire for their children to eat more produce, regardless of their children's current level of FV intake. One caregiver shared, "I don't want my kids to get stuck on junk food and candy … I want them to be able to have FV in their system" [Participant 19]. Some children were described as "picky"; however, several caregivers reported that they tried to encourage produce consumption through modeling and regularly offering a variety of FV.

An Ideal Food Program Would Be Delivery-Based, Low or No Cost, and Provide Supplemental Resources About Produce

When asked to describe an ideal food program aimed at increasing produce access, most caregivers highlighted the need for a delivery-based program to address barriers to grocery shopping. One caregiver stated, "For a lot of people, delivery would be better. Because sometimes it's hard for a lot of low-income people to travel … [delivery] would help a lot of families" [Participant 25]. However, some described that it may be better to offer a pickup option to allow for produce self-selection and further engagement for children by learning about different types of FV.

Regarding cost, most participants felt the produce should be free or covered by benefits. However, some did suggest use of a sliding scale or donation system with a small fee of $5 to $20 for those who can afford it. One described, "It all depends on the income and if they don't get that much, they shouldn't have to pay that much" [Participant 17].

Caregivers highlighted that offering a wide variety of FV could help expose families to new produce options. There were mixed opinions about who should select the produce. Some participants felt it was fine to receive a preselected mix of produce and others preferred that families pick out the produce because of cultural, taste, and dietary preferences. Most caregivers also highlighted the importance of engaging children with produce through age-appropriate activities and educating caregivers by providing recipes and cooking classes.

DISCUSSION

Federal food programs, such as WIC, play a key role in improving nutrition among low-income families. However, WIC benefits are significantly underused, and the COVID-19 pandemic created additional barriers in accessing these benefits because of office closures, communication barriers, and mail delays.[20,31,32] Our study adds key insights to the literature by exploring experiences with produce access among WIC-eligible families during the COVID-19 pandemic. Additionally, we describe caregiver preferences for food assistance programs that can help inform future programming aimed at increasing WIC use and produce access.

We identified barriers to produce access for WIC-eligible participants, many of which were consistent with earlier literature.[33–37] Major barriers included limited availability, lack of convenient purchasing options, higher relative cost, difficulty shopping with young children, and time constraints. Because Pennsylvania selected offline EBT benefit reloading, participants also described challenges with the transition to EBT in the setting of the COVID-19 pandemic and inability to reload benefits electronically.[38–40] Challenges exacerbated by the COVID-19 pandemic included worsened produce shortages, lack of childcare, and decreased access to WIC benefits because of office closures. Consistent with previous literature, owning a vehicle and receiving both SNAP and WIC benefits were described as facilitators to purchasing produce.[41]

Participants described that an ideal food program would include an option for delivery, a wide variety of FV, and provision of recipes and produce-oriented children's activities. Previous studies that piloted online ordering and home delivery demonstrate high acceptability among WIC-eligible participants.[39,42–44] Additionally, participants suggested that a program would be most helpful if free or covered by benefits. Based on our findings, expansion of delivery-based grocery options that are covered wholly or partially by WIC benefits is an ideal next step in facilitating access to fresh produce and addressing FI among WIC-eligible families.[45,46] Delivery-based services are especially needed during emergencies such as the COVID-19 pandemic because they promote social distancing and allow participation by families with young children who face additional barriers to grocery shopping. There is also an opportunity to engage children through education initiatives paired with produce delivery and affect children's food preferences for FV as they grow into adolescence and adulthood.

A major strength of our study is the focus on obtaining direct, actionable feedback from WIC-eligible caregivers on barriers to use of benefits and how to optimize benefit use to increase produce access. Rather than assuming participant needs and desires, our study allows the voice of the community to drive future intervention and policy change. In addition, this is among the first studies to describe barriers to use of FMNP vouchers during the COVID-19 pandemic. Despite these strengths, our study has several limitations. The generalizability of our findings may be limited as our participants were drawn from English-speaking WIC-eligible caregivers in West Philadelphia. Although rates of WIC participation in Philadelphia (48.4%) were similar to statewide (52.7%) rates in early 2021, most WIC participants in Philadelphia identified as African American (52%), whereas statewide they identified as white (71%).[47] Additionally, although WIC is a national program, it is administered at the state level, leading to variation in operations across states.[48,49] Our findings may be particularly applicable to states that have selected offline WIC benefit reloading and to other metropolitan areas, which account for 85% of households experiencing FI nationally.[40,50] Because of resource limitations, non–English-speaking families were excluded from our study. Given the interview-based nature of our study and potential sensitivity of questions, participant answers may have been affected by social desirability bias, although the interviewers encouraged honesty, refrained from judgment, and took measures to preserve participant anonymity.

Concurrent timing with the WIC EBT transition and the COVID-19 pandemic is both a strength and limitation of our study. This allowed for discovery of key insights that can help optimize the payment transition and address food access during a national emergency. However, participants may have difficulty separating their experiences with WIC during COVID-19 from those before, despite specific prompts on relevant timeframe to consider for each question.

CONCLUSIONS

Our study demonstrates a desire for better access to fresh produce among WIC-eligible families and highlights multiple barriers, which have been worsened by the COVID-19 pandemic. Caregivers described a preference for delivery-based, low-cost food programs covered by federal benefits, with inclusion of recipes and children's activities to increase produce intake among children. Informed by caregiver preferences for food programs identified in this qualitative study, we partnered with local community organizations to create a low-cost produce delivery program. Future study will evaluate the effect of price on participation in a produce delivery program for WIC-eligible families as well as the program's impact on produce consumption. Future larger scale studies on acceptability, feasibility, and effectiveness of produce delivery options to increase produce access and use of benefits among WIC-eligible families are needed to inform federal food benefit programs and improve long-term health among this population.

ACKNOWLEDGMENTS

We thank all the caregivers who shared their time and voices with us. We also thank the staff at N.O.R.T.H. Inc. of the Philadelphia WIC Program and at the Children's Hospital of Philadelphia Care Network - Cobbs Creek for their ongoing efforts in serving the children of Philadelphia. We also thank Dr. Cynthia Mollen who provided thoughtful feedback on our manuscript.

ABBREVIATIONS

FI: food insecurity
EBT: electronic benefit transfer
FMNP: Farmers' Market Nutrition Program
FV: fruits and vegetables
SNAP: Supplemental Nutrition Assistance Program
WIC: Special Supplemental Nutrition Program for Women, Infants, and Children

FUNDING: This project was supported by the Community Access to Child Health resident grant program through the American Academy of Pediatrics.

CONFLICT OF INTEREST DISCLOSURES: The authors have indicated they have no potential conflicts of interest to disclose.

REFERENCES

1. National Cancer Institute. Usual dietary intakes: food intakes, U.S. population, 2007–10. Available at: https://epi.grants.cancer.gov/diet/usualintakes/national-data-usual-dietary-intakes-2007-to-2010.pdf. Accessed November 21, 2022

2. Kim SA, Moore LV, Galuska D, et al; Division of Nutrition, Physical Activity, and Obesity, National Center for Chronic Disease Prevention and Health Promotion, CDC. Vital signs: fruit and vegetable intake among children - United States, 2003-2010. *MMWR Morb Mortal Wkly Rep.* 2014; 63(31):671–676

3. Liberali R, Kupek E, Assis MAA. Dietary patterns and childhood obesity risk: a systematic review. *Child Obes.* 2020; 16(2):70–85

4. Lock K, Pomerleau J, Causer L, Altmann DR, McKee M. The global burden of disease attributable to low consumption of fruit and vegetables: implications for the global strategy on diet. *Bull World Health Organ.* 2005;83(2):100–108

5. World Health Organization. Global Status Report on Non Communicable Diseases 2010. Available at: https://apps.who.int/iris/handle/10665/44579. Accessed December 8, 2022

6. Craigie AM, Lake AA, Kelly SA, Adamson AJ, Mathers JC. Tracking of obesity-related behaviours from childhood to adulthood: a systematic review. *Maturitas.* 2011;70(3):266–284

7. Larson N, Laska MN, Story M, Neumark-Sztainer D. Predictors of fruit and vegetable intake in young adulthood. *J Acad Nutr Diet.* 2012; 112(8):1216–1222

8. Maynard M, Gunnell D, Emmett P, Frankel S, Davey Smith G. Fruit, vegetables, and antioxidants in childhood and risk of adult cancer: the Boyd Orr cohort. *J Epidemiol Community Health.* 2003;57(3):218–225

9. Ness AR, Maynard M, Frankel S, et al. Diet in childhood and adult cardiovascular and all cause mortality: the Boyd Orr cohort. *Heart.* 2005;91(7):894–898

10. Kamphuis CBM, Giskes K, de Bruijn GJ, Wendel-Vos W, Brug J, van Lenthe FJ. Environmental determinants of fruit and vegetable consumption among adults: a systematic review. *Br J Nutr.* 2006;96(4):620–635

11. Di Noia J, Byrd-Bredbenner C. Determinants of fruit and vegetable intake in low-income children and adolescents. *Nutr Rev.* 2014; 72(9):575–590

12. Kumar S, Kelly AS. Review of childhood obesity: from epidemiology, etiology, and comorbidities to clinical assessment and treatment. *Mayo Clin Proc.* 2017;92(2):251–265

13. Rossen LM, Schoendorf KC. Measuring health disparities: trends in racial-ethnic and socioeconomic disparities in obesity among 2- to 18-year old youth in the United States, 2001-2010. *Ann Epidemiol.* 2012;22(10):698–704

14. Nord M, Andrews M, Carlson S. Household food security in the United States, 2005. Available at: https://www.ers.usda.gov/webdocs/publications/45655/29206_err29_002.pdf?v=0. Accessed November 21, 2022

15. Feeding America. Map the meal gap. Child food insecurity in Philadelphia County. Available at: https://map.feedingamerica.org/county/2018/

overall/pennsylvania/county/philadelphia. Accessed February 20, 2021

16. Odoms-Young AM, Kong A, Schiffer LA, et al. Evaluating the initial impact of the revised Special Supplemental Nutrition Program for Women, Infants, and Children (WIC) food packages on dietary intake and home food availability in African-American and Hispanic families. *Public Health Nutr.* 2014;17(1):83–93

17. Hillier A, McLaughlin J, Cannuscio CC, Chilton M, Krasny S, Karpyn A. The impact of WIC food package changes on access to healthful food in 2 low-income urban neighborhoods. *J Nutr Educ Behav.* 2012;44(3):210–216

18. Wozniak A, Willey J, Benz J, Hart N. COVID-19 impact survey: version 1. Available at: https://www.covid-impact.org/results. Accessed December 31, 2021

19. Coleman-Jensen A, Rabbitt MP, Gregory CA, Singh A. Household food security in the United States in 2019. Available at: www.ers.usda.gov/publications/pub-details/?pubid=99281. Accessed February 19, 2021

20. USDA Food and Nutrition Service. WIC 2017 eligibility and coverage rates. Available at: https://www.fns.usda.gov/wic-2017-eligibility-and-coverage-rates. Accessed January 3, 2022

21. National Academies of Sciences, Engineering, and Medicine. *Review of WIC Food Packages: Improving Balance and Choice: Final Report.* Washington, DC: National Academies Press; 2017.

22. USDA, Food and Nutrition Service. WIC Farmers' Market Nutrition Program. Available at: https://www.fns.usda.gov/fmnp/fact-sheet-2021. Accessed March 1, 2022

23. US Department of Agriculture, Food and Nutrition Service. WIC FMNP Fiscal Year 2018 Food Nutrition Service 203 Report. Available at: https://www.usda.gov/sites/default/files/documents/32fnsex-notes2018.pdf. Accessed December 8, 2022

24. Anderson JV, Bybee DI, Brown RM, et al. 5 a day fruit and vegetable intervention improves consumption in a low income population. *J Am Diet Assoc.* 2001; 101(2):195–202

25. Kropf ML, Holben DH, Holcomb JP Jr, Anderson H. Food security status and produce intake and behaviors of Special Supplemental Nutrition Program for Women, Infants, and Children and Farmers' Market Nutrition Program participants. *J Am Diet Assoc.* 2007; 107(11):1903–1908

26. Di Noia J, Monica D, Sikorskii A, Nelson J. Pilot study of a Farm-to-Special Supplemental Nutrition Program for Women, Infants, and Children (WIC) intervention promoting vegetable consumption. *J Acad Nutr Diet.* 2021; 121(10):2035–2045

27. DeCuir-Gunby JT, Marshall PL, McCulloch AW. Developing and using a codebook for the analysis of interview data: an example from a professional development research project. *Field Methods.* 2011;23(2):136–155

28. Hager ER, Quigg AM, Black MM, et al. Development and validity of a 2-item screen to identify families at risk for food insecurity. *Pediatrics.* 2010;126(1):e26–e32

29. Maternal & Family Health Services. Farmers' Market Nutrition Program. https://www.mfhs.org/programs/wic-nutrition/wic-farmers-market/. Accessed September 14, 2022

30. Pennsylvania WIC. Farmers' Market Nutrition Program (FMNP). Available at: https://www.pawic.com/FarmerMarket-NutritionProgram.aspx. Accessed September 14, 2022

31. Ventura AK, Martinez CE, Whaley SE. WIC participants' perceptions of COVID-19-related changes to WIC recertification and service delivery. *J Community Health.* 2022;47(2):184–192

32. McElrone M, Zimmer MC, Anderson Steeves ET. A qualitative exploration of predominantly white non-Hispanic Tennessee WIC participants' food retail and WIC clinic experiences during COVID-19. *J Acad Nutr Diet.* 2021; 121(8):1454–1462

33. Woelfel ML, Abusabha R, Pruzek R, Stratton H, Chen SG, Edmunds LS. Barriers to the use of WIC services. *J Am Diet Assoc.* 2004;104(5):736–743

34. Liu CH, Liu H. Concerns and structural barriers associated with WIC participation among WIC-eligible women. *Public Health Nurs.* 2016;33(5):395–402

35. Bertmann FMW, Barroso C, Ohri-Vachaspati P, Hampl JS, Sell K, Wharton CM. Women, infants, and children cash value voucher (CVV) use in Arizona: a qualitative exploration of barriers and strategies related to fruit and vegetable purchases. *J Nutr Educ Behav.* 2014;46(3 suppl):S53–S58

36. Gago CM, Wynne JO, Moore MJ, et al. Caregiver perspectives on underutilization of WIC: a qualitative study. *Pediatrics.* 2022;149(2):e2021053889

37. Seidel M, Brink L, Hamilton M, Gordon L. Increasing WIC Farmers' Market Nutrition Program redemption rates: results and policy recommendations. *Prog Community Health Partnersh.* 2018;12(4):431–439

38. Hanks AS, Gunther C, Lillard D, Scharff RL. From paper to plastic: understanding the impact of eWIC on WIC recipient behavior. *Food Policy.* 2019;83:83–91

39. Zimmer MC, Beaird J, Steeves ETA. WIC participants' perspectives about online ordering and technology in the WIC program. *J Nutr Educ Behav.* 2021;53(7):602–307

40. Vasan A, Kenyon CC, Roberto CA, Fiks AG, Venkataramani AS. Association of remote vs in-person benefit delivery with WIC participation during the COVID-19 pandemic. *JAMA.* 2021;326(15):1531–1533

41. Herman DR. Ensuring access to fruits and vegetables for the nation's most vulnerable – contributions of WIC and SNAP. *Econ Voice.* 2017;14(1)

42. Zimmer M, McElrone M, Anderson Steeves ET. Feasibility and acceptability of a "Click & Collect" WIC online ordering pilot. *J Acad Nutr Diet.* 2021; 121(12):2464–2474.e1

43. Zhang Q, Park K, Zhang J, Tang C. The online ordering behaviors among participants in the Oklahoma Women, Infants, and Children Program: a cross-sectional analysis. *Int J Environ Res Public Health.* 2022;19(3):1805

44. Jilcott Pitts SB, Ng SW, Blitstein JL, et al. Perceived advantages and disadvantages of online grocery shopping among Special Supplemental Nutrition Program for Women, Infants, and Children (WIC) participants in eastern North Carolina. *Curr Dev Nutr.* 2020; 4(5):nzaa076

45. Poblacion A, Cook J, Ettinger de Cuba S, et al. Can food insecurity be reduced in the United States by improving SNAP, WIC, and the community eligibility provision?

Can food insecurity be reduced? *World Med Health Policy.* 2017;9(4):435–455

46. Nagata JM, Seligman HK, Weiser SD. Perspective: the convergence of coronavirus disease 2019 (COVID-19) and food insecurity in the United States. *Adv Nutr.* 2021;12(2):287–290

47. Thriving PA. Women, Infants and Children (WIC) Program. Available at: https://www.papartnerships.org/wp-content/uploads/2022/06/Philadelphia-WIC-Fact-Sheet-2022.pdf. Accessed November 21, 2022

48. Thriving PA. A Time to Thrive: Growing Pennsylvania WIC's Impact on Children and Families. Available at: https://www.papartnerships.org/wp-content/uploads/2021/05/A-Time-to-Thrive-WIC-Policy-Brief.pdf. Accessed February 4, 2022

49. United States Census Bureau. Women, Infants, and Children (WIC) Program Eligibility and Participation. Available at: https://www.census.gov/library/visualizations/interactive/wic-eligibility-participation.html#:~:text=A%20recent%20report%20found%20that,population%20is%20participating%20in%20WIC. Accessed February 4, 2022

50. Coleman-Jensen A, Rabbitt M, Gregory C, Singh A. Household Food Security in the United States in 2020. Available at: https://www.ers.usda.gov/publications/pub-details/?pubid=102075. Accessed November 21, 2022

Caregiver Perspectives on Improving Government Nutrition Benefit Programs

DanaRose Negro, BS,[a,b] Mishaal Yazdani, BS,[b] Lindsay Benitez, BS,[b,c] Chén C. Kenyon, MD, MSHP,[a,b] Alexander G. Fiks, MD, MSCE,[a,b] Aditi Vasan, MD, MSHP[a,b]

OBJECTIVES: The Special Supplemental Nutrition Program for Women, Infants, and Children (WIC) and Supplemental Nutrition Assistance Program (SNAP) provide essential nutrition support for low-income families. However, many eligible families do not receive or fully redeem these benefits. We aimed to understand current and former WIC and SNAP beneficiaries' perceptions of and suggestions for improving both programs.

METHODS: We conducted semistructured phone interviews with caregivers of pediatric patients who were current or former WIC and SNAP beneficiaries at 2 academic pediatric primary care clinics. Interviews were recorded, transcribed, and coded by 2 independent coders using thematic analysis, resolving discrepancies by consensus. Interviews continued until data saturation was reached.

RESULTS: We interviewed 40 caregivers who were predominantly Black (88%) mothers (90%), with 53% and 83% currently using WIC and SNAP, respectively. We identified 4 themes related to participation barriers: (1) limited product variety available through WIC, (2) inconvenience and stigma associated with purchasing WIC products, (3) SNAP income-based eligibility criteria, and (4) burdensome SNAP enrollment and recertification processes. We identified 3 themes related to suggestions for improvement: (a) decreasing stigma associated with participation, (b) allowing online or phone-based enrollment, and (c) improving coordination with health care systems.

CONCLUSIONS: WIC and SNAP beneficiaries identified several modifiable barriers to enrollment and benefits redemption. Pediatric providers should advocate for programmatic improvements that make it easier for families to access and redeem benefits and should consider implementing innovative cross-sector interventions like medical–financial partnerships, direct WIC and SNAP referrals, and data sharing with government assistance offices.

[a]Department of Pediatrics, Perelman School of Medicine, University of Pennsylvania, Philadelphia, Pennsylvania; [b]PolicyLab and Clinical Futures, Children's Hospital of Philadelphia, Philadelphia, Pennsylvania; and [c]Sidney Kimmel Medical College at Jefferson University, Philadelphia, Pennsylvania

Ms Negro conceptualized and designed the study, collected data, conducted initial analyses, and drafted the initial manuscript; Ms Yazdani conceptualized and designed the study, collected data, and conducted initial analyses; Ms Benitez conceptualized and designed the study and collected data; Drs Kenyon and Fiks supervised conceptualization and design of the study; Dr Vasan conceptualized and designed the study and coordinated and supervised data collection and analysis; and all authors critically reviewed and revised the final manuscript, approved the final manuscript as submitted, and agree to be accountable for all aspects of the work.

DOI: https://doi.org/10.1542/peds.2024-067012

Accepted for publication Aug 21, 2024

Address correspondence to Aditi Vasan, MD, MSHP, Roberts Center for Pediatric Research, Children's Hospital of Philadelphia, 2716 South St, Philadelphia, PA 19146. E-mail: vasana@chop.edu

PEDIATRICS (ISSN Numbers: Print, 0031-4005; Online, 1098-4275).

WHAT'S KNOWN ON THIS SUBJECT: The Special Supplemental Nutrition Program for Women, Infants, and Children (WIC) and Supplemental Nutrition Assistance Program (SNAP) are government benefit programs that provide nutrition support for low-income families. Previous studies have identified barriers to participation in either WIC or SNAP.

WHAT THIS STUDY ADDS: This study explores caregiver perspectives on WIC and SNAP simultaneously. Through qualitative interviews with current and former beneficiaries of both programs, we identify several modifiable barriers to participation and highlight cross-cutting strategies for improving program enrollment and benefit redemption.

To cite: Negro DR, Yazdani M, Benitez L, et al. Caregiver Perspectives on Improving Government Nutrition Benefit Programs. *Pediatrics.* 2024;154(5):e2024067012

ARTICLE

Childhood food insecurity is highly prevalent in the United States, affecting 8.8% of households with children in 2022.[1] The American Academy of Pediatrics encourages pediatricians to screen for food insecurity and refer patients to community resources, as highlighted in the 2022 White House Strategy for Hunger, Nutrition, and Health.[2] One set of resources pediatricians can offer are referrals to government nutrition benefit programs, including the Special Supplemental Nutrition Program for Women, Infants, and Children (WIC) and the Supplemental Nutrition Assistance Program (SNAP).

WIC participation is associated with improved birth outcomes and decreased infant mortality.[3] SNAP participation also has demonstrated health benefits, including decreased food insecurity, improved caregiver-reported child health, and decreased developmental risk.[4,5] However, many eligible families do not participate in these programs. There has been a consistent decline in the national WIC coverage rate since 2016, and in 2021, only 51% of WIC-eligible individuals received benefits.[6] The national SNAP coverage rate was only 78% in 2020, with wide variation across states.[7] Some eligible families might choose not to enroll in WIC and SNAP, whereas others may be interested in receiving benefits but have trouble accessing these programs.[8-10]

Previous qualitative studies have explored pediatric caregiver perspectives on either WIC or SNAP and barriers to utilizing each of these programs. Barriers to WIC utilization include food package inflexibility, decreased perceived value after children reach age 1, instore shopping and checkout challenges, difficulty attending appointments, and stigma encountered in the WIC office.[11-16] Recent WIC modernization efforts, including transitioning from paper vouchers to electronic benefits transfer debit cards, providing shopping support via smartphone apps, and initiation of remote certification appointments and remote benefits reloading have been positively received by participants.[11,17-19] SNAP recipients' perspectives and barriers to participation have also been investigated, although to a lesser extent, revealing dissatisfaction with income limits,[20] customer service, and the complex application and benefits determination processes.[8,9]

Because low-income caregivers of young children are often eligible for both WIC and SNAP, understanding caregiver perspectives on both programs could help inform improvements in program design and boost participation synergistically. In this study, we aimed to understand perceptions of WIC and SNAP program benefits, participation barriers, and suggestions for improvement among pediatric caregivers who were current or former WIC and SNAP beneficiaries, with the ultimate goal of identifying cross-cutting strategies for improving both programs.

METHODS

Study Design and Participants

We recruited a convenience sample of parents and caregivers from 2 academic primary care practices within the Children's Hospital of Philadelphia Pediatric Resource Consortium, a primary care practice-based research network.[21] Both practices are in West Philadelphia and serve a predominantly Black (81%) and Medicaid-insured (86%) population.

Participants initially completed a survey regarding preferences for clinic-based food resources and participation in nutrition benefit programs.[22] Demographic information, including self-reported race and ethnicity, was also collected. At the end of the survey, caregivers indicated whether they were interested in participating in a subsequent phone interview exploring their perceptions of clinic-based food resources and their suggestions for improving government nutrition benefit programs.

Inclusion criteria included being 18 years of age or older, able to communicate in English, and having at least 1 child aged <5 years. We focused on English-speaking caregivers because both study practices serve a predominantly English-speaking population and because our semistructured interview guide was developed and pilot-tested in English. We focused on caregivers of children aged <5 because they would be potentially eligible for both WIC and SNAP.

Of caregivers who indicated interest in an interview, we purposively sampled current or former WIC and SNAP beneficiaries. A study team member contacted caregivers by phone to confirm eligibility and schedule a subsequent phone interview. Caregivers provided verbal informed consent before each interview and received a $25 gift card as compensation.

This study was designed to comply with Consolidated Criteria for Reporting Qualitative Research guidelines[23] and approved after expedited review by our institutional review board.

Data Collection

Through review of the literature and pilot testing with caregivers who were current or former WIC and SNAP beneficiaries, we developed an interview guide (Supplemental Information) that included open-ended questions regarding the WIC and SNAP user experience. We first asked about participants' general experiences with each program, and then inquired about suggestions for improving both programs. We also asked how clinics could support families in improving enrollment and redemption across both programs. Interviews were conducted in July and August 2022.

Research Team and Reflexivity

Study team members who conducted interviews (D.N., M.Y., and L.B.) included 2 second-year medical students and 1 clinical research assistant, all with bachelor's degrees and structured training in conducting qualitative research. All interviewers were female; 1 identified as non-Hispanic white, 1 as Hispanic, and 1 as South Asian. The other 3 coinvestigators were pediatricians and health services researchers with masters-level research training and several years of experience caring for food-insecure families in clinical practice. Research team members had no preexisting relationships with participants. Throughout the data collection, analysis, and manuscript preparation process, our team considered how our identities and life experiences may have impacted research conduct and interpretation of findings, consistent with Consolidated Criteria for Reporting Qualitative Research guidelines.[23,24]

Data Analysis

Interviews were audio-recorded and professionally transcribed. Transcripts were reviewed, deidentified, and entered into NVivo (QSR International, Burlington, MA) for analysis. We used a thematic analysis approach to code interview transcripts. Three study team members (A.V., D.N., and M.Y.) initially open-coded 5 transcripts to develop a preliminary coding scheme and dictionary. We used a priori topics from the interview guide to inform codebook development deductively, and then added new codes inductively. Codes were evaluated and revised after each coding session, consistent with a constant comparative method.[25] All interviews were then coded independently by 2 study team members, and intercoder agreement was measured using the κ coefficient, to help ensure a consistent approach to coding across our study team.[26] We met after each set of 5 transcripts was coded, identified codes with a $κ < 0.8$, and resolved discrepancies by consensus. Interviews were continued until our team felt we had reached data saturation, meaning we had captured data that were sufficiently rich and complex to address our study objectives.[25,27,28]

RESULTS

We attempted to contact 63 caregivers and completed 40 interviews, for a response rate of 63%. The 23 caregivers who did not complete interviews either could not be reached by phone after 3 attempts, or initially agreed to be interviewed but could not be reached on subsequent call attempts.

Caregivers' mean age was 32.3 years and the mean age of their youngest child was 1.5 years (Table 1). Caregivers were predominantly Black (88%) and 5% were Hispanic or Latine, similar to the overall population served by the study clinics. All caregivers had experience using both WIC and SNAP, with 52% and 85% currently receiving WIC and SNAP, respectively.

TABLE 1 Demographic Characteristics

	Caregivers ($n = 40$)
Caregiver age, mean	32.3 y
Child age, mean	1.5 y
Relationship to child	
Mother	36 (90%)
Grandmother	3 (8%)
Other relative or legal guardian	1 (2%)
Caregiver race	
Black or African American	35 (88%)
Asian American	1 (2%)
White	1 (2%)
Native American or Alaskan Native	2 (5%)
Other	2 (5%)
Caregiver ethnicity	
Hispanic or Latino/Latinx	2 (5%)
Non-Hispanic or Latino/Latinx	38 (95%)
Caregivers' highest level of education completed	
Some high school	4 (10%)
Graduated high school or received GED	18 (45%)
Some college or associate's degree	14 (35%)
Bachelor's degree	4 (10%)
Current benefit program use	
SNAP and WIC	20 (50%)
SNAP only	14 (35%)
WIC only	1 (2%)
Neither WIC nor SNAP	5 (13%)
Low Income Home Energy Assistance Program	4 (10%)
Temporary Assistance for Needy Families	3 (8%)
Supplemental Security Income	4 (10%)
Previous benefit program use	
SNAP	40 (100%)
WIC	40 (100%)
LIHEAP	13 (33%)
TANF	12 (30%)
SSI	6 (15%)

GED, General Education Development; LIHEAP, Low Income Home Energy Assistance Program; SSI, Supplemental Security Income; TANF, Temporary Assistance for Needy Families.

We identified 2 themes related to benefits of participation (Table 2), 4 themes related to barriers to participation (Table 3), and 3 themes related to suggestions for improvement (Table 4).

Benefits of WIC Participation

Caregivers expressed appreciation for the range of services provided by WIC. Caregivers liked that WIC encouraged nutritious food choices. One mother shared, "We get to get foods that we don't normally eat, which is good for us because it's much healthier. I get to expose my family to wheat bread ... more produce, more fruits, and stuff like that" (participant 28, former WIC and SNAP participant). Caregivers also appreciated WIC's nutrition education and support programs, including breastfeeding support, nutrition brochures, recipes, and Farmers Market Nutrition Program

TABLE 2 Benefits of WIC and SNAP Participation: Themes and Representative Quotes

WIC Theme	Quotes
1. Caregivers appreciate WIC's provision of infant formula, nutritious food, and nutrition and breastfeeding education.	"I like that [WIC] gives you the option to get nutritional food, because sometimes the nutritional food costs more than the fast food. I like that I'm able to get fresh vegetables and not just fresh vegetables, but [also] canned fruit, fruit cups, and things like that for the kids." Participant 10 (current WIC and SNAP participant)
	"The WIC program actually offered more than just food. I remember when I first had my 3-year-old, and I was trying to breastfeed but he really wouldn't latch on or he would and he would only drink for 2 minutes and then stop, and I was just frustrated, not knowing what was going on. They also offered breastfeeding classes and stuff like that. So, I'm not going to lie, they actually did help me get better at breastfeeding and understanding the infant's emotion and stuff like that during breastfeeding. So, I like that it's just not food, but it's also, they offer other services. Because the lady that I was speaking to, she actually helped me understand how to breastfeed better." Participant 30 (former WIC participant, current SNAP participant)

SNAP Theme	Quotes
2. Caregivers appreciate being able to use SNAP benefits to purchase a variety of food items.	"I like SNAP because we can get whatever we want. I can go full grocery shopping and get meals that'll last for weeks, and not have to pick and choose, or try to figure out how many ounces is this meat, or if I can get this meat because of the ounce size or the quantity. And I can just buy whatever I want...As long as it's cold, and as long as it's approved by EBT, I can get it. I can get my kids whatever milk I want them to drink. It doesn't have to be cow's milk. I get them oat milk. I can get them whatever juice, and it doesn't have to be a sugary beverage. It can be whatever beverage I want my kids to drink." Participant 7 (former WIC participant, current SNAP participant)
	"If you need [SNAP], it's great because it can literally fill your house with food … You can go to the store, you can go to literally a corner store, if your child is hungry, and buy them a sandwich." Participant 20 (former WIC participant, current SNAP participant)
	"[Using SNAP benefits has] been great. No problems because with SNAP, as long as it's anything foodwise you purchase, as long as it's not anything that's already cooked or anything like that. So, it's plenty of things that you could buy as long as it's food items." Participant 39 (former WIC participant, current SNAP participant)

EBT, electronic benefits transfer.

vouchers. One caregiver noted how WIC's nutrition education had benefited her family, "[WIC] gave me different ideas of different meals to make for the kids to keep them healthy" (participant 12, former WIC participant, current SNAP participant).

Benefits of SNAP Participation

Caregivers valued the autonomy and flexibility provided in making food purchases using SNAP, allowing them to account for their families' preferences and dietary restrictions. One caregiver noted, "All products are really SNAP products, unless it's cooked [food]" (participant 10, current WIC and SNAP participant). Caregivers positively contrasted this flexibility with WIC's product, brand, and size restrictions. Many caregivers shared that the freedom associated with SNAP facilitated an easy shopping experience and convenient redemption of benefits.

Barriers to WIC Participation

WIC Product Restrictions Can Make It Challenging to Use These Benefits

Participants noted numerous ways in which WIC's strict product restrictions led to underutilization of benefits. Caregivers particularly highlighted limitations related to product size, formulation, and brand restrictions, which were exacerbated during the 2022 formula shortage. Some participants also described difficulty navigating WIC accommodations for their children's food allergies. One parent shared, "I'm like, 'my son is allergic to [dairy].' And [WIC] just took it off, as opposed to giving us more [benefits] in a different area" (Participant 13, current WIC and SNAP participant). Additionally, some caregivers noted that WIC coverage of 100% juice felt inconsistent with their pediatrician's recommendation to limit juice intake.

Families Commonly Encounter Challenges When Redeeming WIC, Including Absent Product Labels and Stigmatizing Checkout Experiences

Caregivers also shared challenges associated with WIC redemption. Many caregivers reported difficulty identifying WIC products. One caregiver noted, "Finding which products [are covered] takes time … you have to literally look at the weights, look at the actual names, the flavors" (participant 22, current WIC and SNAP participant). Caregivers also described sometimes feeling embarrassed when making purchases using WIC, particularly if they were forced to return or exchange products they had believed were WIC-eligible.

Barriers to SNAP Participation

SNAP's Income-Based Eligibility Criteria Can Be a Barrier to Participation for Working Families

Some caregivers described no longer meeting SNAP income eligibility criteria, which are often more stringent

TABLE 3 Barriers to WIC and SNAP Participation: Themes and Representative Quotes

WIC Themes	Quotes
1. WIC product restrictions can make it challenging to use these benefits.	"If they actually surveyed more people in the community who used WIC, then they would know what [products] to give us. Because they're just going off a broad list. Not what's in our community. If you base stuff off of people in the suburbs or in the outskirts that don't live in our neighborhood, you're not giving [us] exactly what we need. Or when they do cover [products], they give us more of what we don't need and less of what we could use." Participant 3 (current WIC and SNAP Participant)
	"Like right now, because we're in the shortage of formula, it's very, very hard for me as a grandparent with looking for formula, and because of the WIC guidelines, they limit the amount and the allotted form of the formula when you do find it. So, if you find it, right? In a store that may have it, you're still limited to that [amount] because of the guidelines that WIC has on certain formulas... the limitations. So, it makes it harder for us." Participant 4 (current WIC and SNAP participant)
	"So, WIC has been an up-and-down experience, because, for my child … he has a lot of food allergies. And WIC is very black and white. So like, the things like the fish and the eggs and the milk and things that my son is allergic to, they will not give me alternatives...he can't get the tuna, so why we can't make that instead money for fruits and vegetables? … They don't really consider the children with food allergies, and that's kind of like a hindrance to me." Participant 13 (current WIC and SNAP participant)
2. Families commonly encounter challenges when redeeming WIC, including absent product labels and stigmatizing checkout experiences.	"Finding [WIC products] in stores has been a struggle. Even just for instance, for cereal … I really feel like it if there was a WIC section [in stores], it would be easier. Because sometimes, you get to the register and they're like, 'Well, this is not a part of our WIC program at this location.' And it's just like, 'Well, this is difficult, because I just stood and looked at these aisles for 45 min just looking at cereal to make sure that I'm getting the cereal that fits in the criteria of what I need.'" Participant 22 (current WIC and SNAP participant)
	"[Finding WIC products] was a little difficult because certain stores doesn't have, 'Oh, this is a WIC product.' And then some stores does have WIC products labeled in bright yellow, which was very convenient and very much easier, instead of me assuming that 1 product is a WIC product and then going up to the register and then it ends up being not, and then you hold up a whole line. So, it would be very much more helpful and convenient if all stores would just label their product as a WIC product." Participant 28 (former WIC and SNAP participant)
	"The checkout process can be, No. 1, embarrassing for the person getting these products because maybe they don't want everyone to know that they're getting these benefits. And No. 2, frustrating for the cashier as well, because now they have a line for the people and they have to stop what they're doing to go find the proper qualifying items for the customer that's in line. So, it's just the convenience of it all and the privacy of it all, too. Like, I don't want everybody to know that I am receiving these benefits, because it's honestly nobody's business." Participant 18 (former WIC participant, current SNAP participant)
SNAP Themes	**Quotes**
3. SNAP's income-based eligibility criteria can be a barrier to participation for working families.	"The [SNAP] income limits are just too low. They're just entirely too low. There's an entire population of people that are struggling paycheck to paycheck … trying to figure out how to feed their kids based off of working with minimum-wage jobs or maybe getting paid a little bit more than minimum wage, but still income ineligible. You're still in that grocery store trying to make $20 into $100, but you're just not eligible." – Participant 16 (current WIC participant, former SNAP participant)
	"If you're working, and I go apply for SNAP, and I can't get it… I think some of the parents out here that's working should be able to get SNAP to help feed their children. Because you've got bills to pay. And then, you've got to think about, 'Wow, now, I have to go shopping for food and I really don't have that money.' But you spend it. Because you have to eat to survive." Participant 23 (former WIC participant, current SNAP participant)
	"They sit there and be like, 'Oh, because I make $14.50 [an hour], that my food stamps should go down a bit because I can technically financially afford it. I'm like, 'No. Just because I'm making this amount of money, that's literally providing rent, bills, car [insurance], all that for my kids. That has nothing to do with food.' If I then have to kick out money for food, I'm really struggling. My food stamps should not go lower just because I'm making a little bit more money." Participant 36 (current WIC and SNAP participant)
4. SNAP enrollment and recertification processes can be burdensome and lead to unexpected loss of benefits.	"So, my main issue with SNAP is, I was on the program, and I guess it's because I didn't submit something or something, and then they automatically...They just stop your benefit, especially in times when you really need them." Participant 12 (former WIC participant, current SNAP participant)
	"It's just, recently, my [SNAP] benefits were cut off and I didn't get a notification or nobody called me. Nobody sent me a letter. They just cut them off because they said that I needed to send them some type of paper, but I didn't get a notification of it that they were getting cut off... I didn't have a job and we didn't have any money, so we were trying to scramble around to find ways to get for food for my daughter." Participant 27 (current WIC and SNAP participant)
	"It is a headache with the food stamps, the caseworkers, they don't always put everything in the computer right. And so then sometimes, they cut your food stamp and stuff like that, and then you don't know why and have to try to figure it out … Sometimes, you send the information in wrong and then it's confusing. And then, they're also just constantly switching off working without calling you or letting you know." Participant 29 (current WIC and SNAP participant)

TABLE 4 Suggestions for Improving Both the WIC and SNAP Programs: Themes and Representative Quotes

Cross-Cutting Themes	Quotes
1. Both WIC and SNAP enrollment processes could be improved by decreasing stigma associated with program participation.	"Just to me, a lot of the workers need to be trained better to make people feel [SNAP] is a program that can help you instead of making them feel like they're less than because they're on this program." Participant 25 (former WIC and SNAP participant)
	"[WIC is] okay the way that it is, I would just want better customer service inside the WIC offices, and more people who are inclined to actually help the customers that walk in there… In terms of actually helping people, like the food stamp office, the WIC offices, a lot of those people don't even really care about the people that come in … And this is why a lot of people find it difficult to even get [applications] done, because you already have a lot of things going on, and the people that you're going to really don't want to help you, they'll literally treat you like trash." Participant 35 (former WIC participant, current SNAP participant)
2. Online and phone-based benefits enrollment and redemption support could improve the WIC and SNAP user experience.	"They need to continue to push online enrollment. They have been doing that since the pandemic and they need to continue. They need to continue to try to support the online system, that telephone system to help with making that process easier because you get, that attention is different when you get someone over the phone that's calling just to talk to you and it's not the chaos of everything going on around you in the [county assistance] office that's often times like I said, very negative, disheveled, disorganized, dysfunctional, and aggressive." Participant 16 (current WIC participant, former SNAP participant)
	"I do have the [WIC] app, and I wish they would send me messages like, 'Okay, it's in 2 wk that we're going to reload your card' … I wish they would inform me like, 'Okay, [this benefit] is about to expire. Use it now or your card will be reloaded again on this date' … It [would] probably be better to give me an estimate time on when things are about to expire, when things are going to reload, and what necessary information that I need to provide them to keep my benefits." Participant 28 (former WIC and SNAP participant)
	"Rather than getting, having to actually go to the 1 WIC office in your district or in your area, maybe it can be a virtual appointment, some type of virtual checkup, or something of that nature, because everybody can't get to those offices." Participant 38 (former WIC participant, current SNAP participant)
3. Improved coordination between health care providers and WIC and SNAP could boost participation.	"If somebody [in clinic] can volunteer and help families with a tablet or a laptop and help them sign up for [benefits], I think that would be great because you feel more connected and safer. And the hospital, the clinic is a little, some people are a little more personable than how the SNAP people are in the office." Participant 19 (former WIC participant, current SNAP participant)
	"It was a little difficult for me to go back to the [WIC] office and get my WIC loaded back on my card. So, it would be more convenient for me to go to my children's health care provider and just get it done there all at once." Participant 28 (former WIC and SNAP participant)
	"I just feel like they just need to make [WIC] more convenient for people, because it's a mess and it's all over the place. It's not structured right. I think it should really go through the doctors. Listen, when I had my son, he got weighed and then I went to WIC a day later or 2, just a couple days after I came from the doctor's office from getting weighed, getting his measurements and all that. You having to go to the WIC to do the same thing? I feel like that's silly. I feel like it's not worth it." Participant 34 (former WIC participant, current SNAP participant)

than WIC criteria, despite experiencing food insecurity. Caregivers voiced frustration that the program did not consider other essential expenses, like rent, in eligibility determination. One caregiver shared, "They keep going off your income, but they don't understand that you have bills that you have to pay… People have to put gas in their cars …They don't calculate none of that" (participant 14, current WIC and SNAP participant). Another caregiver shared her experience just missing the eligibility threshold: "[It feels like] they want me to cut my hours at work to be approved for the program, and I don't see the benefit in that for my children" (participant 15, former WIC and SNAP participant).

SNAP Enrollment and Recertification Processes Can Be Burdensome and Lead to Unexpected Loss of Benefits

Many caregivers encountered obstacles during SNAP enrollment and recertification, including delays in receiving or renewing benefits. Caregivers also shared experiences

of losing benefits, often without previous notification and sometimes because of case worker error. One caregiver said, "It's the keeping SNAP [benefits] that's hard. It's like, as soon as you get a job or you do something and you get a little more money, they cut everything off. Or somebody does something in the system and messes up your entire application, [and then] you have to redo [it]" (participant 3, current WIC and SNAP participant).

Improving WIC and SNAP Enrollment and Redemption

Both WIC and SNAP Enrollment Processes Could Be Improved by Decreasing Stigma Associated With Program Participation

Caregivers described stigma encountered in WIC and county assistance offices, as well as broader societal misconceptions around program participation. One caregiver shared, "It's not good to already be in a stressful life situation and then have to go into these atmospheres where the workers aren't friendly, too. So maybe more training for the workers to learn how to deal with people in high-stress situations in a more professional and courteous manner" (participant 18, former WIC participant, current SNAP participant).

Online and Phone-Based Benefits Enrollment and Redemption Support Could Improve the WIC and SNAP User Experience

Many caregivers discussed the convenience of online and phone-based enrollment applications, compared with in-person or mail applications. One caregiver shared, "I feel like more people would enroll [in WIC] if they didn't have to physically go down there and be interviewed" (participant 21, former WIC participant, current SNAP participant). Another caregiver highlighted the value of the WIC smartphone application for identifying eligible products, "If I'm not sure about something, I can check the WIC app to see what qualifies for it" (participant 10, current WIC and SNAP participant).

Improved Coordination Between Health Care Providers and WIC and SNAP Could Boost Participation

Multiple caregivers suggested improved coordination between WIC, SNAP, and medical offices as a potential strategy for increasing enrollment and retention. One caregiver said, "They should have a WIC department inside of the hospital ... so when people have their infants, they can sign up for WIC right then and there" (participant 33, current WIC and SNAP participant). Caregivers also suggested that clinics should provide families with help enrolling in WIC and SNAP, and that sharing children's measurements and laboratory values with WIC could minimize the need for redundant testing.

DISCUSSION

This study is among the first to simultaneously examine perspectives on WIC and SNAP among a population of low-income caregivers with experience using both programs. Participants valued WIC's provision of infant formula, breastfeeding support, and subsidies for nutritious food, but disliked stringent product restrictions and associated in-store shopping challenges. These findings are consistent with previous reports on barriers to WIC participation.[11–16] Regarding SNAP, participants valued the flexibility of benefits, but noted the sometimes limiting nature of income-based eligibility criteria and highlighted the need to reduce administrative burdens associated with maintaining benefits. In line with this suggestion, previous research on the SNAP program has shown improved retention in the setting of policies that simplify recertification and reduce the burden of interim eligibility reporting requirements.[29,30]

Across both programs, caregivers discussed stigma encountered in program offices and opportunities for technology to improve the user experience. Importantly, improved coordination with clinics and health care providers emerged as a key strategy for improving enrollment and retention. Participants noted that parts of their children's WIC appointments, like measurements of height, weight, and hemoglobin levels, could feel redundant with well-child visits and viewed this as an opportunity for improved data sharing to reduce redundancy. Participants also supported creating standardized processes for WIC and SNAP enrollment in clinical settings, like having a benefits enrollment navigator available to families during primary care visits.

The themes identified in this study highlight the need for clinicians and health systems to support families in accessing and using WIC and SNAP. Several pediatric primary care clinics have started working toward improved coordination with WIC through colocation, electronic health record integration, and even coenrollment at concurrent primary care and WIC visits.[31–35] The concurrent care model allows families to complete WIC enrollment and receive WIC nutrition and lactation counseling during primary care visits, resulting in improved convenience, reduced redundancy, and decreased transportation costs.[35] Our findings provide support for scaling these approaches, which could mitigate the sometimes duplicative nature of pediatric and WIC office visits. Some clinics have also begun providing colocated benefits enrollment support through medical–financial partnerships, and our findings support this approach to both addressing food insecurity and boosting government nutrition program participation.[36–38]

Our findings also highlight potential strategies for federal and state policymakers seeking to improve WIC and SNAP to better meet families' needs. In April 2024, the USDA's Food and Nutrition Service announced several changes to the WIC food package, including soy-based substitutions for dairy products and an increased fruit and vegetable allowance.[39] Although these changes are promising, our findings suggest that future WIC innovations should also focus on minimizing size and packaging restrictions and ensuring vendor compliance with labeling of WIC-eligible products. In addition, our findings support continued implementation of virtual options for WIC certification, benefits reloading, and nutrition education.[40] Studies have shown that applications like WIC Shopper are associated with increased benefit redemption, and our findings support broader awareness and adoption of these applications.[41,42] The challenges described by caregivers of children with food allergies also highlight the importance of clear communication of WIC policies to beneficiaries, because WIC does allow some food substitutions with physician attestation of an allergy.

Food and Nutrition Service also published its reevaluation of the Thrifty Food Plan in 2022, resulting in a 21% increase in SNAP benefits.[43] Our findings support this expansion, given the many competing expenses faced by working families. Our findings also suggest that modifying

SNAP to only cover foods that are deemed nutritious, as has been proposed in Congress,[44] may have the unintended consequence of reducing the flexibility, autonomy, and ease of redemption that beneficiaries currently value. If policies that restrict SNAP purchases to nutritious products are implemented, our findings suggest that policymakers should focus on ensuring clear labeling requirements that facilitate easy identification of SNAP-eligible products and optimize the in-store experience for beneficiaries. Across both programs, state agencies should ensure staff are trained to minimize stigma associated with receiving benefits and to treat all applicants and beneficiaries with dignity and respect.

Our study has several limitations. As a qualitative study of a low-income English-speaking primary care population in West Philadelphia, we acknowledge that the themes that emerged may not be generalizable to other settings. Although there are national standards for both programs, administration of WIC and SNAP varies widely by state. Health systems and state policymakers should therefore consider conducting similar qualitative studies focused on their own patients and constituents. In addition, future studies should include caregivers who speak languages other than English, because these individuals likely have unique experiences not captured in this study.

CONCLUSIONS

Current and former WIC and SNAP participants suggested several improvements to boost program participation, including reducing stigma in the enrollment process, decreasing administrative burdens in the renewal process, and improved coordination with health care providers. To help close the eligibility/enrollment gap, pediatric providers should consider partnering with local assistance offices and federal and state policymakers to provide health system-based benefits enrollment support, improve data sharing to reduce redundancy for participants, and advocate for WIC and SNAP programmatic improvements.

ACKNOWLEDGMENTS

We thank the network of primary care clinicians and their patients and families for their contributions to this project and to all clinical research facilitated through the Pediatric Research Consortium at Children's Hospital of Philadelphia.

ABBREVIATIONS

SNAP: Supplemental Nutrition Assistance Program
WIC: Special Supplemental Nutrition Program for Women, Infants, and Children

---

FUNDING: Dr Vasan's work on this project was supported by the Academic Pediatric Association (2021 Young Investigator Award) and the Agency for Healthcare Research and Quality (grants F32HS02855 and K08HS029396). Dr Kenyon's work on this project was supported by National Institutes of Health grant K23HL136842. The other authors received no additional funding. The Academic Pediatric Association, the Agency for Healthcare Research and Quality, and National Institutes of Health did not participate in the design or conduct of this study.

CONFLICT OF INTEREST DISCLOSURES: The authors have indicated they have no conflicts of interest to disclose.

REFERENCES

1. Rabbitt MP, Hales LJ, Burke MP, Coleman-Jensen A. US Department of Agriculture Economic Research Service. Household food security in the United States in 2022. Available at: https://www.ers.usda.gov/publications/pub-details/?pubid=107702. Accessed January 2, 2024

2. Biden-Harris. Administration national strategy on hunger, nutrition, and health. Available at: https://www.whitehouse.gov/wp-content/uploads/2022/09/White-House-National-Strategy-on-Hunger-Nutrition-and-Health-FINAL.pdf. Accessed January 2, 2024

3. Venkataramani M, Ogunwole SM, Caulfield LE, et al. Maternal, infant, and child health outcomes associated with the Special Supplemental Nutrition Program for Women, Infants, and Children. *Ann Intern Med.* 2022;175(10):1411–1422

4. Mabli J, Worthington J. Supplemental Nutrition Assistance Program participation and child food security. *Pediatrics.* 2014;133(4):610–619

5. Ettinger de Cuba SA, Bovell-Ammon AR, Cook JT, et al. SNAP, young children's health, and family food security and health care access. *Am J Prev Med.* 2019;57(4):525–532

6. US Department of Agriculture Food and Nutrition Service. National- and state-level estimates of WIC eligibility and program reach in 2021. *Available at:* https://www.fns.usda.gov/research/wic/eligibility-and-program-reach-estimates-2021. Accessed January 2, 2024

7. Cunnyngham K. Empirical Bayes shrinkage estimates of state Supplemental Nutrition Assistance Program participation rates: fiscal year 2018 to fiscal year 2020. Available at: https://fns-prod.azureedge.us/sites/default/files/resource-files/snap-participation-2020-tech-report.pdf. Accessed January 2, 2024

8. Haynes-Maslow L, Hardison-Moody A, Patton-Lopez M, et al. Examining rural food-insecure families' perceptions of the Supplemental Nutrition Assistance Program: a qualitative study. *Int J Environ Res Public Health.* 2020;17(17):6390

9. Robbins S, Ettinger AK, Keefe C, Riley A, Surkan PJ. Low-Income urban mothers' experiences with the Supplemental Nutrition Assistance Program. *J Acad Nutr Diet.* 2017;117(10):1538–1553

10. Lora KR, Hodges L, Ryan C, Ver Ploeg M, Guthrie J. Factors that influence children's exits from the Special Supplemental Nutrition

Program for Women, Infants, and Children: a systematic review. *Nutrients.* 2023;15(3):766

11. Gago CM, Wynne JO, Moore MJ, et al. Caregiver perspectives on underutilization of WIC: a qualitative study. *Pediatrics.* 2022;149(2):e2021053889

12. Panzera AD, Bryant CA, Hawkins F, et al. Mapping a WIC mother's journey: a preliminary analysis. *Soc Mark Q.* 2017;23(2):137–154

13. Weber S, Uesugi K, Greene H, Bess S, Reese L, Odoms-Young A. Preferences and perceived value of WIC foods among WIC caregivers. *J Nutr Educ Behav.* 2018;50(7):695–704

14. Weber SJ, Wichelecki J, Chavez N, Bess S, Reese L, Odoms-Young A. Understanding the factors influencing low-income caregivers' perceived value of a federal nutrition program, the Special Supplemental Nutrition Program for Women, Infants, and Children (WIC). *Public Health Nutr.* 2019;22(6):1056–1065

15. Barnes C, Halpern-Meekin S, Hoiting J. "I used to get WIC … but then I stopped": how WIC participants perceive the value and burdens of maintaining benefits. *RSF.* 2023;9(5):32–55

16. Chauvenet C, De Marco M, Barnes C, Ammerman AS. WIC recipients in the retail environment: a qualitative study assessing customer experience and satisfaction. *J Acad Nutr Diet.* 2019;119(3):416–424.e2

17. US Department of Agriculture Food and Nutrition Service. Leveraging the White House conference to promote and elevate nutrition security: the role of the USDA Food and Nutrition Service. Available at: https://www.fns.usda.gov/nutrition-security/fns-role. Accessed January 2, 2024

18. US Department of Agriculture Food and Nutrition Service. WIC modernization. Available at: https://www.fns.usda.gov/wic/modernization. Accessed January 2, 2024

19. Vasan A, Kenyon CC, Roberto CA, Fiks AG, Venkataramani AS. Association of remote versus in-person benefit delivery with WIC participation during the COVID-19 pandemic. *JAMA.* 2021;326(15):1531–1533

20. Caspi CE, De Marco M, Welle E, et al. A qualitative analysis of SNAP and minimum wage policies as experienced by workers with lower incomes. *J Hunger Environ Nutr.* 2022;17(4):521–539

21. Fiks AG, Grundmeier RW, Margolis B, et al. Comparative effectiveness research using the electronic medical record: an emerging area of investigation in pediatric primary care. *J Pediatr.* 2012;160(5):719–724

22. Vasan A, Negro D, Yazdani M, et al. Caregiver preferences for primary care clinic-based food assistance: a discrete choice experiment. *Acad Pediatr.* 2024;24(4):619–626

23. Tong A, Sainsbury P, Craig J. Consolidated criteria for reporting qualitative research (COREQ): a 32-item checklist for interviews and focus groups. *Int J Qual Health Care.* 2007;19(6):349–357

24. Mays N, Pope C. Assessing quality in qualitative research. *BMJ.* 2000;320(7226):50–52

25. Glaser BG. The constant comparative method of qualitative analysis. *Soc Probl.* 1965;12(4):436–445

26. O'Connor C, Joffe H. Intercoder reliability in qualitative research: debates and practical guidelines. *Int J Qual Methods.* 2020;19:160940691989922

27. Saunders B, Sim J, Kingstone T, et al. Saturation in qualitative research: exploring its conceptualization and operationalization. *Qual Quant.* 2018;52(4):1893–1907

28. Braun V, Clarke V. To saturate or not to saturate? Questioning data saturation as a useful concept for thematic analysis and sample-size rationales. *Qual Res Sport Exerc Health.* 2021;13(2):201–216

29. Kenney EL, Soto MJ, Fubini M, Carleton A, Lee M, Bleich SN. Simplification of Supplemental Nutrition Assistance Program recertification processes and association with uninterrupted access to benefits among participants with young children. *JAMA Netw Open.* 2022;5(9):e2230150

30. Gray C. Leaving benefits on the table: evidence from SNAP. *J Public Econ.* 2019;179:104054

31. Monroe BS, Rengifo LM, Wingler MR, et al. Assessing and improving WIC enrollment in the primary care setting: a quality initiative. *Pediatrics.* 2023;152(2):e2022057613

32. Bailey-Davis L, Kling SMR, Cochran WJ, et al. Integrating and coordinating care between the Women, Infants, and Children Program and pediatricians to improve patient-centered preventive care for healthy growth. *Transl Behav Med.* 2018;8(6):944–952

33. Morris G, Bailey-Davis L, Cochran W, et al. Perceptions about care coordination between pediatricians and Women, Infants and Children (WIC) for early childhood obesity prevention. *Pediatrics.* 2018;141(1_MeetingAbstract):590

34. Kling SM, Harris HA, Marini M, et al. Advanced health information technologies to engage parents, clinicians, and community nutritionists in coordinating responsive parenting care: descriptive case series of the women, infants, and children enhancements to Early Healthy Lifestyles for Baby (WEE Baby) Care Randomized Controlled Trial. *JMIR Pediatr Parent.* 2020;3(2):e22121

35. Goldstein B, Steiner A, Vander Wielen L, Bennett K, Tomcho M. Integration of Special Supplemental Nutrition Program for Woman, Infants, and Children (WIC) in primary care settings. *J Community Health.* 2024;49(2):330–337

36. Dalembert G, Fiks AG, O'Neill G, Rosin R, Jenssen BP. Impacting poverty with medical financial partnerships focused on tax incentives. *NEJM Catal.* 2021;2(4)

37. Bell ON, Hole MK, Johnson K, Marcil LE, Solomon BS, Schickedanz A. Medical–financial partnerships: cross-sector collaborations between medical and financial services to improve health. *Acad Pediatr.* 2020;20(2):166–174

38. Vasan A, Beatty B, DiFiore G, et al. Connecting families to benefit programs through a standardized nutrition screener. *Ann Fam Med.* 2024;22(3):259

39. Federal Register. Special Supplemental Nutrition Program for Women, Infants, and Children (WIC): revisions in the WIC food packages. Available at: https://www.federalregister.gov/documents/2024/04/18/2024-07437/special-supplemental-nutrition-program-for-

women-infants-and-children-wic-revisions-in-the-wic-food. Accessed July 8, 2024

40. Ventura AK, Martinez CE, Whaley SE. WIC participants' perceptions of COVID-19–related changes to WIC recertification and service delivery. *J Community Health*. 2022;47(2): 184–192

41. Zhang Q, Zhang J, Park K, Tang C. App usage associated with full redemption of WIC food benefits: a propensity score approach. *J Nutr Educ Behav*. 2021;53(9):779–786

42. Zhang Q, Zhang J, Park K, Tang C. Association between usage of an app to redeem prescribed food benefits and redemption behaviors among the Special Supplemental Nutrition Program for Women, Infants, and Children participants: cross-sectional study. *JMIR Mhealth Uhealth*. 2020;8(10):e20720

43. US Department of Agriculture Food and Nutrition Service. USDA modernizes the Thrifty Food Plan, updates SNAP benefits. Available at: https://www.fns.usda.gov/news-item/usda-0179.21. Accessed January 10, 2024

44. US Senator Cory Booker of New Jersey. Booker, Rubio introduce bipartisan SNAP legislation to measure and improve nutrition security and diet quality. Available at: https://www.booker.senate. gov/news/press/booker-rubio-introduce-bipartisan-snap-legislation-to-measure-and-improve-nutrition-security-and-diet-quality. Accessed March 4, 2024

Caregiver Perspectives on Underutilization of WIC: A Qualitative Study

Cristina M. Gago, MPH,[a] Jhordan O. Wynne, MPH,[a] Maggie J. Moore, MS,[a] Alejandra Cantu-Aldana, MD,[a] Kelsey Vercammen, PhD, MSc,[b] Laura Y. Zatz, ScD, MPH,[a,c] Kelley May, MPH,[d] Tina Andrade,[d] Terri Mendoza,[d] Sarah L. Stone, PhD,[d] Josiemer Mattei, PhD,[a] Kirsten K. Davison, PhD,[e] Eric B. Rimm, ScD,[a,b,f] Rachel Colchamiro, MPH,[d] Erica L. Kenney, ScD[a]

OBJECTIVES: The Special Supplemental Nutrition Program for Women, Infants, and Children (WIC) is a federal program that improves the health of low-income women (pregnant and postpartum) and children up to 5 years of age in the United States. However, participation is suboptimal. We explored reasons for incomplete redemption of benefits and early dropout from WIC.

METHODS: In 2020–2021, we conducted semistructured interviews to explore factors that influenced WIC program utilization among current WIC caregivers ($n = 20$) and caregivers choosing to leave while still eligible ($n = 17$) in Massachusetts. By using a deductive analytic approach, we developed a codebook grounded in the Consolidated Framework for Implementation Research.

RESULTS: Themes across both current and early-leaving participants included positive feelings about social support from the WIC clinic staff and savings offered through the food package. Participants described reduced satisfaction related to insufficient funds for fruits and vegetables, food benefits inflexibility, concerns about in-clinic health tests, and in-store item mislabeling. Participants described how electronic benefit transfer cards and smartphone apps eased the use of benefits and reduced stigma during shopping. Some participants attributed leaving early to a belief that they were taking benefits from others.

CONCLUSIONS: Current and early-leaving participants shared positive WIC experiences, but barriers to full participation exist. Food package modification may lead to improved redemption and retention, including increasing the cash value benefit for fruits and vegetables and diversifying food options. Research is needed regarding the misperception that participation means "taking" benefits away from someone else in need.

abstract

Full article can be found online at www.pediatrics.org/cgi/doi/10.1542/peds.2021-053889

Departments of [a]Nutrition, [b]Epidemiology, and [c]Social and Behavioral Sciences, Harvard T.H. Chan School of Public Health, Boston, Massachusetts; [d]Massachusetts Department of Public Health, Boston, Massachusetts; [f]Channing Division of Network Medicine, Brigham and Women's Hospital, Harvard Medical School, Boston, Massachusetts; and [e]School of Social Work, Boston College, Chestnut Hill, Massachusetts

Ms Gago conceptualized and designed the study, designed the data collection instruments, coordinated and supervised data collection, collected data, contributed to the primary and secondary rounds of coding, designed and revised the codebook, drafted the initial manuscript, and reviewed and revised the manuscript; Ms Wynne contributed to the primary and secondary rounds of coding, reviewed and revised the codebook, contributed to data interpretation and theme development, and reviewed and revised the manuscript; Ms Moore coordinated and supervised data collection, collected data, contributed to the primary and secondary rounds of coding, reviewed and revised the codebook, contributed to data interpretation and theme development, and reviewed and revised the manuscript; Dr Cantu-Aldana collected data, contributed to the primary and secondary rounds of coding, reviewed and revised the codebook, interpreted data, contributed to theme development, and reviewed and revised the manuscript; Drs Vercammen and Zatz conceptualized and designed the study, critically reviewed

WHAT IS KNOWN ON THIS SUBJECT Previous research suggests several factors contribute to early drop-out, including dissatisfaction with the food package, reduction in food benefit value at the child's first birthday, lack of time and transportation to access appointments, common misconceptions around eligibility, and cultural barriers.

WHAT THIS STUDY ADDS No researchers have examined or compared the facilitators and barriers identified by both current and early-leaving, though eligible, WIC caregivers after the implementation of novel innovations to facilitate shopping and clinical experiences.

To cite: Gago CM, Wynne JO, Moore MJ, et al. Caregiver Perspectives on Underutilization of WIC: A Qualitative Study. *Pediatrics.* 2022;149(2):e2021053889

ARTICLE

The Special Supplemental Nutrition Program for Women, Infants, and Children (WIC) is a federal nutrition program that provides millions of low-income women, infants, and children with nutrition education, breastfeeding support, and health care services.[1] WIC also provides benefits in the form of either paper vouchers or electronic benefits transfer (EBT) cards, which act like debit cards for purchase of eligible foods from WIC-approved retailers.[2] The quantity and type of foods in each food package depend on participant age and stage but generally include staple foods, such as milk, whole grains, and fruits and vegetables (F&V).

Although 14 million people are eligible for WIC, less than half are enrolled.[3] Of those enrolled, many do not use the full extent of services offered.[4,5] Suboptimal retention and redemption patterns reveal that many participants face barriers to full participation.[4,5] Underutilization of WIC[3] is a pediatric health concern, given the well-documented benefits of WIC for nutrition,[6,7] health,[8] cognition,[9] and access to care[10–13] during an important developmental period.[14,15] An urgent need exists to identify opportunities to better facilitate participation.

Previous researchers have attributed suboptimal engagement to dissatisfaction with the WIC food package[16,17]; lack of time,[18,19] transportation,[20] and/or childcare for appointments[18,21]; increased income[19,22]; linguistic barriers[23]; and misinformation.[24,25] However, most studies on early termination and low redemption were conducted before the 2009 food package update,[26] which, among many changes, added F&V and whole grains to better align with the Dietary Guidelines for Americans.[27] Most studies also preceded recent changes to program delivery,

including the introduction, in many states, of electronic tools like EBT cards and smartphone shopping apps,[17–19,21,22] which can be used in stores to scan and identify WIC-eligible products. Furthermore, few researchers have investigated the perspectives of families who dropped out of the program early despite still being eligible. By using the Consolidated Framework for Implementation Research (CFIR),[28] we documented the perspectives of current WIC enrollees and those who dropped out of the program early to identify key aspects of program structure and delivery that may be related to program underutilization.[3,20]

METHODS

Study Design

This qualitative study was conducted in Massachusetts in partnership with the state WIC office, which served ~110 000 to 113 000 individuals in a given month during the study period (August 2020 to January 2021).[29] We spoke to caregivers of WIC-eligible children under the age of 5 years who were currently enrolled in WIC (current participants) or recently (ie, 6–24 months before the date of the interview) chose to leave WIC for reasons other than ineligibility (early-leaving participants). To participate in this study, caregivers also had to be age >18 years; live in Massachusetts; speak English, Spanish, or Portuguese; have a WIC-eligible child under the age of 5 years; and have participated in WIC for at least 6 months.

Recruitment

Study flyers were as the primary method of recruitment; directors of local WIC clinic and community organizations (eg, Head Start, libraries, pantries, schools) posted electronic flyers to their social

media sites and newsletters. We also posted paper flyers at the end of checkout lanes and diaper aisles in grocery stores that accept WIC. The Massachusetts WIC office used administrative records to identify early-leaving caregivers and mailed them a study flyer. We screened 62 caregivers, spanning urban and rural Massachusetts, of whom 41 were eligible and 21 ineligible (Fig 1). Of the 41 eligible caregivers, 4 withdrew and 37 were interviewed (20 current participants, 17 early-leaving participants) between August 2020 and January 2021.

Semistructured Interviews and Online Demographic Survey

Underutilization is an undesirable outcome of program implementation. We used an implementation science perspective to consider multiple levels of WIC's implementation—its structure and delivery—that may affect program utilization. Informed by CFIR[28] and previous investigations into determinants of poor redemption and retention,[16,19,30–34] we developed a demographic survey (Supplemental Data 1 and 2) and interview guide (Supplemental Data 3 and 4). Areas of inquiry, including general WIC experience, food benefits, WIC at home, shopping experiences, and appropriateness of WIC in context, were mapped onto CFIR constructs[28] and thus organized into intervention characteristics, process, and outer setting (Fig 2). Trained qualitative researchers conducted and audio recorded 45-minute phone interviews with current ($n = 20$) and early-leaving ($n = 17$) participants in English, Spanish, and Portuguese. Before each interview, caregivers were asked to complete the anonymous online demographic survey (18 current participants; 17 early-leaving participants). After completing the survey and the

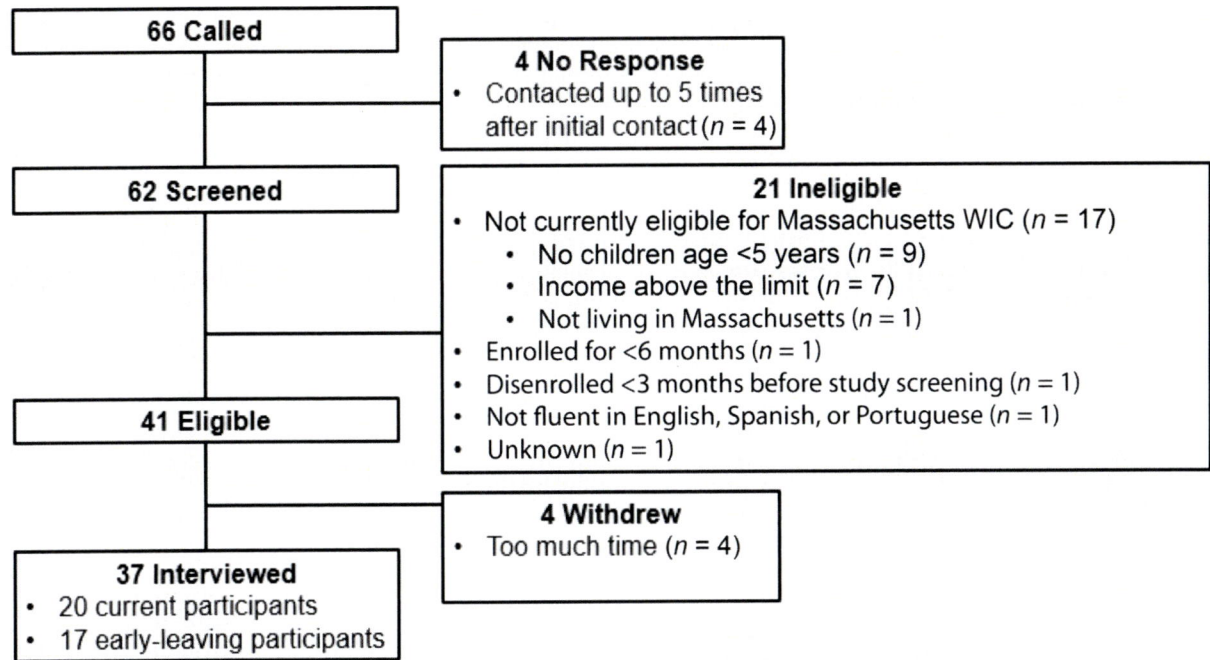

FIGURE 1
Flow diagram documenting recruitment and enrollment.

Analysis

The short demographic survey data were downloaded as a comma-separated values file from Qualtrics. We used Excel to calculate the frequency of responses for each question, stratified by WIC enrollment status. We ran χ^2 tests to examine differences by WIC enrollment status.

The interviews were audio recorded and transcribed verbatim. English and Spanish transcripts were analyzed in their original languages; Portuguese transcripts were professionally translated to English for analysis. All quotes included in the article have been translated into English; illustrative quotes (Table 2) were selected through a final review of all codes after theme generation. Before analysis, C.M.G. created a preliminary codebook, deductively informed by CFIR, with codes

related to the 5 main CFIR constructs listed above.

Trained qualitative researchers (C.M.G., J.O.W., M.J.M., and A.C.-A.) were involved in developing the guides and conducting the interviews. In their collection, analysis, and interpretation of the data, these researchers brought salient identities, including, but not limited to, their gender, race and ethnicity, language preference, and family composition. C.M.G. is white Hispanic American, bilingual (English and Spanish), and childless. M.J.M. is white American and a native English speaker; she has biological and stepchildren aged 2 to 24 years. A.C.-A. is white Mexican, bilingual (Spanish and English), and childless. J.O.W. is Black American, native English and proficient Spanish speaker, childless, and a former child recipient of WIC.

Current and early-leaving participant transcripts were coded independently before theme

generation, allowing for potential differences in codes to inductively arise for current versus early-leaving participants, should different codes prove relevant to each sample. Given that similar codes were identified for the 2 groups, a single codebook was used with all codes applicable to both groups, although themes were generated separately among current versus early-leaving participants. Next, researchers independently coded the same 3 transcripts, met over video to compare codes, arrived at an agreement on differing codes through discussion, and updated the codebook to address inconsistencies (Supplemental Table 4). This revision involved no conceptual changes but rather clarification of specifics and collapse of redundant or unnecessary codes. Seven of the remaining transcripts were double coded by 2 independent reviewers for comparison to ensure consistency in coding using the updated codebook; subsequently, the team met to reconcile differences and reach agreement through

FIGURE 2
Conceptual framework informed by the CFIR: why does WIC exhibit suboptimal implementation?

discussion.[35,36] All coding differences were due to the representation of multiple codes in 1 segment; no conceptual differences in code meaning were noted. With confidence that coding was conceptually consistent across the research team, the remaining 28 transcripts were coded by single reviewers; all uncertainties were brought to the coding team for agreement through video discussion. NVivo version 12 (QSR International) was used to organize and analyze coded data.

RESULTS

Sample Characteristics

Most of our sample was female (97%), age >30 years (70%), with up to 3 children ($n = 30$, 86%;

Table 1). Participants were most likely to identify as Hispanic (63%) and white (47%). Approximately half joined WIC before 2014 (43%) and were referred by their doctor (51%). Compared with early-leaving participants, significantly more current participants identified as Hispanic (67% vs 59%), married (78% vs 35%), enrolled before 2014 (59% vs 23%), and never enrolled in the Supplemental Nutrition Assistance Program (SNAP; 61% vs 29%). Fewer current participants reported being recipients of formula through WIC either presently or in the past (22% vs 82%).

Theme 1: F&V Benefits Are Insufficient

A key theme that arose in both current and early-leaving

participants was related to the package's perceived value, which is characterized as an "intervention characteristic" critical to implementation success (Fig 2). Regardless of enrollment status, caregivers reported general satisfaction with the food benefits package (Table 2). Caregivers unanimously reported that WIC performed well at "covering the basics," such as milk, eggs, and bread. F&V were among the most important offerings; many reported buying and consuming more F&V over time. Some even mentioned that the F&V allowance was the main motivation for continued enrollment. However, most caregivers found the cash value benefit to be insufficient, set at $11 per month in Massachusetts per

TABLE 1 Sample Characteristics of Participants Currently or Previously Enrolled (ie, Early-Leaving) in WIC, 2020–2021 ($n = 37$)

	Participants			P^c
	Total ($n = 35$)	Current ($n = 18$)[a]	Early-leaving ($n = 17$)[b]	
Demographics and socioeconomic status				
Interview language				.6
English	46	40	53	
Spanish	38	45	29	
Portuguese	16	15	18	
Age, years[d]				.2
18–29	29	17	44	
30–34	32	39	25	
35–44	38	44	31	
Race[d]				.9
Black	18	18	18	
White	47	47	47	
Other	35	35	35	
Hispanic (vs not)	63	67	59	.04
Completed high school (vs not)[e]	73	67	80	.4
Employed (vs other)[f]	43	27	60	.07
SNAP				.02
Currently enrolled	34	33	35	
Enrolled in the past	14	6	24	
Never enrolled	46	61	29	
Food insecure (vs not)[g]	49	39	59	.2
Household				
Married (vs not)[h]	57	78	35	.01
Number of children at home				.1
1	31	17	47	
2	31	33	29	
≥3	37	50	24	
History with WIC				
First enrolled before 2014	43	59	23	.05
Referred by a doctor (vs other)	51	44	59	.3
Knew someone in WIC before joining	59	50	69	.3
Told others about WIC since joining	86	83	88	.7
Receive(d) formula (vs no)	51	22	82	<.001

Shown are the frequencies as percentages. Because of missing data, some categories may not sum to 100% of the study sample.

[a] Two participants (current WIC caregivers) chose not to complete the anonymous demographic survey; additionally, 1–2 participants chose not to respond to specific survey questions, including those on race, employment status, and date of first enrollment.

[b] One to 4 early-leaving participants chose not to respond to specific survey questions, including those on age, educational attainment, employment status, food security, date of first enrollment in WIC, and whether they knew someone in WIC before joining.

[c] Significant differences by WIC enrollment status (current or early-leaving) were determined from χ^2 tests.

[d] Options included Black or African American, white, American Indian, Asian American, multiracial/multiethnic, and other (open response).

[e] Options included less than a high school degree, high school degree or equivalent, some college but no degree, associate degree, bachelor's degree, and graduate degree.

[f] Options included employed and working part time, employed and working full time, unemployed, and prefer not to say. Prefer not to say was counted as missing.

[g] Those who responded agreed to 1 or both of the following questions included in the food insecure frequency: (1) Since the start of the COVID-19 pandemic (February 2020), we worried about whether our food would run out before we got money to buy more (may not add up to 20 because of missing data or incomplete surveys) and/or (2) since the start of the COVID-19 pandemic (February 2020), the food we bought just did not last, and we did not have money to get more.

[h] Those who reported living with a partner were included in the married frequency.

woman and child (age 1–5 years) at the time of the interviews. Although struggling to acquire enough F&V each month, caregivers reported an overabundance of other benefits (eg, dairy, cereal). Early-leaving participants were also more likely to report receiving formula and commented on its high financial value.

Theme 2: Food Benefits' Inflexibility Prevents Full Redemption

The low adaptability of the food package (in relation to allergies, cultural appropriateness, and individual preferences) also arose as a key barrier to successful implementation (Fig 2). Participants reported challenges in acquiring proof of allergies, and many paid for alternatives out of pocket. Additionally, some immigrants in our sample cited unprocessed whole grains (alongside F&V) as culturally appropriate and foundational and argued that WIC does not offer enough quantity and variety. Individual preferences were most often reported in relation to dislike of dairy, yogurt flavors, and whole-

TABLE 2 Illustrative Quotations Stratified by WIC Current and Early-Leaving Participants

	Current Participants	Early-Leaving Participants
Theme 1: F&V benefits are insufficient.		
Insufficient F&V	"It gives about 10%. For example, they pay $11 for fruits and vegetables ... [but] I spend more than that every time." (record 19)	"They give you $11 worth of fruits and vegetables, but that was all that I was using ... I didn't think it was worth it." (record 65)
	"I just asked if we could get more money like allowance for actual fruit or veggies ... they gave me 4 more dollars for fruits and...it's not enough." (record 7)	"We did buy the veggies, but it's not [a] big amount ... we always bought more than that...we want more veggies." (record 72)
Theme 2: Food benefits' inflexibility prevents full redemption.		
Benefits' inflexibility	"They just don't give you a lot of alternatives ... even if it's for another healthy [food]." (record 19)	"[I want for WIC] to give a little bit more freedom for a different kind of bread ... so you can use it." (record 59)
Allergies	"WIC didn't want to change his milk because it was a special formula, even with the form from the doctor asking for a new formula." (record 21)	"I told them that it wasn't working, that my son was allergic, and ... I had to take what they gave me." (record 71)
Preferences	"But it's a personal preference. I prefer to have almond milk over Lactaid." (record 17)	"I just noticed a lot of the benefits that they were offering, I wasn't really using, so I slowly just stopped using them." (record 65)
Cultures	"One of the foods that we have missed the most ... [was] our Brazilian rice, Tio João ... these things, we pay them in cash." (record 21)	"We're not from US originally ... [and] the way we cook and the meals we are used to are a little different from American." (record 71)
Theme 3: EBT cards and smartphone apps improve the shopping experience; however, in-store item mislabeling is still linked with embarrassment at checkout.		
EBT cards	"I think it's a lot easier because I was around with my older kids when they had the paper checks. So, I think it's a lot easier." (record 13)	"I was more embarrassed that it would take so much time when it was the ... checks and ... this time around I was like, 'Oh my God, it's like a credit card.'" (record 27)
Smartphone shopping apps	"The app keeps track of what is left for the month. It reminds ... so [you can] try to use up whatever you have left." (record 14)	"The app was the best thing ever." (record 69)
Checkout	"I was having trouble at the register, and I tried like 4 different stores [which is] like a lot of work for the employees as well." (record 14)	"It was always a problem ... and it's embarrassing ... are you going to leave all your stuff and go find the right one?" (record 31)
Theme 4: Both current and early-leaving participants reported positive clinical experiences; however, barriers to care were more often reported by early-leaving participants.		
Positive experience	"I don't have any bad experiences; I've had really good ones. I feel like it helps me." (record 24)	"The service is good, the communication is good, the support is good, the help is good. There are no complaints." (record 62)
Wait times	"The appointments were quick." (record 21)	"They ended up taking their walk-ins before their scheduled appointments." (record 65)
Ability to reschedule	"I am close to the WIC office, and they have availability and everything ... it has been easy for me." (record 10)	"Let's say if I missed 1 appointment, it will cost me the whole month because I will get the other appointment in 3 weeks." (record 53)
Recertification	"I don't think it's difficult to apply for WIC if you're qualified." (record 25)	"I feel like they should've been more understanding ... [and] given me more time [to gather the required documents]." (record 31)
Theme 5: Caregivers will not accept benefits that they do not need.		
Consideration of need	"I use it because I need it. And it helps out a lot." (record 24)	"I am lucky enough to be blessed enough with having a mom that was able to help me with everything ... I wouldn't want to take away from somebody else if they needed it more than I do." (record 69)
	"But if I had a better job, if my financial situation was better, I wouldn't use it because I'm not the kind of person that just wants things for free if you're not in need." (record 25)	"I don't really need it because I get food stamps. When I did run out of milk and stuff like that and the eggs, WIC was that backup." (record 62)

wheat bread. As a result of benefits' limited acceptability, caregivers wasted food, shared extras with others, and left benefits unspent.

Theme 3: EBT Cards and Smartphone Apps Improve the Shopping Experience; However, In-Store Item Mislabeling Is Still Linked With Embarrassment at Checkout

Electronic tools have proved invaluable to the process of WIC service delivery. Participants reported positive experiences with paying with EBT cards and using smartphone shopping apps to identify eligible items and available benefits (Table 2). Those with older children reflected on the fundamental change they experienced while transitioning from paper vouchers to EBT cards, reporting reductions in stigma, administrative burden, and stress. Embarrassment was still reported, with checkout challenges resulting from in-store label mistakes (ie, products were labeled as "WIC eligible" when they were not). Almost all caregivers used smartphone shopping apps; those who did not use them blamed poor in-store Internet access/cell service, which prevented access to pictures and label scanning.

Theme 4: Both Current and Early-Leaving Participants Reported Positive Clinical Experiences; However, Barriers to Care Were More Often Reported by Early-Leaving Participants

Almost all participants reported positive clinical experiences (Table 2). Only current participants reported having a specific advocate at their local clinic (ie, someone they trusted and had gotten to know over time). These advocates or "champions" emerged as a critical catalyst for promoting better retention by building and maintaining trust with their assigned WIC caregivers. This important resource is part of WIC's implementation process (Fig 2). WIC participants who were aware of the

clinical, therapeutic, and nutritional services offered rated them highly; however, many were not aware that these services are universally provided. Most negative feedback, usually cited by early-leaving participants, was related to administrative barriers, including lack of clarity in requirements for certification, challenges rescheduling appointments, long wait times, and challenges with transportation to and from appointments. In response, some participants requested that appointments move online to save time and avoid transportation issues; others requested the opportunity to submit recertification paperwork online to avoid issues on appointment day. Several early-leaving participants also described clinical requirements as unnecessary, redundant, and/or burdensome; examples included WIC staff repeating clinic measurements when they may be available through records offered by pediatricians, testing iron levels, and requesting child vaccination records.

Theme 5: Caregivers Will Not Accept Benefits That They Do Not Need

Consideration of participant needs and resources is essential for successful implementation (Fig 2). When enrolling, current and early-leaving WIC caregivers made a clear distinction between eligibility for WIC and need for WIC benefits. Those who believed that WIC was unnecessary stopped recertifying, regardless of whether they were still eligible (Table 2). In their definition of need (described as fluid and transient), current participants often cited employment, housing, social services (eg, SNAP), partnership stability, immigration status, and food security as less stable compared with early-leaving participants. Participants also defined need as a concept relative to those around them; some reported leaving, or considering leaving, out of fear that participation would take resources from someone more in

need. Of those who identified a sense of need, some paired it with feelings of shame, which they described as being related to a lack of self-sufficiency and as being highly visible to others.

DISCUSSION

Our study was one of the first to examine the perspectives of both current WIC caregivers and those who were eligible but left the program early. Previous studies were largely limited to the current caregiver experience,[16,37,38] with that of the early-leaving caregivers nearly absent from the peer-reviewed literature. Informed by CFIR, we studied WIC implementation to identify unique opportunities to promote service adoption. We identified key themes across different levels of the WIC experience, many of which were consistent with earlier literature. Study participants were disappointed by the insufficiency of F&V benefits[16,30] and described low adaptability of the food package,[16] high satisfaction with WIC technologies,[39] and positive feelings toward clinic staff.[31] Current and early-leaving participants differed in their level of satisfaction with clinical services, perceived level of need, and degree of social connection with WIC staff.

Study participants reported a link between their perceptions of the benefits' value, acceptability, and appropriateness and their own redemption behaviors and retention in the program. Consistent with previous literature stating that formula is a key driver of participation during infancy,[34] the early-leaving participants were much more likely to report formula receipt during their period of enrollment and commented on the financial incentive to continue enrollment through infancy for that reason. Low package adaptability meant that participants were unable to make desired modifications to fit their needs. The US Department of Agriculture (USDA) should consider increasing food package flexibility,[16] beyond the current substitutions allowed through waivers[40] or medical documentation,[41] while maintaining healthful standards. WIC may be able to diversify food package options on the basis of patterns derived from redemption data and cultural preferences.[16] Perceived value may increase through an expansion of the monthly F&V allowance. Study participants were clear: $11 per month for F&V is not enough. The temporary increase to $35 per month, as part of the American Rescue Plan of 2021, should be evaluated and, if successful, made permanent, as it could encourage greater availability of F&V at local retailers[42] and consumption among participants.[43–48]

Improving shopping and checkout experiences is also important; EBT cards and smartphone shopping apps have proved invaluable in this regard. Common complaints about the shopping experience were related to transaction errors at checkout,[49,50] followed by limited in-store selection.[33,38,51–54] The USDA should continue to invest in EBT cards[50] and smartphone shopping apps,[39] which have led to increased redemption and reduced in-store stigma.[50] To address adoption challenges and to optimize app use, WIC staff may continue to offer enrollees ongoing technical assistance; however, careful consideration must be given to the potential to exacerbate inequities for participants without access to smartphones. Additional recommendations offered by study participants include training grocery store staff on WIC-approved items, creating in-store spaces to highlight approved items, and developing peer-to-peer learning spaces for caregivers to share shopping strategies with one another.

Most participants (even early-leavers) cited positive experiences with their WIC clinic; however, only current participants could name a specific in-clinic champion. WIC clinics may help to foster consistency and familiarity in care by scheduling families with the same nutrition staff member for each appointment. WIC agencies can use this good rapport to better engage caregivers with resources and services beyond the food benefits, such as lactation consultations, nutrition education, and cooking demonstrations. Although these services are delivered to all WIC participants, many did not recognize or highly value service receipt. Those who acknowledged these as "services," as opposed to "requirements," seemed to rank them highly.

Caregivers who cited a high degree of coordination between their doctor and the WIC clinic reported higher in-clinic satisfaction; those who rated their in-clinic services poorly did so out of frustration with clinical requirements, which they regarded as unnecessary or repetitive (eg, iron testing, assessment of child vaccination records). Key areas for improvement include offering a clear explanation for the need and utility behind these requirements and streamlining health record data transfer between pediatricians and WIC clinics.[55] Health care providers are also in the position to offer careful communication around WIC eligibility, perceived need, and potential for financial security, with obstetrician and pediatrician's offices serving as a caregiver's first point of contact with WIC.

WIC leaders should also consider continuing to build on technologies that support remote[56] nutrition service delivery (eg, online nutrition education, telehealth) while still promoting the development of

personal relationships by assigning families the same nutrition staff member for each appointment. By building off lessons, WIC administrators have learned through the past year of implementing COVID-19 waivers that a need exists to support flexibility in child nutrition authorization tied to physical presence requirements.

Even with significant advancements in the shopping experience, caregivers still reported shame with the acceptance of assistance, as has been documented for decades.[20] As with previous studies,[16,57,58] many in our sample justified WIC as a temporary service—something to leave as soon as possible to allow room for others. Addressing misperceptions about availability and eligibility, limiting barriers to entry, reducing administrative burden,[59,60] and expanding eligibility[61–63] are key strategies that warrant future research. Although caregivers reported leaving to open space for others more in need, the early-leaving participants reported high rates of food insecurity and continued enrollment in SNAP; therefore, additional examination of the relationship between perceived need and the decision to disenroll from WIC is needed.

The present study has several strengths. Our research team is one of the first to summarize the feedback of both current and eligible, although early-leaving, WIC caregivers. Our timing provided the opportunity to examine the effects of several recent innovations, including increased uptake of EBT cards and smartphone shopping apps. Although these changes likely had an impact on retention,[50] the extent of that impact is not yet fully reflected in the literature. Remote data collection methods also allowed us to reach caregivers from across the state, spanning rural and urban clinics.

TABLE 3 Actionable Recommendations Addressing Key Facilitators and Barriers to Full Program Participation, as Described by Current and Early-Leaving Participants

Theme	Recommendations
Theme 1: F&V benefits are too small.	At a national level, USDA should consider increasing the F&V allowance. More broadly, the USDA should consider expanding the food package flexibility, while keeping the program's focus on nutritional adequacy.
Theme 2: Food benefit inflexibility prevents full redemption.	
Theme 3: Electronic tools improve the shopping experience.	EBT cards[50] and WIC smartphone apps[39] have increased redemption and reduced in-store stigma.[50] WIC should continue investing in these technologies, which make benefits use easier.
Theme 4: Clinical and administrative requirements can be burdensome.	WIC leaders could consider promoting stronger relationships between WIC caregivers and staff, making more services and administrative processes available remotely,[56] and streamlining health record data transfer between pediatricians and clinics.
Theme 5: Caregivers will disenroll early if not in need.	At time of referral and recertification, health care providers can offer careful communication around WIC eligibility, perceived need, and potential for financial security.[65] In terms of policy, expansion or universalization of eligibility[61] (eg, Community Eligibility Provision[62,63]) may reduce barriers to entry and help to shift public perception around government assistance.

Because the timing of our study (August 2020 to January 2021) was during the COVID-19 pandemic, some limitations were introduced. Participants may have had difficulty separating their experiences with WIC during COVID-19 from their experiences before, although interviewers offered reminders to think about prepandemic experiences. Limitations to the representativeness and generalizability of our findings may be associated with our relatively small sample size, common in qualitative research, and sampling from Massachusetts, where WIC coverage is higher than the national average. However, examination of national- and state-level data[3,64] revealed that our sample of current WIC caregivers is relatively representative, and many of our findings are consistent with those from studies conducted in other states.[16,57,58] Finally, social desirability bias may have been introduced by our format; to counter this, interviewers started each interview by emphasizing that there were no wrong answers.

The possible demographic differences between the current and early-leaving caregivers warrant additional research to better understand their role in WIC retention. Investigators should explore communication strategies to mitigate the comparison of relative need, which may be a barrier to enrollment. An urgent need exists for implementation and evaluation of reform at the policy, retail, and clinic level to combat barriers to redemption and retention, including low acceptability and flexibility of the food benefits, mixed feelings about clinical requirements, and administrative barriers to maintaining appointments (Table 3).

CONCLUSIONS

Our study team is one of the first to describe the experiences of both current and early-leaving WIC caregivers. The findings reveal that caregivers highly value F&V benefits, desire more autonomy in food choices, benefit from social connectedness with clinic staff, and prefer more opportunities to fulfill administrative requirements remotely. Some participants who left early did so because they believed that they would free their spot for someone more in need. Providers who refer families to WIC, such as obstetricians and pediatricians, may help to shift understanding around WIC eligibility by communicating that there are enough benefits for everyone who is eligible; improved care coordination with WIC clinics may also facilitate continued enrollment.

ACKNOWLEDGMENTS

We thank all the caregivers who shared their voices and feedback with us; they are essential contributors in the movement to continue improving services for future WIC families. We also thank all WIC clinic staff members and clinicians who work tirelessly to serve families nationally. This study was made possible by the invaluable efforts of our trained qualitative interviewers, Fernanda Antunes and Vivian Ortiz.

ABBREVIATIONS

CFIR: Consolidated Framework for Implementation Research
EBT: electronic benefits transfer
F&V: fruits and vegetables
SNAP: Supplemental Nutrition Assistance Program
USDA: US Department of Agriculture
WIC: Special Supplemental Nutrition Program for Women, Infants, and Children

and revised the data collection instruments, and reviewed and revised the manuscript; Ms May and Dr Stone conceptualized and designed the study, critically reviewed and revised the data collection instruments, coordinated contact and communication with partners at local clinics, and reviewed and revised the manuscript; Ms Andrade, Ms Mendoza, and Drs Mattei and Davison critically reviewed the manuscript for important intellectual content; Drs Rimm and Kenney and Ms Colchamiro conceptualized and designed the study, reviewed and revised the data collection instruments, supervised data collection and analysis, and critically reviewed the manuscript for important intellectual content; and all authors approved the final manuscript as submitted and agree to be accountable for all aspects of the work.

DOI: https://doi.org/10.1542/peds.2021-053889

Accepted for publication Oct 28, 2021

Address correspondence to Erica L. Kenney, ScD, Department of Nutrition, Harvard T.H. Chan School of Public Health, 677 Huntington Ave, Boston, MA 02115. E-mail: ekenney@hsph.harvard.edu

PEDIATRICS (ISSN Numbers: Print, 0031-4005; Online, 1098-4275).

Copyright © 2022 by the American Academy of Pediatrics

FINANCIAL DISCLOSURE: The authors have indicated they have no financial relationships relevant to this article to disclose.

FUNDING: This work was supported by Harvard Catalyst | The Harvard Clinical and Translational Science Center (National Center for Advancing Translational Sciences, National Institutes of Health award UL 1TR002541) and financial contributions from Harvard University and its affiliated academic health care centers. The content is solely the responsibility of the authors and does not represent the official views of Harvard Catalyst, Harvard University and its affiliated academic health care centers, or the National Institutes of Health. Ms Gago was supported by the Harvard T32 Education Program in Cancer Prevention (training grant 5T32CA057711) from the National Institutes of Health. Dr Vercammen was supported by a Canadian Institute of Health Research doctoral foreign study award (0492002603). The Harvard Catalyst grant provided feedback on the initial proposal via consultation with a Community Advocacy Board. The National Institutes of Health and the Canadian Institute of Health Research had no role in the design and conduct of the study. Funded by the National Institutes of Health (NIH).

POTENTIAL CONFLICT OF INTEREST: The authors have indicated they have no potential conflicts of interest to disclose.

REFERENCES

1. Food and Nutrition Service, US Department of Agriculture. About WIC. Available from: https://www.fns.usda.gov/wic/about-wic. Accessed February 22, 2021

2. Food and Nutrition Service, US Department of Agriculture. WIC Food Packages - Regulatory Requirements for WIC-Eligible Foods. Available from: https://www.fns.usda.gov/wic/wic-food-packages-regulatory-requirements-wic-eligible-foods. Accessed February 22, 2021

3. Food and Nutrition Service, US Department of Agriculture. WIC 2017 Eligibility and Coverage Rates. Available from: https://www.fns.usda.gov/wic-2017-eligibility-and-coverage-rates. Accessed February 22, 2021

4. National Academies of Sciences, Engineering, and Medicine; Health and Medicine Division; Food and Nutrition Board; Committee to Review WIC Food Packages. *Review of WIC Food Packages: Improving Balance and Choice: Final Report.* Washington, DC: National Academies Press; 2017

5. Food and Nutrition Service, US Department of Agriculture. WIC Eligibility and Coverage Rates - 2018. Available at: https://www.fns.usda.gov/wic/eligibility-and-coverage-rates-2018. Accessed February 22, 2021

6. Jun S, Catellier DJ, Eldridge AL, Dwyer JT, Eicher-Miller HA, Bailey RL. Usual nutrient intakes from the diets of US children by WIC participation and income: findings from the Feeding Infants and Toddlers Study (FITS) 2016. *J Nutr.* 2018;148(9S):1567S–1574S

7. Schneider JM, Fujii ML, Lamp CL, Lönnerdal B, Dewey KG, Zidenberg-Cherr S. The use of multiple logistic regression to identify risk factors associated with anemia and iron deficiency in a convenience sample of 12-36-mo-old children from low-income families. *Am J Clin Nutr.* 2008;87(3):614–620

8. Lee BJ, Mackey-Bilaver L. Effects of WIC and Food Stamp Program participation on child outcomes. *Child Youth Serv Rev.* 2007;29(4):501–517

9. Jackson MI. Early childhood WIC participation, cognitive development and academic achievement. *Soc Sci Med.* 2015; 126:145–153

10. Buescher PA, Horton SJ, Devaney BL, et al. Child participation in WIC: Medicaid costs and use of health care services. *Am J Public Health.* 2003;93(1):145–150

11. Thomas TN, Kolasa MS, Zhang F, Shefer AM. Assessing immunization interventions in the Women, Infants, and Children (WIC) program. *Am J Prev Med.* 2014;47(5):624–628

12. Bersak T, Sonchak L. The impact of WIC on infant immunizations and health care utilization. *Health Serv Res.* 2018; 53(suppl 1):2952–2969

13. Lee JY, Rozier RG, Norton EC, Kotch JB, Vann WF Jr. Effects of WIC participation on children's use of oral health services. *Am J Public Health.* 2004;94(5): 772–777

14. Grimm KA, Kim SA, Yaroch AL, Scanlon KS. Fruit and vegetable intake during infancy and early childhood. *Pediatrics.* 2014;134(suppl 1):S63–S69

15. Perrine CG, Galuska DA, Thompson FE, Scanlon KS. Breastfeeding duration is associated with child diet at 6 years. *Pediatrics.* 2014;134(suppl 1):S50–S55

16. Weber S, Uesugi K, Greene H, Bess S, Reese L, Odoms-Young A. Preferences and perceived value of WIC foods

among WIC caregivers. *J Nutr Educ Behav.* 2018;50(7):695–704

17. Hammad TA, Havas S, Damron D, Langenberg P. Withdrawal rates for infants and children participating in WIC in Maryland. *J Am Diet Assoc.* 1997;97(8):893–895

18. Woelfel ML, Abusabha R, Pruzek R, Stratton H, Chen SG, Edmunds LS. Barriers to the use of WIC services. *J Am Diet Assoc.* 2004;104(5):736–743

19. Rosenberg TJ, Alperen JK, Chiasson MA. Why do WIC participants fail to pick up their checks? An urban study in the wake of welfare reform. *Am J Public Health.* 2003;93(3):477–481

20. Liu CH, Liu H. Concerns and structural barriers associated with WIC participation among WIC-eligible women. *Public Health Nurs.* 2016;33(5):395–402

21. Damron D, Langenberg P, Anliker J, Ballesteros M, Feldman R, Havas S. Factors associated with attendance in a voluntary nutrition education program. *Am J Health Promot.* 1999;13(5):268–275

22. Schneiders B, Thacker W. *Increasing the Utilization of WIC Program Benefits in Virginia. Final Report.* Richmond, VA: Virginia Department of Health, Division of Public Health and Nutrition; 1995

23. Sekhobo JP, Peck SR, Byun Y, et al. Use of a mixed-method approach to evaluate the implementation of retention promotion strategies in the New York State WIC program. *Eval Program Plann.* 2017;63:7–17

24. Vargas ED, Pirog MA. Mixed-status families and WIC uptake: The effects of risk of deportation on program use. *Soc Sci Q.* 2016;97(3):555–572

25. Pelto DJ, Ocampo A, Garduño-Ortega O, et al. The nutrition benefits participation gap: barriers to uptake of SNAP and WIC among Latinx American immigrant families. *J Community Health.* 2019;45(3):488–491

26. Tester JM, Leung CW, Crawford PB. Revised WIC food package and children's diet quality. *Pediatrics.* 2016;137(5):e20153557

27. US Department of Agriculture and US Department of Health and Human Services. Dietary Guidelines for Americans, 2020–2025. 9th Edition. December 2020.

Available at: DietaryGuidelines.gov. Accessed December 20, 2021

28. Damschroder LJ, Aron DC, Keith RE, Kirsh SR, Alexander JA, Lowery JC. Fostering implementation of health services research findings into practice: a consolidated framework for advancing implementation science. *Implement Sci.* 2009;4(1):50

29. Food and Nutrition Service, US Department of Agriculture. WIC Data Tables: Monthly Data – State Level Participation by Category and Program Costs. FY 2021 (preliminary). https://www.fns.usda.gov/pd/wic-program. Accessed May 28, 2021

30. Bertmann FM, Barroso C, Ohri-Vachaspati P, Hampl JS, Sell K, Wharton CM. Women, infants, and children cash value voucher (CVV) use in Arizona: a qualitative exploration of barriers and strategies related to fruit and vegetable purchases. *J Nutr Educ Behav.* 2014;46(3 suppl):S53–S58

31. Christie C, Watkins JA, Martin A, Jackson H, Perkin JE, Fraser J. Assessment of client satisfaction in six urban WIC clinics, 2006. Available at: https://digitalcommons.unf.edu/cgi/viewcontent.cgi?article=1001&context=hnut_facpub. Accessed February 22, 2021

32. Gleason S, McGuire D, Morgan R. *Opportunities to Enhance American Indian Access to the WIC Food Package: Evidence From Three Case Studies.* Portland, ME: Altarum Institute; 2014

33. Najjar SK. *Barriers to WIC Benefits Redemption Among Participants in Washington State* [master's thesis]. Seattle, WA: University of Washington; 2014

34. Whaley SE, Whaley M, Au LE, Gurzo K, Ritchie LD. Breastfeeding is associated with higher retention in WIC after age 1. *J Nutr Educ Behav.* 2017;49(10):810–816.e1

35. Bryman A, Burgess RG. Developments in qualitative data analysis: an introduction. In: Bryman A, Burgess RG, eds. *Analyzing Qualitative Data.* Oxfordshire, UK: Routledge; 1994:1–17

36. McDonald N, Schoenebeck S, Forte A. Reliability and inter-rater reliability in qualitative research: norms and guidelines for CSCW and HCI practice. *Proceedings of the ACM on Human-*

Computer Interaction. 2019;3(CSCW):1–23

37. Weinfield NS, Borger C, Au LE, Whaley SE, Berman D, Ritchie LD. Longer participation in WIC is associated with better diet quality in 24-month-old children. *J Acad Nutr Diet.* 2020;120(6):963–971

38. Chauvenet C, De Marco M, Barnes C, Ammerman AS. WIC recipients in the retail environment: a qualitative study assessing customer experience and satisfaction. *J Acad Nutr Diet.* 2019;119(3):416–424.e2

39. Zhang Q, Zhang J, Park K, Tang C. Association between usage of an app to redeem prescribed food benefits and redemption behaviors among the Special Supplemental Nutrition Program for Women, Infants, and Children participants: cross-sectional study. *JMIR Mhealth Uhealth.* 2020;8(10):e20720

40. Food and Nutrition Service, US Department of Agriculture. WIC - Food Package Substitution Waiver. Available at: https://www.fns.usda.gov/wic/food-package-substitution-waiver. Accessed July 13, 2021

41. Food and Nutrition Service, US Department of Agriculture. WIC - Food Package Medical Documentation. Available at: https://www.fns.usda.gov/wic/food-package-medical-documentation. Accessed July 13, 2021

42. Hillier A, McLaughlin J, Cannuscio CC, Chilton M, Krasny S, Karpyn A. The impact of WIC food package changes on access to healthful food in 2 low-income urban neighborhoods. *J Nutr Educ Behav.* 2012;44(3):210–216

43. Zhang Q, Alsuliman MA, Wright M, Wang Y, Cheng X. Fruit and vegetable purchases and consumption among WIC participants after the 2009 WIC food package revision: a systematic review. *Adv Nutr.* 2020;11(6):1646–1662

44. Herman DR, Harrison GG, Jenks E. Choices made by low-income women provided with an economic supplement for fresh fruit and vegetable purchase. *J Am Diet Assoc.* 2006;106(5):740–744

45. Herman DR. Ensuring access to fruits and vegetables for the nation's most vulnerable – contributions of WIC and SNAP. *Economists Voice.* 2017;14(1):1–8

46. Durward CM, Savoie-Roskos M, Atoloye A, et al. Double Up Food Bucks participation is associated with increased fruit and vegetable consumption and food security among low-income adults. *J Nutr Educ Behav.* 2019;51(3):342–347

47. Wielenga V, Franzen-Castle L, Toney A, Dingman H. Nebraska Double Up Food Bucks increases purchases of fresh fruits and vegetables among SNAP users. *Curr Dev Nutr.* 2020;4(suppl 2):731–731

48. Garner JA, Coombs C, Savoie-Roskos MR, Durward C, Seguin-Fowler RA. A qualitative evaluation of Double Up Food Bucks farmers' market incentive program access. *J Nutr Educ Behav.* 2020;52(7):705–712

49. Zimmer MC, Beaird J, Steeves EA. WIC participants' perspectives of facilitators and barriers to shopping with eWIC compared with paper vouchers. *J Nutr Educ Behav.* 2021;53(3):195–203

50. Hanks AS, Gunther C, Lillard D, Scharff RL. From paper to plastic: understanding the impact of eWIC on WIC recipient behavior. *Food Policy.* 2019;83:83–91

51. Gleason S, McGuire D, Morgan R. *Opportunities to Enhance American Indian Access to the WIC Food Package: Evidence from Three Case Studies.* Portland, ME: Altarum Institute; 2014

52. Okeke JO, Ekanayake RM, Santorelli ML. Effects of a 2014 statewide policy change on cash-value voucher redemptions for fruits/vegetables among participants in the Supplemental Nutrition Program for Women, Infants, and Children (WIC). *Matern Child Health J.* 2017;21(10):1874–1879

53. Phillips D, Bell L, Morgan R, Pooler J. *Transition to EBT in WIC: Review of Impact and Examination of Participant Redemption Patterns: Final Report.* Portland, ME: Altarum Institute; 2014

54. Black MM, Hurley KM, Oberlander SE, et al. Participants' comments on changes in the revised special supplemental nutrition program for women, infants, and children food packages: the Maryland Food Preference Study. *J Am Diet Assoc.* 2009;109(1):116–123

55. Morris G, Bailey-Davis L, Cochran W, et al. Perceptions about care coordination between pediatricians and Women, Infants and Children (WIC) for early childhood obesity prevention. *Pediatrics.* 2018;141(1 MeetingAbstract):590

56. Weber SJ, Dawson D, Greene H, Hull PC. Mobile phone apps for low-income participants in a public health nutrition program for Women, Infants, and Children (WIC): review and analysis of features. *JMIR Mhealth Uhealth.* 2018;6(11):e12261

57. Maslow AH. *Motivation and Personality.* Delhi, India: Prabhat Prakashan; 1981

58. Shue H. *Basic Rights: Subsistence, Affluence, and US Foreign Policy.* Princeton, NJ: Princeton University Press; 2020

59. Moynihan D, Herd P, Harvey H. Administrative burden: learning, psychological, and compliance costs in citizen-state interactions. *J Public Adm Res Theory.* 2015;25(1):43–69

60. Barnes CY. "It takes a while to get used to": the costs of redeeming public benefits. *J Public Adm Res Theory.* 2021;31(2):295–310

61. Nianogo RA, Wang MC, Basurto-Davila R, et al. Economic evaluation of California prenatal participation in the Special Supplemental Nutrition Program for Women, Infants and Children (WIC) to prevent preterm birth. *Prev Med.* 2019;124:42–49

62. Hecht AA. *Universal Free School Meals: Implementation of the Community Eligibility Provision and Impacts on Student Nutrition, Behavior and Academic Performance.* Baltimore, MD: Johns Hopkins University; 2020

63. Bartfeld JS. The Community Eligibility Provision: continuing the century-long debate over universal free school meals. *Am J Public Health.* 2020;110(9):1272–1273

64. Food and Nutrition Service, US Department of Agriculture. WIC Racial-Ethnic Group Enrollment Data 2016. Available at: https://www.fns.usda.gov/wic/wic-racial-ethnic-group-enrollment-data-2016. Accessed September 17, 2021

65. Poblacion A, Cook J, Ettinger de Cuba S, et al. Can food insecurity be reduced in the United States by improving SNAP, WIC, and the community eligibility provision? *World Med Health Policy.* 2017;9(4):435–455

Assessing and Improving WIC Enrollment in the Primary Care Setting: A Quality Initiative

Bryan S. Monroe, MD,[a] Lina M. Rengifo, MD,[a] Meagan R. Wingler, MD,[a] Jeanna R. Auriemma, MD,[a] Alysha J. Taxter, MD, MSCE,[b] Brenda Ramirez, MS,[a] Laurie W. Albertini, MD,[a] Kimberly G. Montez, MD, MPH[a]

BACKGROUND AND OBJECTIVES: The Special Supplemental Nutrition Program for Women, Infants, and Children (WIC) provides food and other resources to mitigate the harmful effects of food insecurity on child and maternal health. From a 2009 peak, nationwide WIC participation declined through 2020. Our objectives were to understand factors influencing WIC engagement and improve WIC enrollment through novel, primary care-based quality improvement interventions.

METHODS: Plan-do-study-act cycles were implemented at a majority Medicaid-insured pediatric primary care clinic. Universal WIC screening at <5-year-old well-child visits was initiated, with counseling and referrals offered to nonparticipants. Clinic providers received WIC education. WIC screening, counseling reminders, and referrals were streamlined via the electronic health record. Families were surveyed on WIC participation barriers. Patient demographic data were analyzed for predictors of WIC participation.

RESULTS: Mean new WIC enrollments increased significantly (42%) compared with baseline, with sustained special cause variation after study interventions. Provider WIC knowledge improved significantly at study end ($P <.001$). Rates of WIC screening, counseling, and referrals remained stable for >1 year after study interventions. The most common family-reported barriers to WIC participation were "Access problems" and "WIC knowledge gap." Factors associated with decreased WIC participation in multivariable analysis were increasing age ($P <.001$), and non-Medicaid insurance status ($P = .03$).

CONCLUSIONS: We demonstrate feasible primary care-based screening, education, and referral interventions that appear to improve WIC enrollment. We identify knowledge gap and access problems as major potentially modifiable barriers to WIC participation. The expansion of similar low-cost interventions into other settings has the potential to benefit under-resourced children and families.

[a]Wake Forest University School of Medicine, Winston-Salem, North Carolina; and [b]Nationwide Children's Hospital, Columbus, Ohio

Dr Monroe conceptualized and designed the study, designed the data collection instruments, collected data, supervised the data collection, cleaning, and analysis, and drafted the initial manuscript; Drs Rengifo and Wingler conceptualized and designed the study, designed the data collection instruments, collected data, and drafted portions of the initial manuscript; Drs Auriemma and Montez contributed to the conceptualization and design of the study and data collection instrument; Dr Taxter contributed to the design and implementation of study interventions involving the electronic health record; Ms Ramirez contributed to data acquisition; Dr Albertini contributed to study design and data acquisition; and all authors reviewed and revised the manuscript, approved the final manuscript as submitted, and agree to be accountable for all aspects of the work.

DOI: https://doi.org/10.1542/peds.2022-057613

Accepted for publication Apr 21, 2023

Address correspondence to Bryan S. Monroe, MD, Department of Pediatrics, Duke University Health, 2301 Erwin Rd, Durham, NC 27710. E-mail: bryan.monroe@duke.edu

PEDIATRICS (ISSN Numbers: Print, 0031-4005; Online, 1098-4275).

FUNDING: No external funding.

CONFLICT OF INTEREST DISCLOSURES: The authors have indicated they have no potential conflicts of interest relevant to this article to disclose.

To cite: Monroe BS, Rengifo LM, Wingler MR, et al. Assessing and Improving WIC Enrollment in the Primary Care Setting: A Quality Initiative. *Pediatrics.* 2023;152(2):e2022057613

Food insecurity (FI), the lack of dependable access to sufficient food for an active and healthy life, has significant detrimental impacts on child and maternal health.[1] The presence of FI prenatally and in early childhood has been linked to low birth weight, poor health status, impaired development and higher rates of hospitalization, emergency department visits, and maternal depression.[2,3] To mitigate early childhood FI, the Special Supplemental Nutrition Program for Women, Infants, and Children (WIC) provides nutritious foods, breastfeeding support, nutrition education, and health care referrals to low-income pregnant and postpartum individuals and children <5 years old.[4] WIC benefits are linked to decreased rates of low birth weight, infant mortality, and FI and improved maternal prenatal care, anemia, and

QUALITY REPORT

obesity.[5–7] WIC also improves breastfeeding initiation, children's vocabulary, memory, immunization rates, and likelihood of receiving routine well-child care.[8,9]

Despite WIC's benefits, national data reveal that the total number of WIC participants declined from a 2009 peak of 9.2 million to 6.3 million in 2020, while the percentage of eligible families enrolled in WIC declined from 63.5% in 2011 to 56.9% in 2018.[10,11] Children aged 1 to 4 years have the lowest coverage rate; only 44.3% of eligible children participated in 2018 compared with 97.8% of infants (<12 months) and 84.4% of postpartum individuals.[11] This national decline in WIC participation is reflected locally in Forsyth County, North Carolina. Mean monthly WIC participation declined by 26% county-wide from 2015 to 2019, with a 33% decline at the WIC office evaluated in this study.[12]

Numerous barriers influence WIC attrition: problems with access, transportation, and enrollment, food choice restrictions, and ignorance of WIC, among others.[7,13–15] Caregivers may leave WIC when they stop receiving infant formula, contributing to a large participation decline after infancy.[16,17] Additionally, more restrictive immigration enforcement and the 2018 expanded federal public charge rule created a suppressive effect on public benefit usage among Hispanic immigrants.[18,19] The Hispanic population is the largest WIC-participating group but had a disproportionate decline in WIC use relative to other racial/ethnic groups from 2016 to 2018.[11]

The primary care setting may be ideal for improving WIC participation. Implementing screening and referrals for federal nutrition programs may identify unmet social needs missed by standard FI screening.[20] FI is often transitory and may be missed by periodic well-child visit screens, highlighting the importance of connecting families with resources accessible between visits.[14,21] Despite the potential for primary care to connect families to FI resources, scant research evaluates primary care strategies to improve WIC participation.

The purpose of this quality improvement (QI) study was to implement primary care-based interventions to improve WIC enrollment. The primary aim was to increase WIC enrollment at our co-located WIC office by ≥10% by December 2021. We targeted a 10% increase because of the novelty of the interventions and concern for impact mitigation from significantly reduced patient clinic volumes during the coronavirus disease 2019 (COVID-19) pandemic.[22] The secondary aim was to assess factors influencing WIC participation to better comprehend the local decline in WIC participation mirrored nationally and inform potential QI interventions.

METHODS

Study Context and Design

The study was conducted at Atrium Health Wake Forest Baptist's Downtown Health Plaza Pediatric Clinic, an academic primary care clinic located in Winston-Salem, Forsyth County, NC. In 2014 and 2015, Winston-Salem ranked fourth in the nation for the prevalence of children experiencing food hardship, and children served at the clinic reside in zip codes with the highest prevalence of unmet health needs in Forsyth County.[23,24] The clinic serves >14 000 children, with >19 000 total visits per year. In 2019, the patient population was majority Medicaid-insured (92%) and Hispanic-identifying (65%); 45% preferred speaking Spanish, and 14.1% reported FI.[25] The clinic contains co-located offices for pediatrics, obstetrics/gynecology, internal medicine, and WIC. The WIC office only serves patients of the co-located clinics. WIC enrollment appointments grant same-day benefit access. These appointments transitioned from in-person to telephone in April 2020 because of COVID-19.

Data collection occurred from June 2020 to December 2021. To achieve the primary aim of improving WIC enrollment, several key drivers (Fig 1) were identified with action items for each. Action items were implemented via 3 plan-do-study-act (PDSA) cycles.

Study Sample

All patients <5 years old presenting for a well-child visit between July 29, 2020 and December 31, 2021 were eligible for inclusion. Any patient <5 years old presenting for a non-well-child visit and all patients ≥5 years old were excluded. All providers caring for clinic patients were included in the provider educational intervention.

PDSA 1 (June 2020 to September 2020): Provider Education, WIC Screening, Counseling, and Referral

During the month preceding patient interventions, providers were assessed on their actual and perceived baseline WIC knowledge and counseling; correct answers and explanations were provided post-assessment. Shortly after, education about WIC and upcoming QI interventions was disseminated via a resident didactic session, an E-mail to all providers, and posted in provider workrooms. Providers were reassessed with the same test after the implementation of all PDSA cycles 10 months later.

The clinic already screened social drivers of health, including FI, housing, and transportation insecurity, but did not screen WIC enrollment. Screening questions for caregiver reports of WIC enrollment and WIC interest were embedded into the electronic health record (EHR) note templates used to guide <5-year-old well-child visits. These questions identified WIC non-participants and WIC-interested non-participants, respectively. A bilingual (English/Spanish) 3-item paper questionnaire was provided to all families surveying for WIC participation barriers and referral interest/consent. This was voluntarily completed during visits and later collected by the project team; all who consented were referred. Providers were instructed to counsel WIC-interested non-participants

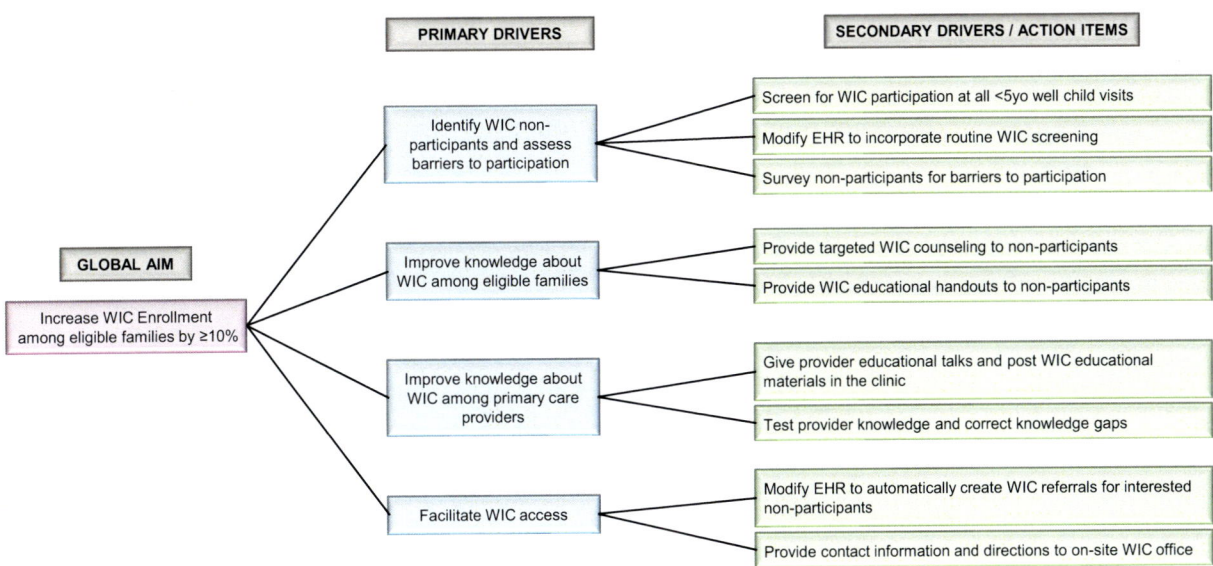

FIGURE 1
Legend, project driver diagram.

either by (1) educating them about WIC services, eligibility, and enrollment verbally and/or with a bilingual informational handout or (2) referring same-visit to a bilingual food resource specialist (who provided WIC education). Interpreters were used to screen and counsel non-English-speaking families. We estimate screening alone added an average of 5 to 10 seconds to the visit time, whereas additional counseling added 15 to 30 seconds.

PDSA 2 (September 2020 to November 2020): Provider Reeducation

More extensive provider educational activities (interactive presentation during resident didactics, e-mail educating all providers about project interventions) were implemented to reach more providers and reinforce WIC counseling.

PDSA 3 (November 2020 to December 31, 2021): EHR WIC Referrals

EHR note templates were modified to ask WIC nonparticipants about referral interest/consent. If referral interest/consent was documented, a referral was sent automatically to a clinic staff member who facilitated referral to WIC; this system replaced paper referral consent. To improve tracking of provider counseling, a prompt was embedded in the EHR note template to document WIC counseling.

Measures

The primary outcome measure was a monthly count of new WIC enrollments at the co-located WIC office. New enrollments were thought to be more sensitive to interventions targeting nonparticipants compared with total WIC participation, which included those already enrolled. The deidentified data were provided directly by Forsyth County WIC from 2019 to 2021.

Three clinic-based process measures were tracked: WIC screening percentage, counseling percentage, and referral count. Screening tracked the percentage of all <5-year-old well-child visits with a completed EHR screening. Counseling tracked the percentage of WIC-interested nonparticipants with a documented counseling or food resource specialist referral. Counseling began with PDSA 1 but was not reliably recorded and trackable until PDSA 3 (November 2020). Referrals tracked a count because referral percentage was always 100%; referral interest/consent (denominator) always triggered referral (numerator) by design. The number of "WIC-interested" was not used as the referral denominator because some families consented to referral that were overall undecided on WIC-interest, leading to more referrals than expressed WIC interest. All screening, counseling, and referral data were EHR-derived. None of these functions occurred before the study; thus, no baseline data existed for comparison.

A fourth process measure was provider knowledge. We compared provider perceived and actual WIC knowledge, WIC counseling confidence, and counseling frequency before and 10 months after initial provider education.

New WIC enrollments data were plotted on a c-type statistical process control chart by using established rules and practices.[26,27] Microsoft Excel v16.0 was used to create the control chart and plot run charts for WIC screening, counseling, and referral process measures. Provider perception of WIC knowledge and counseling

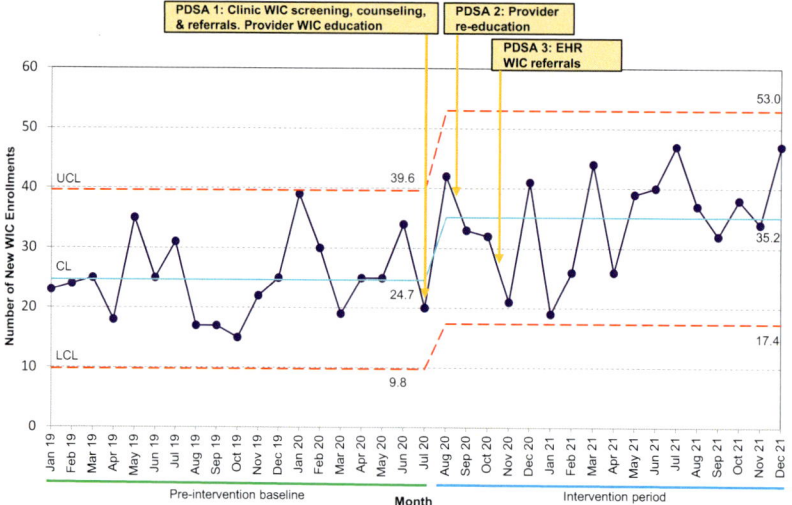

FIGURE 2

Legend, WIC new enrollments at the co-located WIC office.
UCL, upper control limit; LCL, lower control limit; C, mean.

before and after education were compared by using Fisher's exact test; provider WIC knowledge test scores were compared with a 2-sample *t* test.

Secondary Analyses on WIC Participation Barriers and Predictors

Barriers to WIC participation data came from completed self-report surveys administered from July 2020 to February 2021. Patient demographic and clinical EHR data were extracted during this period to test for predictors of WIC participation. These data were not obtained after February 2021, so only the July 2020 to February 2021 subpopulation was used for this secondary analysis. Variables hypothesized to have associations with WIC participation were chosen, including age, sex, race/ethnicity (evaluated as 1 variable), preferred language, self-reported FI, insurance status, and growth percentiles (body-mass-index [BMI] for ≥2 years old and weight-for-length [WFL] for <2 years old).

Predictors of WIC participation were examined by using univariable and multivariable logistic regression. All variables were used to control one another in multivariable analysis because all had plausible potential associations with WIC participation. Statistical analysis was completed with SPSS v26. The study was approved by the Wake Forest University School of Medicine Institutional Review Board (IRB 00064032).

RESULTS

Outcome and Process Measures

New WIC enrollments at the co-located WIC office (Fig 2) reveal a pattern of improved WIC enrollment with sustained special cause variation after project interventions. The centerline was fixed during the preintervention baseline period when the system is thought to have been stable. Special cause variation corresponding to interventions was noted after August 2020 with several months >3-σ limits (upper control limit) from the preintervention centerline. New enrollments increased by 42.5%, from a monthly mean of 24.7 during the baseline period to 35.2 after interventions.

Process measure data were tracked from July 2020 to December 2021. Of 4740 total well-child encounters, 4072 were WIC-screened (85.9%), 3171 reported WIC enrollment (77.8% of those screened), and 197 of 248 WIC-interested nonparticipants were counseled (79.4%). WIC screening and counseling rates (Fig 3) did not show sustained change after interventions; both had medians of 85% or greater. A total of 386 families consented to WIC referral. Referrals showed an unsustained increase after EHR referral integration (PDSA 3) and a June 2021 to November 2021 decrease that returned to near the median by December 2021.

Provider knowledge is shown in Table 1. There were 37 and 21 respondents to the initial and follow-up surveys, respectively, which were composed of 65% to 70% women, 40% first-year residents, 40% to 45% upper-year residents, and 15% to 20% attending physicians in both surveys. Both perceived and actual WIC knowledge improved significantly (*P* <.001) after educational interventions; additionally, providers reported significant improvement in their WIC counseling confidence (*P* = .002) and frequency (*P* <.001).

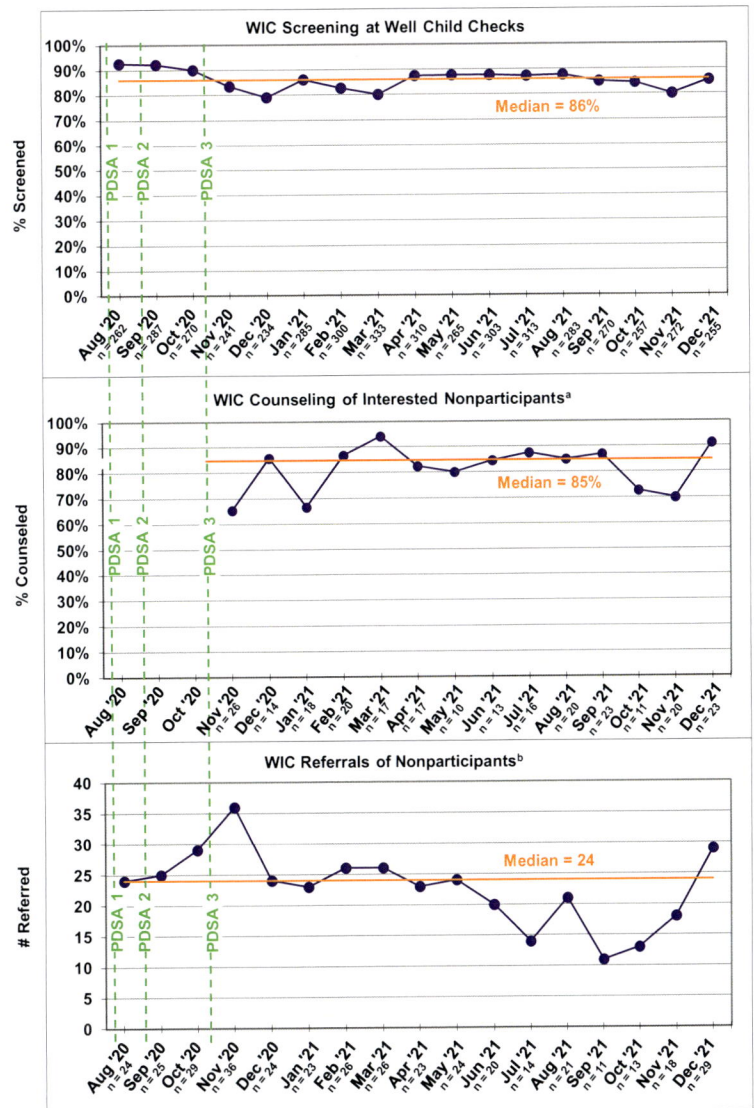

FIGURE 3

Legend, process measures: WIC screening, counseling, and referrals.

[a] No data available before PDSA 3.

[b] Count reported because referral rate did not vary during study.

Secondary Analyses on WIC Participation Barriers and Predictors

There were 1801 total well-child encounters extracted from July 2020 to February 2021. We eliminated 500 same-patient return encounters to ensure 1 encounter per patient (preferencing the encounter with the most complete data or first encounter if equal) and 130 encounters missing WIC participation data, leaving 1171 encounters for analysis. This population self-identified as 55.2% Hispanic, 26.1% Black, 5.2% white, and 12.6% "Other" race/ethnicity (Table 2). The vast majority (91.8%) of patients were Medicaid-insured while 5.8% had no insurance. The majority (74.3%) reported WIC enrollment and 11.7% reported FI.

A total of 190 WIC nonparticipating families completed the survey on barriers to participation. The 3 most common barriers were "Access problems" (32.6%), "WIC knowledge gap" (31.1%), and "Don't need WIC" (30.5%). "Access problems" and "WIC knowledge gap" represent groupings of several similar barriers that are listed in Table 3. "Fear/worry about using government benefits" was reported by 7.9% of respondents, all of whom identified as Hispanic (14.7% of Hispanic respondents).

TABLE 1 Provider Perceived and Actual WIC Knowledge

	Pre-education, No. (%) (*n* = 37)	Post-education, No. (%) (*n* = 21)	OR (95% CI)	*P*
Perceived knowledge of WIC benefits				
Good/excellent	22 (59)	21 (100)	1.68 (1.29 to 2.19)	<.001
Neutral/fair/poor	15 (41)	0 (0)		
Perceived knowledge of WIC eligibility				
Good/excellent	11 (30)	18 (86)	2.88 (1.71 to 4.88)	<.001
Neutral/fair/poor	26 (70)	3 (14)		
Confidence in WIC counseling				
Good/excellent	16 (43)	18 (86)	1.98 (1.32 to 2.98)	.002
Neutral/fair/poor	21 (57)	3 (14)		
Frequency discussing WIC in visits				
Always/often	14 (38)	20 (95)	2.52 (1.65 to 3.85)	<.001
Sometimes/rarely/never	23 (62)	1 (5)		
Actual WIC knowledge				
Overall average % correct[a]	62.4	77.1	−0.15 (−0.21 to −0.09)[b]	<.001

[a] Out of a 10-question knowledge test.
[b] Mean difference (95% CI).

Analysis for the predictors of WIC participation revealed significant associations of child age and insurance status with WIC participation that persisted when controlling for other variables (Table 4). As child age

TABLE 2 Demographic Characteristics of Participants

Characteristic	No. (%) of Participants (*n* = 1171)
Sex	
Male	621 (53.0)
Female	550 (47.0)
Age, y	
<1	484 (41.3)
1	257 (21.9)
2	144 (12.3)
3	135 (11.5)
4	151 (12.9)
Race/ethnicity	
Hispanic	646 (55.2)
Black	306 (26.1)
Other	148 (12.6)
White	61 (5.2)
Asian/Polynesian	9 (0.8)
Missing data	1 (0.1)
Preferred language	
English	705 (60.2)
Spanish	450 (38.4)
Other	16 (1.4)
Insurance	
Medicaid	1075 (91.8)
None	68 (5.8)
Private	28 (2.4)
FI	137 (11.7)
WIC status	
Participant	870 (74.3)
Nonparticipant	301 (25.7)

increased, the odds of WIC participation decreased (odds ratio [OR] 0.62, 95% confidence interval [CI] 0.57–0.69). Privately insured or uninsured families had lower odds of WIC participation than Medicaid-insured families (OR 0.54, 95% CI 0.31–0.93). Race/ethnicity and growth percentiles had significant associations with WIC participation in univariable analysis that did not persist when controlling for other variables. The "Other" racial/ethnic group had lower odds of WIC participation compared with all other groups (OR 1.60, 95% CI 1.09–2.33). As BMI and WFL percentiles increased, the odds of WIC participation decreased (OR 0.99, 95% CI 0.99–1.00). Self-reported FI and preferred language (English/Spanish) had no associations with WIC participation.

DISCUSSION

Our findings indicate a measurable and sustainable benefit of relatively simple and inexpensive screening, education, and referral strategies on WIC enrollment. We demonstrated the feasibility of incorporating these interventions into an existing clinic framework. This study contributes to a clearer understanding of barriers to WIC participation, identifying WIC knowledge gaps and access problems as significant potentially modifiable barriers. We also identified several predictors of lower WIC participation, the most robust being older child age and non-Medicaid insurance status, with weaker effects seen for "Other" race/ethnicity and higher growth percentiles. Overall, this study provides a better understanding of factors influencing WIC engagement and reveals strategies to enhance enrollment.

The potential for primary care practices to impact WIC enrollment is apparent when considering the unparalleled contact pediatric providers have with families during their child's early years. Previous efforts to tap this

TABLE 3 Barriers to WIC Participation

Barriers	No. (%) Respondents[a] (n = 190)
Access problems	62 (32.6)
Don't have time	24 (12.6)
Forgot/need to reapply	15 (7.9)
Problems with WIC card/applying	10 (5.3)
Problems using WIC at stores	8 (4.2)
Transportation problem	5 (2.6)
WIC knowledge gap	59 (31.1)
Don't know how to apply	29 (15.3)
Thought I wasn't eligible	24 (12.6)
Didn't know about WIC	6 (3.2)
Don't need WIC	58 (30.5)
Fear/worry about COVID-19	23 (12.1)
Fear/worry about using government benefits	15 (7.9)

[a] Respondents could select multiple applicable barriers.

potential include toolkits promoting collaborative strategies between primary care and WIC, and studies investigating the feasibility of information-sharing between WIC and primary care.[28–31] To our knowledge, this study is the first to directly measure the impact and sustainability of primary care site QI interventions on WIC enrollment. Our screening, counseling, and referral rates remained remarkably stable throughout the study period, which may be attributable to the power of EHR-integrated processes (screening and counseling reminders built-in to EHR workflow and automated referrals). The early strength and sustained impact of EHR-integrated interventions may explain the improvement in the WIC enrollments outcome despite no improvement in our processes after implementation. The improvement in WIC enrollment represented by sustained special cause variation coincident with study interventions speaks to the potential of these interventions. These findings argue for further application in other settings to maximize benefits to under-resourced families and children at a low cost to the medical system.

Our study sheds new light on knowledge gap as a major barrier to WIC participation. Previous studies focus on access problems as barriers to participation (also noted in our study), but rarely identify knowledge deficiency.[7,15,32] We suspect WIC knowledge deficiency exists in most populations and, perhaps was unmasked by improved WIC access over time. Compared with myriad access problems that can interfere with WIC engagement, knowledge gaps may be more easily modifiable through simple educational interventions. Our study's interventions were designed to proactively target both knowledge and access barriers with focused education and direct WIC referral. We also gained revealing insights into immigrant-specific barriers to WIC because of our majority Hispanic population. A proportion of nonparticipating Hispanic families attributed WIC avoidance to concerns about using government

benefits; this may be an underestimate if some families were too wary to respond to surveys or attend clinic visits. This finding suggests that policies like the 2018 expanded federal public charge rule have lingering suppressive effects on immigrant public benefit usage and supports targeted education efforts to dispel fears that WIC impacts immigration status.[18,19]

Beyond barriers to WIC, several patient characteristics predicted WIC participation. A lower likelihood of WIC involvement as children age and in non-Medicaid-insured families are concordant with national data, suggesting why these findings were most robust.[11] Future interventions targeting children ≥1 year old may be most effective at improving WIC participation. The "Other" racial/ethnic group was least likely to participate in WIC, a predictive factor not found in a previous study.[33] This group preferred Spanish more than White/Black groups, but less than the Hispanic group; they might represent families with more distant Hispanic ancestry (second generation or later) who are less likely to report Hispanic identity.[34] Further investigation to characterize this group is warranted. Despite the disproportionate decline in Hispanic WIC participation nationally and impacts from federal public charge, we did not detect lower odds of WIC participation among Hispanic patients and thus chose not to pursue Hispanic-specific interventions.[11] Higher WFL and BMI percentiles predicted lower odds of WIC participation, which may be suggestive of healthier diets in WIC-participating families, a trend well-supported by the literature.[35]

TABLE 4 Predictors of WIC Participation

Predictor	Univariable Analysis		Multivariable Analysis[a]	
	OR (95% CI)	P	OR (95% CI)	P
Age, mo	0.63 (0.57 to 0.69)	<.001	0.62 (0.57 to 0.69)	<.001
Race/ethnicity				
Hispanic vs other	1.60 (1.09 to 2.33)	.01	1.04 (0.66 to 1.63)	.87
White vs other	2.61 (1.25 to 5.44)	.01	1.94 (0.85 to 4.40)	.11
Black vs other	2.24 (1.45 to 3.47)	<.001	1.42 (0.88 to 2.31)	.15
White vs Hispanic	1.63 (0.83 to 3.20)	.16	1.85 (0.84 to 4.09)	.13
Black vs Hispanic	1.40 (1.01 to 1.94)	.047	1.36 (0.89 to 2.08)	.16
Black vs white	0.86 (0.42 to 1.75)	.57	0.74 (0.33 to 1.61)	.44
Insurance				
Private vs Medicaid	0.11 (0.05 to 0.27)	<.001	0.09 (0.04 to 0.23)	<.001
None vs Medicaid	0.57 (0.34 to 0.95)	.03	0.54 (0.31 to 0.93)	.03
Preferred language				
Spanish vs English	0.79 (0.60 to 1.03)	.08	1.03 (0.72 to 1.49)	.86
Other vs English	0.35 (0.13 to 0.99)	.048	0.31 (0.08 to 1.15)	.08
BMI or WFL percentile[b]	0.99 (0.99 to 1.00)	.04	0.99 (0.99 to 1.00)	.60
FI	1.06 (0.70 to 1.59)	.80	1.04 (0.66 to 1.62)	.87

[a] Each measure adjusted for all other variables (age, race/ethnicity, insurance, language, BMI or WFL percentile, food insecurity).
[b] WFL percentile used for <2-year-old, BMI percentile used for ≥2-year-old.

There are several limitations to our study. Our interventions are well-suited for clinics with substantial under-resourced populations; however, the interventions may require adaptation for clinics serving populations with lower WIC eligibility. Having a WIC office co-located with a pediatric practice is uncommon, although as with most practices, there was no previous collaboration with WIC, allowing for the potential generalizability of our interventions. We did not assess WIC eligibility because income questions would likely have complicated and discouraged participation in screening. We estimate WIC-ineligibility as <2% because 92% of our population was eligible via Medicaid and 6% were uninsured and largely eligible via income. We included all insurance statuses in the analysis to examine insurance as a WIC predictor, recognizing that a small contingent of WIC-ineligible families was included. We could not include balancing measures examining project impact on WIC appointment wait times or well-child visit time because of COVID-19 ending WIC in-person appointments and high variability in well-child visits, respectively. WIC's COVID-19-mediated transition from in-person to telephone enrollment appointments starting in April 2020 may have made it easier for some families to enroll, potentially resulting in increased enrollments. For 4 months after this change, however, new enrollments remained near the baseline period mean, with the first marked enrollment increase coincident with PDSA 1. COVID-19-related rises in unemployment and FI may also have contributed to shifts in WIC participation, although this impact may have been partially ameliorated by federal assistance during the study period.[36,37]

CONCLUSIONS

In a clinic serving a majority of WIC-eligible families, the implementation of WIC screening, family and provider education, and referrals was associated with increased WIC enrollment. Provider WIC knowledge also increased after these interventions, and WIC screening, counseling, and referral rates remained robust for >1 year after interventions. Family knowledge gaps about WIC eligibility and enrollment may be a significant barrier preventing WIC participation. The substantial evidence that WIC improves health and growth outcomes for young children of under-resourced families argues for clinic-based initiatives to promote participation. Feasible clinic interventions may advance that goal, empowering primary pediatric providers to connect families with available nutritional resources to protect child health.

ACKNOWLEDGMENTS

The authors would like to acknowledge Danielle M. Weber, PhD, for statistical consultation in conducting data analysis and assisting in interpretation and Mayte Grundseth, MEd, RD, for the provision of key study data and assisting in study design.

ABBREVIATIONS

BMI: body mass index
CI: confidence interval
COVID-19: coronavirus disease 2019
EHR: electronic health record
FI: food insecurity
OR: odds ratio
PDSA: Plan-Do-Study-Act
QI: quality improvement
WFL: weight-for-length
WIC: Special Supplemental Nutrition Program for Women, Infants, and Children

REFERENCES

1. Coleman-Jensen A, Rabbitt MP, Gregory CA, Singh A; Economic Research Service, US Department of Agriculture. Household food security in the United States in 2020. Available at: https://www.ers.usda.gov/webdocs/publications/102076/err-298.pdf. Accessed September 1, 2021

2. Cook JT, Frank DA. Food security, poverty, and human development in the United States. *Ann N Y Acad Sci.* 2008;1136(1):193–209

3. Thomas MMC, Miller DP, Morrissey TW. Food insecurity and child health. *Pediatrics.* 2019;144(4):e20190397

4. US Department of Agriculture, Food and Nutrition Service. Special Supplemental Nutrition Program for Women, Infants, and Children (WIC). Available at: https://www.fns.usda.gov/wic. Accessed November 30, 2021

5. Kotelchuck M, Schwartz JB, Anderka MT, Finison KS. WIC participation and pregnancy outcomes: Massachusetts Statewide Evaluation Project. *Am J Public Health.* 1984;74(10):1086–1092

6. Caan B, Horgen DM, Margen S, et al. Benefits associated with WIC supplemental feeding during the interpregnancy interval. *Am J Clin Nutr.* 1987;45(1):29–41

7. Black MM, Cutts DB, Frank DA, et al; Children's Sentinel Nutritional Assessment Program Study Group. Special Supplemental Nutrition Program for Women, Infants, and Children participation and infants' growth and health: a multisite surveillance study. *Pediatrics.* 2004;114(1):169–176

8. Ryan AS, Wenjun Z, Acosta A. Breastfeeding continues to increase into the new millennium. *Pediatrics.* 2002;110(6):1103–1109

9. Rush D, Horvitz DG, Seaver WB, et al. The National WIC Evaluation: evaluation of the Special Supplemental Food Program for Women, Infants, and Children. I. Background and introduction. *Am J Clin Nutr.* 1988;48(2 Suppl):389–393

10. US Department of Agriculture, Food and Nutrition Service. WIC data tables: national level annual summary. Available at: https://www.fns.usda.gov/pd/wic-program. Accessed September 1, 2021

11. US Department of Agriculture, Food and Nutrition Service. National WIC eligibility and participation 2005–2018. Available at: https://www.fns.usda.gov/wic/eligibility-and-coverage-rates-2018. Accessed September 1, 2021

12. Forsyth County Department of Public Health. Forsyth County, NC WIC participation data; 2020. Accessed September 1, 2021

13. Liu CH, Liu H. Concerns and structural barriers associated with WIC participation among WIC-eligible women. *Public Health Nurs.* 2016;33(5):395–402

14. Orr CJ, Chauvenet C, Ozgun H, et al. Caregivers' experiences with food insecurity screening and impact of food insecurity resources. *Clin Pediatr (Phila).* 2019;58(14):1484–1492

15. Woelfel ML, Abusabha R, Pruzek R, et al. Barriers to the use of WIC services. *J Am Diet Assoc.* 2004;104(5):736–743

16. Weber S, Uesugi K, Greene H, et al. Preferences and perceived value of WIC foods among WIC caregivers. *J Nutr Educ Behav.* 2018;50(7):695–704

17. US Department of Agriculture, Food and Nutrition Service. Summary of WIC state agency strategies for increasing child retention July 2014. Available at: https://wicworks.fns.usda.gov/resources/summary-wic-state-agency-strategies-increasing-child-retention. Accessed September 1, 2021

18. Perreira KM, Yoshikawa H, Oberlander J. A new threat to immigrants' health - the public-charge rule. *N Engl J Med.* 2018;379(10):901–903

19. Haley JM, Kenney GM, Bernstein H, Gonzalez D. One in five adults in immigrant families with children reported chilling effects on public benefit receipt in 2019: urban institute. Available at: https://www.urban.org/research/publication/one-five-adults-immigrant-families-children-reported-chilling-effects-public-benefit-receipt-2019. Accessed September 1, 2021

20. Bottino CJ, Rhodes ET, Kreatsoulas C, et al. Food insecurity screening in pediatric primary care: can offering referrals help identify families in need? *Acad Pediatr.* 2017;17(5):497–503

21. Tablazon IL, Palakshappa D, OBrian F, et al. Perspectives of caregivers experiencing persistent food insecurity at an academic primary care clinic. *Acad Pediatr.* 2021;S1876-2859(21):00390–00399

22. Brown CL, Montez K, Amati JB, et al. Impact of COVID-19 on pediatric primary care visits at four academic institutions in the Carolinas. *Int J Environ Res Public Health.* 2021;18(11):5734

23. Forsyth County Department of Public Health, Epidemiology Division. Forsyth County community health assessment report. Accessed September 1, 2021

24. Food Research and Action Center. Food hardship in America: households with children especially hard hit. Available at: https://frac.org/research/resource-library/food-hardship-america-households-children-especially-hard-hit-september-2016. Accessed September 1, 2021

25. Montez K, Brown CL, Garg A, et al. Trends in food insecurity rates at an academic primary care clinic: a retrospective cohort study. *BMC Pediatr.* 2021;21(1):364

26. Carey RG. *Improving Healthcare with Control Charts: Basic and Advance SPC Methods and Case Studies.* Milwaukee, WI: ASQ Quality Press; 2003

27. Gupta M, Kaplan HC. Measurement for quality improvement: using data to drive change. *J Perinatol.* 2020;40(6):962–971

28. Council on Community Pediatrics; Committee on Nutrition. Promoting food security for all children. *Pediatrics.* 2015;136(5):e1431–e1438

29. Food Research and Action Center. Making WIC work better: strategies to reach more women and children and strengthen benefits use. Available at: https://frac.org/research/resource-library/making-wic-work-better-strategies-to-reach-more-women-and-children-and-strengthen-benefits-use. Accessed September 1, 2021

30. Bailey-Davis L, Kling SMR, Cochran WJ, et al. Integrating and coordinating care between the Women, Infants, and Children Program and pediatricians to improve patient-centered preventive care for healthy growth. *Transl Behav Med.* 2018;8(6):944–952

31. Kling SM, Harris HA, Marini M, et al. Advanced health information technologies to engage parents, clinicians, and community nutritionists in coordinating responsive parenting care: descriptive case series of the women, infants, and children enhancements to early healthy lifestyles for baby (WEE Baby) care randomized controlled trial. *JMIR Pediatr Parent.* 2020;3(2):e22121

32. Thompson SE, Smith BA, Rees KS. Perceived barriers to participation in a supplemental nutrition program among low-income women on the US/Mexico border. *Calif J Health Promot.* 2005;3(3):24–28

33. Whaley SE, Martinez CE, Paolicelli C, et al. Predictors of WIC participation through 2 years of age. *J Nutr Educ Behav.* 2020;52(7):672–679

34. Lopez MH, Gonzalez-Barrera A, Lopez G. *Hispanic Identity Fades Away Across Generations as Immigrant Connections Fall Away.* Washington, DC: Pew Research Center; 2017

35. Food Research and Action Center. The role of the federal child nutrition programs in improving health and well-being. Available at: https://frac.org/research/resource-library/hunger-health-role-federal-child-nutrition-programs-improving-health-well. Accessed September 1, 2021

36. Niles MT, Bertmann F, Belarmino EH, et al. The early food insecurity impacts of COVID-19. *Nutrients.* 2020;12(7):2096

37. Waxman E, Gupta P, Gonzalez D; Urban Institute. Food insecurity edged back up after COVID-19 relief expired. Available at: https://www.urban.org/research/publication/food-insecurity-edged-back-after-covid-19-relief-expired. Accessed September 1, 2021

Health Care as a Partner in Federal Nutrition Programs: Call for Advocacy

Laura M. Plencner, MD,[a] Molly Krager, MD,[a] Danielle Cullen, MD, MPH, MSHP[b]

Food insecurity (FI), already common in the United States, was further exacerbated by the coronavirus disease 2019 (COVID-19) pandemic through individual and structural-level pathways. Childhood FI is associated with adverse health outcomes, including increased rates of hospitalization, anxiety and aggression, and poorer overall health.[1–3] By taking an active role in addressing FI, children's hospitals can be a key partner in meeting the needs of their communities and promoting health equity. There is growing evidence supporting the feasibility and acceptability of health care-based programs to address FI by integrating within clinical care, particularly for children and families. Simultaneously, there are systemic barriers that may prevent or limit the ability of the health care sector to engage in this space. This is the case for federal nutrition programs, many of which are intended to improve the food security of children but are not specifically designed for implementation within the health care setting. In addition to leveraging federal nutrition programs to directly assist patients experiencing FI, health care systems can have an even more broad and sustainable impact by fostering a policy environment that enables or incentivizes cross-sector collaboration. We use the exemplar of the United States Department of Agriculture's (USDA) Summer Food Service Program (SFSP) to demonstrate that (1) it is feasible for health care systems to leverage federal nutrition programs; (2) patients and families benefit when health care systems participate in these programs; and (3) advocacy for more inclusive and flexible policies regulating these programs is essential to facilitating health care's participation.

The USDA's SFSP has been successfully implemented in health care systems since at least 2015. The SFSP is a federally funded, state-administered program providing children with access to free, nutritious meals in summer months when schools are not in session and during unanticipated school closures.[4] The SFSP is underutilized, serving <15% of children who receive free and reduced-price lunch during the school year nationally, and the health care setting has been proven as a potential point of entry to expand programmatic reach.[5] Both Children's Mercy Kansas City (CMKC) and Children's Hospital of

[a]University of Missouri Kansas City, Kansas City, Missouri; and
[b]University of Pennsylvania, Philadelphia, Pennsylvania

Drs Plencner, Krager, and Cullen led the advocacy work at Children's Mercy Kansas City and Children's Hospital of Philadelphia, drafted the manuscript, and reviewed and revised the manuscript; and all authors approved the final manuscript as submitted and agree to be accountable for all aspects of the work.

DOI: https://doi.org/10.1542/peds.2022-057027

Accepted for publication Sep 6, 2022

Address correspondence to Laura M. Plencner, MD, Department of Pediatrics, Children's Mercy Kansas City, 2401 Gillham Rd, Kansas City, MO 64108. E-mail: lmplencner@cmh.edu

PEDIATRICS (ISSN Numbers: Print, 0031-4005; Online, 1098-4275).

FUNDING: No external funding.

CONFLICT OF INTEREST DISCLAIMER: Dr Plencner serves on national advisory group for No Kid Hungry Early Childhood Team and received an honorarium for her time and service. All other authors have indicated they have no conflicts of interest relevant to this article to disclose.

To cite: Plencner LM, Krager M, Cullen D. Health Care as a Partner in Federal Nutrition Programs: Call for Advocacy. *Pediatrics.* 2022;150(6):e2022057027

Philadelphia (CHOP) have been operating successful SFSP programs since 2016 and 2017, respectively, with increasing numbers of participating meal distribution sites and children served each year. Collectively, the hospital systems served 24 757 meals in the 10-week summer of 2019. Though SFSP implementation in health care has been demonstrated to be feasible and effective in terms of meal provision at the point of clinical care, connecting families to other community resources, and building positive experiences to increase comfort in accessing community sites, there are few health care-based SFSP sites. This may stem from challenges with integrating the program regulations into the unique setting of health care. For example, SFSP meals must be eaten on-site in a congregate setting at a standard meal service time. Although these regulations make sense at a more traditional settling like a summer camp, they are problematic for clinical areas that do not have a dedicated cafeteria or clinic visits that do not take place over the lunch hour. Flexibility to tailor the program to the unique clinical setting is needed to increase the feasibility of health care participation and expand the reach and impact of the program.

The importance of the health care system's role in addressing FI, and serving as an SFSP site, was further underscored during the pandemic. As a trusted and safe community institution that remained open during the early pandemic, the health care setting served as an important point-of-entry into community supports including food programs. In the spring of 2020, the federal government passed the Families First Coronavirus Response Act, granting the USDA authority to issue nationwide waivers supporting access to federal nutrition programs including the SFSP.[6] The Child Nutrition Response waivers allowed flexibility to standard SFSP regulations to adapt the program to the increased need in the community, as well as increase safety of program operations with infection prevention measures and social distancing. With the streamlined procedures and operational flexibility offered by the waivers, both CMKC and CHOP were able to not only successfully operate during the COVID-19 pandemic, but also overcome some prepandemic challenges. Allowing meals to be eaten outside of traditional mealtimes, grab-and-go meal service and extended weeks of meal service amplified the impact of their programs, serving more than 150 000 meals collectively from March 2020 to August 2021, a >600% increase from the previous year.

As SFSP sites began to plan for summer 2022, the original Child Nutrition Response waivers were gradually being phased out. This left many programs in a state of uncertainty as they continued to struggle with downstream effects of the COVID-19 pandemic, such as supply chain shortages and increased food prices. Health care-based SFSP sites faced the additional barrier of continued increased infection prevention and control measures, still necessary to protect their vulnerable patients, even if their surrounding communities had loosened or eliminated all restrictions. In short, a return to prepandemic hospital operations was not possible, and thus a return to pre-pandemic SFSP operations in the health care setting was not possible. Ultimately, just days before the final Child Nutrition Response waivers were due to expire, Congress passed a bill including a new set of more limited, temporary waivers.[7] The decision of whether to "opt in" to these waivers was left to individual state agencies. Since uptake varies by state, access to SFSP is inconsistent and operational challenges remain for many programs. For example, although CHOP was able to continue utilizing 2 of the key waivers that allowed the program to operate safely and effectively during the pandemic, CMKC was not able to use any waivers. With differences in waiver uptake by state in the summer of 2022, the consequences of health care-based programs operating under waivers compared with prepandemic operations may become more evident.

Our experience demonstrates that children's hospitals are uniquely positioned to address FI by leveraging federal nutrition programs and underscores the important role of advocacy at the state and federal level to enhance programmatic flexibility, and thereby increase health care system participation. By temporarily allowing for more streamlined operations, the Child Nutrition Response Waivers illustrated the largely untapped potential of the health care system to improve access to federal nutrition programs without compromising program integrity. Additional policies allowing for health care-specific implementation and the flexibility to integrate these programs within the clinical workflow could lead to increased collaboration with community organizations and improvements in child health. Children's hospitals are urgently needed to craft innovative solutions to address FI now, such as participation in SFSP, and to advocate for policies that will increase the positive impact that health care systems can have in the future. Advocacy is timely because the federal government has elevated the issue of FI with acknowledgment of its health effects and prioritization of solutions with the White House Conference on Hunger, Nutrition, and Health in the fall of 2022, as well as the ongoing child nutrition program reauthorization. It is essential for policymakers to hear from children's hospitals when making decisions about how to administer, regulate, and fund these programs to successfully implement in the health care setting and have the greatest benefit for children.

ABBREVIATIONS

CHOP: Children's Hospital of Philadelphia
CMKC: Children's Mercy Kansas City
COVID-19: coronavirus disease 2019
FI: food insecurity
SFSP: Summer Food Service Program
USDA: United States Department of Agriculture

REFERENCES

1. Map the Meal Gap. Feeding America. Available at: https://map.feedingamerica.org/county/2016/overall/pennsylvania/county/philadelphia/. Accessed July 31, 2022

2. Cook JT, Frank DA, Levenson SM, et al. Child food insecurity increases risks posed by household food insecurity to young children's health. *J Nutr.* 2006; 136(4):1073–1076

3. Whitaker RC, Phillips SM, Orzol SM. Food insecurity and the risks of depression and anxiety in mothers and behavior problems in their preschool-aged children. *Pediatrics.* 2006;118(3): e859–e868

4. USDA Food and Nutrition Service. Summer Food Service Program. Available at: https://www.fns.usda.gov/sfsp/summer-food-service-program. Accessed July 31, 2022

5. Cullen D, Blauch A, Mirth M, Fein J. Complete eats: summer meals offered by the Emergency Department for Food Insecurity. *Pediatrics.* 2019;144(4):e20190201

6. United States Department of Agriculture Food and Nutrition Services Child Nutrition Programs. COVID-19 waivers by state. Available at: https://www.fns.usda.gov/disaster/pandemic/covid-19/cn-waivers-flexibilities. Accessed January 10, 2022

7. Congress.gov. S.2089–Keep Kids Fed Act of 2022. Available at: https://www.congress.gov/bill/117th-congress/senate-bill/2089?loclr=bloglaw. Accessed July 1, 2022

Cost-effectiveness of Improved WIC Food Package for Preventing Childhood Obesity

Erica L. Kenney, ScD, MPH,[a,b] Matthew M. Lee, MS,[a] Jessica L. Barrett, MPH,[b] Zachary J. Ward, PhD, MPH,[c] Michael W. Long, ScD, MPH,[d] Angie L. Cradock, ScD, MPE,[b] David R. Williams, PhD,[b] Steven L. Gortmaker, PhD[b]

BACKGROUND AND OBJECTIVES: The Special Supplemental Nutrition Program for Women, Infants, and Children (WIC) prevents food insecurity and supports nutrition for more than 3 million low-income young children. Our objectives were to determine the cost-effectiveness of changes to WIC's nutrition standards in 2009 for preventing obesity and to estimate impacts on socioeconomic and racial/ethnic inequities.

METHODS: We conducted a cost-effectiveness analysis to estimate impacts from 2010 through 2019 of the 2009 WIC food package change on obesity risk for children aged 2 to 4 years participating in WIC. Microsimulation models estimated the cases of obesity prevented in 2019 and costs per quality-adjusted-life year gained.

RESULTS: An estimated 14.0 million 2- to 4-year old US children (95% uncertainty interval (UI), 13.7–14.2 million) were reached by the updated WIC nutrition standards from 2010 through 2019. In 2019, an estimated 62 700 (95% UI, 53 900–71 100) cases of childhood obesity were prevented, entirely among children from households with low incomes, leading to improved health equity. The update was estimated to cost $10 600 per quality-adjusted-life year gained (95% UI, $9760–$11 700). If WIC had reached all eligible children, more than twice as many cases of childhood obesity would have been prevented.

CONCLUSIONS: Updates to WIC's nutrition standards for young children in 2009 were estimated to be highly cost-effective for preventing childhood obesity and contributed to reducing socioeconomic and racial/ethnic inequities in obesity prevalence. Improving nutrition policies for young children can be a sound public health investment; future research should explore how to improve access to them.

[a]Department of Nutrition, [b]Department of Social and Behavioral Sciences, and [c]Center for Health Decision Science, Harvard T.H. Chan School of Public Health, Boston, Massachusetts; and [d]Department of Prevention and Community Health, Milken Institute School of Public Health, George Washington University, Washington, District of Columbia

Dr Kenney conceptualized the study, developed the analysis plan, supervised analysis, drafted the manuscript, and critically reviewed and revised the manuscript; Mr Lee and Ms Barrett conducted the analysis, contributed to drafting the manuscript, and critically reviewed and revised the manuscript; Dr Ward developed the microsimulation model and critically reviewed the manuscript; Dr Long contributed to the conceptualization of the study and critically reviewed the manuscript; Drs Cradock and Williams critically reviewed and revised the manuscript; Dr Gortmaker contributed to the conceptualization of the study and the development of the microsimulation model and critically reviewed and revised the manuscript; and all authors approved the final manuscript as submitted and agree to be accountable for all aspects of the work.

DOI: https://doi.org/10.1542/peds.2023-063182

Accepted for publication Oct 25, 2023

WHAT'S KNOWN ON THIS SUBJECT: Changes to the Special Supplemental Nutrition Program for Women, Infants and Children (WIC) in 2009 improved diet quality for WIC participants and reduced the risk of obesity for 2- to 4-year-old participants.

WHAT THIS STUDY ADDS: We estimate the cost effectiveness of the 2009 changes for preventing childhood obesity and reducing racial/ethnic and socioeconomic disparities using a microsimulation model over 10 years; we also estimate the hypothetical impact of full WIC participation.

To cite: Kenney EL, Lee MM, Barrett JL, et al. Cost-effectiveness of Improved WIC Food Package for Preventing Childhood Obesity. *Pediatrics.* 2024;153(2):e2023063182

ARTICLE

During the period of rapid development in early childhood, ensuring children can access healthful foods, with the critical nutrients needed for healthy growth, is essential.[1] To protect infants and young children from the nutritional risks associated with poverty, the United States has used, since 1972, the Special Supplemental Nutrition for Women, Infants, and Children (WIC) program.[2] WIC provides nutritional assistance to pregnant, postpartum, and breastfeeding mothers and their children up to age 5 years; to be eligible, families must have household incomes at or below 185% of the federal poverty line (FPL) and be considered at nutritional risk.[3] An estimated 6.2 million people participate in WIC nationwide, approximately 3.4 million of whom are young children[4]; even so, the program is underused, reaching only half of those who are eligible, and participation among eligible individuals varies widely by state.[5] WIC has been associated with improved birth outcomes,[6] better child cognitive and academic outcomes,[7] and a reduced risk of food insecurity.[4,8]

Although WIC was developed in an era when inadequate nutrition was a primary concern, the children whose lower household incomes make them eligible for WIC have been disproportionately at risk for a relatively newer nutrition-related health threat: excess weight gain for healthy growth, or childhood obesity.[9,10] Traditionally, WIC's food package (the list of foods and beverages that could be obtained with WIC vouchers) had been designed to ensure basic nutritional adequacy for young children at low cost, not to prevent obesity. In 2009, however, the US Department of Agriculture (USDA), which administers WIC, modified the WIC food package to promote foods that would continue to support nutritional adequacy while also reducing future chronic disease risk.[11] As a result, the quantities of juice that could be purchased with WIC benefits were decreased, whole grain breads were required, and a cash-value voucher for purchasing fruits and vegetables was added. These changes to the food package led to increases in WIC recipients' fruit and vegetable consumption, reductions in juice consumption, and reductions in caloric intake,[12-16] and were also associated with reductions in childhood obesity risk.[17-19]

However, it is unclear whether these changes were cost-effective for preventing childhood obesity. As further food package changes are considered,[20] it is important to understand the cost-effectiveness of the initial changes, as well as their impact on socioeconomic and racial/ethnic disparities in obesity risk. Additionally, given the substantial declines in retention in WIC as children age and large differences in WIC coverage across states,[21] and the prioritization of addressing underparticipation as a policy goal,[22] it is also important to consider what impact these changes could have had if WIC fully reached all eligible children. This study aims to estimate the implementation costs of the 2009 WIC package change and the cost-effectiveness of the package change for preventing cases of childhood obesity among young children in households with low incomes.

METHODS

Study Design

This cost-effectiveness analysis study used the Childhood Obesity Intervention Cost Effectiveness Study (CHOICES) methodology, which has been applied to assess the cost-effectiveness of several childhood obesity prevention policies and programs.[23-26] The CHOICES approach involves: a key partner engagement process to identify policies and programs for modeling; a systematic evidence review process to identify model inputs for a given policy's or program's effects on child weight, costs to society, and population reach; and a microsimulation model to estimate potential impacts on childhood obesity, population reach, implementation costs, and healthcare cost savings over a 10-year period.

Intervention

Advisory partners suggested evaluating the cost-effectiveness of the 2009 WIC package changes for childhood obesity prevention. Specifically, we evaluated the changes to the WIC food package for 1- to 4-year-old children, which resulted in WIC benefits being directed toward less juice, cheese, and eggs and more whole grains, as well as a change to low-fat or nonfat milk and the addition of a cash value voucher for fruits and vegetables.[11]

Identification of Model Inputs

Effect

Although the food package targets 1- to 4-year olds, we focused on outcomes for 2- to 4-year-old children because obesity prevalence is not calculated by WIC in 1-year-old children. To project the impact of the package changes on childhood obesity risk, we used estimates from a natural experimental study, using an interrupted time series analysis that tested how the introduction of the 2009 package change was associated with changes in time trends in obesity.[17] This analysis found that, although before 2009 the prevalence of obesity among WIC-participating 2- to 4-year olds was increasing steadily (by 0.23 percentage points per year), after the package change was implemented the prevalence of obesity started significantly declining by an estimated −0.34 percentage points per year. These results are consistent with other localized evaluations of the impact of the package change on childhood obesity.[18] We used state-level estimates of the national impact on childhood obesity to account for strong state-by-state variation.

Reach

To estimate the population reached by the package change, we used estimates of the number of children who are eligible for WIC and the number and percentage of eligible children who participate in WIC in each state from administrative data released by USDA Food and Nutrition Services. Given that enrollment in WIC among eligible children varies substantially by child age, race/ethnicity, and state, we used age-, race/ethnicity-, and state-stratified estimates of participation.[27–30] We assumed WIC eligibility among 2- to 4-year-old children based on household income eligibility (ie, children in households with incomes at or below 185% of the FPL were eligible) given that nearly all income-eligible children are classified as being at "nutritional risk."[21,31]

Costs

We used standard costing methodological approaches to estimate the incremental costs associated with implementation of the 2009 WIC food package change compared with no change.[32,33] We used a modified societal perspective, taking into account labor costs, opportunity costs, and equipment costs related to the food package changes. This involved accounting for costs at: (1) the federal level, where the program is partly administered; (2) state WIC agencies, which are largely responsible for implementing WIC policies and programs; and (3) WIC retailers (ie, supermarkets, grocery stores, corner stores, and pharmacies that are eligible to sell foods and beverage to WIC participants).[34] Of note, there was no estimated difference in the cost of the foods themselves for the WIC program given that the 2009 package change, which was designed to be cost-neutral, has not been found to increase the cost of the average recipient's food package.[35] Costs were derived from searches of administrative reports and from personal communications with WIC agency staff. Labor costs were estimated using data from the Bureau of Labor Statistics.[36,37] Costs are discounted at 3% annually, adjusted for inflation, and reported in 2019 US dollars. More details on model inputs can be found in the Supplemental Information.

Microsimulation Model

Using these data on the cost, population reach, and effectiveness of the WIC food package change, we then used the CHOICES microsimulation model to estimate outcomes related to childhood obesity for the US population from 2010 through 2019 associated with the package change, along with estimates of uncertainty for each outcome. The microsimulation model leverages detailed data from multiple nationally representative datasets to simulate the experiences of individuals in the US population related to height/weight trajectories and health, accounting for projected population growth.[38] The model assumes a 1-time effect from the intervention, and then calculates expected body mass index (BMI) trajectories moving forward in childhood from that initial BMI change. The model estimates health care costs associated with each unit change of BMI using age- and sex-specific estimates derived from the Medical Expenditure Panel Survey.[39] The model also estimates gains in quality-adjusted life years (QALYs), which are a measure of health benefit in terms of both quantity and quality of life lived. QALYs are used to estimate a cost-effectiveness metric, cost per

QALY, and enable comparisons with the cost-effectiveness of other interventions. QALYs were estimated using published estimates of the relationship between weight category and health-related quality of life by sex and age group for children[40] and adults.[41,42] For children, a recent meta-analysis[40] calculated the decrement in health-related quality of life weights linked with overweight and obesity using a variety of measures. We also used published[13] adult weights, which use nationally representative health care expenditure data,[41] to calculate weights for children, making use of the strong relationship between child and adult weight status. When compared with the first set of weights, results were similar; thus, we chose to use the weights based on more representative data. More details on the calculation of QALYs can be found elsewhere[43] and in the Supplemental Information. To account for uncertainty in model inputs, we calculated 95% uncertainty intervals (UI), using 1000 Monte Carlo iterations for a simulated nationally representative population of 1 million individuals. Further details on the CHOICES microsimulation model are available in the Supplemental Information.

We used the microsimulation model to estimate 10-year population reach, implementation costs, QALYs gained, health care costs saved per dollar invested, cost-per-QALY, and the number of cases of childhood obesity prevented just in the year 2019, under 2 scenarios: (1) "historical" implementation, in which the benefits of the WIC package change would only accrue to children who actually participated (primary scenario); and (2) "full" implementation, in which we estimated what benefits society could have seen if all eligible children had participated in WIC (secondary scenario). We also projected whether the WIC program might have impacted socioeconomic and income-related racial/ethnic disparities in childhood obesity by comparing the percentage point differences in obesity prevalence between (1) children in poverty and children with household income at or above 350% FPL and (2) non-Hispanic white children compared with non-Hispanic Black and Hispanic children that would have been expected with and without the package change.

RESULTS

Primary Scenario

From 2010 through 2019, the model estimated that 14.0 million 2- to 4-year-old children (95% UI, 13.7–14.2 million), all from households with low income, were reached by the WIC package change (Table 1). The WIC package change is estimated to have prevented 62 700 cases of childhood obesity in the year 2019 alone (95% UI. 53 900–71 100). Combining data on implementation costs with health care cost savings attributable to the prevented cases of childhood obesity, the WIC 2009 package change is estimated to have saved $0.27 in health care costs per dollar invested

TABLE 1 Projected 10-Year Cost-Effectiveness Outcomes (Mean and 95% Uncertainty Intervals) of the 2009 WIC Food Package Change, 2010–2019		
	Historical Model	**Full Participation Model**
Children reached by the intervention (million)[a]	14.0 (13.7–14.2)	29.6 (29.0–30.0)
Implementation costs (million)	$248 ($247–$248)	$248 ($247–$248)
Implementation cost per child reached by the intervention	$17.70 ($17.40–$18.10)	$8.36 ($8.24–$8.52)
Healthcare costs saved (million)	$67.6 ($65.7–$69.6)	$161 ($157–$165)
Health care cost savings per dollar invested	$0.27 ($0.27–$0.28)	$0.65 ($0.63–$0.67)
Net costs (million)	$180 ($178–$182)	$86.8 ($82.7–$90.6)
Total cases of childhood obesity prevented in the year 2019 alone[a]	62 700 (53 900–71 100)	145 000 (125 000–166 000)
Cost per quality-adjusted life year gained	$10 600 ($9760–$11 700)	$2180 ($1980–$2430)

All costs and health outcomes are discounted at 3% annually unless otherwise noted; costs are reported in 2019 US dollars.
[a] Not discounted.

(95% UI, $0.27–$0.28) and cost $10 600 per QALY gained (95% UI, $9760–$11 700).

The WIC 2009 package change is also estimated to have narrowed income-related disparities in childhood obesity prevalence (Fig 1). Because the program is targeted only to children from households with low incomes, the cases of obesity estimated to have been prevented were entirely concentrated among these children, with an estimated 196 cases and 188 cases prevented per 100 000 children for children with household incomes at or below 130% and between 131% to 185% of the FPL, respectively, and no change predicted for the highest income group. This resulted in the gap in obesity prevalence between children in poverty compared with children with family incomes at or above 350% of the FPL shrinking by 4.5%. Similarly, because WIC participants are more likely to identify as Black or Hispanic than white, reductions in disparities by race/ethnicity were also observed, with 126 cases of childhood obesity prevented per 100 000 for Black children and 183 cases prevented per 100 000 for Hispanic children, compared with 33 cases per 100 000 prevented for White children.

Secondary Scenario

Meanwhile, we estimate that if there had been complete participation in WIC among eligible 2- to 4-year olds, 29.6 million children (95% UI, 29.0–30.0 million) (ie, an additional 15.6 million) would have been reached in this 10-year period, and that 145 000 cases of childhood obesity (95% UI, 125 000–166 000) could have been prevented in 2019 (Table 1). Complete participation would have resulted in similar implementation costs to the primary scenario (because most costs were incurred at the agency and retailer levels, and thus would not depend on the number of WIC participants) but with more overall health care cost savings ($161 million; 95% UI, $157–$165 million for full participation compared with $67.6 million; 95% UI, $65.7–$69.6 million for the historical model), resulting in lower net costs to

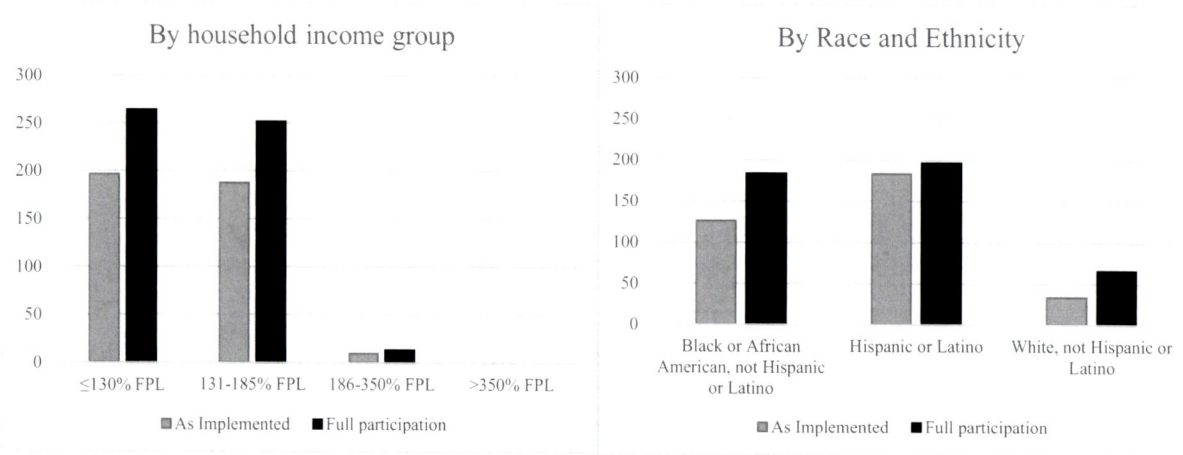

FIGURE 1
Projected cases of childhood obesity prevented per 100 000 people in 2019 attributable to the WIC package change in historical and full participation scenarios, by household income status and race/ethnicity.

society of $86.8 million (95% UI, 82.7–90.6 million). Subsequently, this would have resulted in higher health care cost savings per dollar invested ($0.65; 95% UI, $0.63–$0.67) and a substantially lower cost per QALY gained ($2180 per QALY; 95% UI, $1980–$2430). If all income-eligible children had been reached, the gap in obesity prevalence between children in poverty compared with children with family incomes at or above 350% of the FPL would have shrunk by 6.0%.

DISCUSSION

In this study, we projected that the 2009 changes to the WIC food package were highly cost-effective for preventing childhood obesity and improved health equity. Updating the food package is estimated to have prevented nearly 60 000 cases of childhood obesity in the year 2019 alone, entirely among children living in households with low income, and to have been a good investment for health, at a cost-per-QALY of $10 600. This cost-per-QALY is well below most established willingness-to-pay thresholds, which typically range from $50 000 to $150 000 per QALY in the United States.[44,45] Furthermore, the package change is estimated to have narrowed socioeconomic gaps in obesity prevalence. As policymakers consider strategies to improve health and promote health equity, our analyses show that updating nutrition standards for this critical food assistance program— one that reaches millions of young children with low incomes and provides a range of benefits for healthy development— was likely a beneficial and cost-effective policy.

Furthermore, this study found that the population health benefits could have been more than doubled, while resulting in similar implementation costs, if WIC had been able to reach all eligible 2- to 4-year-old children. In other words, the United States missed out on preventing an additional 82 300 cases of childhood obesity in 2020 because of WIC's not reaching all eligible preschool-aged children. In turn, payers of health care costs in the United States, including public and private insurance and families, missed out on saving an additional $93.4 million in health care costs. Diminished retention in the WIC program as children age, dropping from nearly 100% coverage of eligible infants to only 25% coverage of eligible 4-year olds,[21] is a critical concern for WIC.[22] Children and families cannot receive the numerous economic, health, and developmental benefits of the WIC program if they are not participating in the program in the first place.

Our results suggest 2 key considerations for leveraging WIC to promote eating patterns that help equitably prevent chronic disease and obesity. First, policy efforts to further improve the nutritional quality of the WIC food packages are needed. The results from the 2009 package change for population health are promising. However, surveillance data of obesity in WIC preschool-aged children suggests a leveling off of the decline in obesity prevalence,[46] suggesting

that the 2009 food package changes may have had all of the impact they can. The USDA, using science-based recommendations from the National Academy of Medicine, recently proposed regulations to update the WIC package change further, including making a change introduced during the COVID-19 pandemic to increase the benefit amount for the fruit and vegetable cash-value voucher permanent. Such changes to strengthen WIC's nutritional offerings might further benefit population health. Second, more research and action are needed to better understand how to improve WIC's reach. Existing research suggests that reduced satisfaction with the food package for children plays a role, particularly for families whose cultural food traditions do not align with foods in the package (eg, families who do not consume dairy or cold breakfast cereal).[47,48] Experiencing stigma while shopping with WIC benefits has also been cited as a potential reason, with confusion and mislabeled items in WIC-participating retailers contributing to these experiences.[49] Mechanisms to streamline and use electronic apps and tools for WIC to address some of these issues, such as smartphone apps to help identify WIC-eligible products in-store[47,50] and the use of electronic-benefit-transfer cards,[51] have had promising effects.[52] Further evaluation of strategies to help keep eligible participants enrolled throughout their eligibility period is needed.

There are several limitations to this study. Because it is not possible to randomize children to receive WIC benefits, the evidence we used for the effect of the WIC package change on child BMI is subject to bias. It is possible that the association between the WIC package change and decreased obesity prevalence over time is due to compositional changes in the WIC population or some other population-wide effect. However, the original analysis used for the BMI effect in this paper adjusted for changes in sociodemographic composition of the WIC population over time and also accounted for changes in economic conditions over time[17]; moreover, the findings of a change in dietary intake and weight status related to the 2009 WIC package change have been consistently replicated across multiple studies and contexts.[12–14,18] Other obesity prevention interventions, such as breastfeeding or physical activity interventions, could also have theoretically influenced childhood obesity among WIC 2- to 4-year olds, though such influences have not been quantified. Other limitations related to data availability include a lack of data on whether there were differential effects of the WIC package change by race/ethnicity— our model estimates of disparities changes are based solely on the fact that WIC is used by relatively higher proportions of Black and Hispanic children, not on estimated differences in effect size—and a lack of data about the administrative costs required for increasing WIC participation in our secondary scenario. A further limitation is that this cost-effectiveness model focuses solely on obesity prevention and does not consider other potential impacts on child health that may have resulted from the WIC package change. For example, it is unknown whether the package change had any impacts on children's cognitive development.

CONCLUSIONS

The WIC 2009 food package change is estimated to have reduced childhood obesity for children in households with low income and to be highly cost-effective while improving health equity. WIC's beneficial impact could be expanded by identifying strategies to increase enrollment and improve retention in the program.

Address correspondence to Erica Kenney, ScD, MPH, Department of Nutrition, Harvard T.H. Chan School of Public Health, 665 Huntington Ave, Boston, MA 02115. E-mail: ekenney@hsph.harvard.edu

PEDIATRICS (ISSN Numbers: Print, 0031-4005; Online, 1098-4275).

FUNDING: This study was supported by the National Institutes of Health (R01HL146625 and K01DK125278), The JPB Foundation, and the Centers for Disease Control and Prevention (U48DP006376).

CONFLICT OF INTEREST DISCLOSURES: The authors have indicated they have no potential conflicts of interest to disclose. The findings and conclusions are those of the authors and do not necessarily represent the official position of the National Institutes of Health, the Centers for Disease Control and Prevention, or other funders.

REFERENCES

1. U.S. Department of Agriculture, U.S. Department of Health and Human Services. *Dietary Guidelines for Americans, 2020–2025.* 9th ed. USDA; 2020

2. United States Department of Agriculture Food and Nutrition Services. Special Supplemental Nutrition Program for Women, Infants, and Children (WIC): about WIC. Available at: https://www.fns.usda.gov/wic/about-wic. Accessed June 7, 2022

3. United States Department of Agriculture Food and Nutrition Services. WIC eligibility requirements. Available at: https://www.fns.usda.gov/wic/wic-eligibility-requirements. Accessed June 7, 2022

4. USDA Food and Nutrition Service. WIC program participation and costs. Available at: https://fns-prod.azureedge.us/sites/default/files/resource-files/wisummary-12.pdf. Accessed December 18, 2022

5. United States Department of Agriculture Food and Nutrition Service. WIC 2019 eligibility and coverage rates. Available at: https://www.fns.usda.gov/wic/2019-eligibility-coverage-rates. Accessed January 3, 2023

6. Bitler MP, Currie J. Does WIC work? The effects of WIC on pregnancy and birth outcomes. *J Policy Anal Manage.* 2005;24(1):73–91

7. Jackson MI. Early childhood WIC participation, cognitive development and academic achievement. *Soc Sci Med.* 2015;126:145–153

8. Kreider B, Pepper JV, Roy M. Identifying the effects of WIC on food insecurity among infants and children. *South Econ J.* 2016; 82(4):1106–1122

9. Weaver RG, Brazendale K, Hunt E, Sarzynski MA, Beets MW, White K. Disparities in childhood overweight and obesity by income in the United States: an epidemiological examination using three nationally representative datasets. *Int J Obes.* 2019;43(6): 1210–1222

10. Ogden CL, Carroll MD, Lawman HG, et al. Trends in obesity prevalence among children and adolescents in the United States, 1988-1994 through 2013-2014. *JAMA.* 2016;315(21):2292–2299

11. Institute of Medicine. *WIC Food Packages: Time for a Change.* The National Academies Press; 2005

12. Schultz DJ, Byker Shanks C, Houghtaling B. The impact of the 2009 Special Supplemental Nutrition Program for Women, Infants, and Children Food Package revisions on participants: a systematic review. *J Acad Nutr Diet.* 2015;115(11):1832–1846

13. Ng SW, Hollingsworth BA, Busey EA, Wandell JL, Miles DR, Poti JM. Federal nutrition program revisions impact low-income households' food purchases. *Am J Prev Med.* 2018;54(3):403–412

14. Tester JM, Leung CW, Crawford PB. Revised WIC food package and children's diet quality. *Pediatrics.* 2016;137(5):e20153557

15. Andreyeva T, Tripp AS. The healthfulness of food and beverage purchases after the federal food package revisions: the case of two New England states. *Prev Med.* 2016;91:204–210

16. Andreyeva T, Luedicke J, Tripp AS, Henderson KE. Effects of reduced juice allowances in food packages for the women, infants, and children program. *Pediatrics.* 2013;131(5):919–927

17. Daepp MIG, Gortmaker SL, Wang YC, Long MW, Kenney EL. WIC food package changes: trends in childhood obesity prevalence. *Pediatrics.* 2019;143(5):e20182841

18. Chaparro MP, Crespi CM, Anderson CE, Wang MC, Whaley SE. The 2009 Special Supplemental Nutrition Program for Women, Infants,

and Children (WIC) food package change and children's growth trajectories and obesity in Los Angeles County. *Am J Clin Nutr.* 2019;109(5):1414–1421

19. Pan L, Freedman DS, Sharma AJ, et al. Trends in obesity among participants aged 2-4 years in the Special Supplemental Nutrition Program for Women, Infants, and Children - United States, 2000-2014. *MMWR Morb Mortal Wkly Rep.* 2016;65(45):1256–1260

20. Food and Nutrition Service. Proposed rule: Special Supplemental Nutrition Program for Women, Infants, and Children: Revisions in the Women, Infants, and Children food packages (docket FNS-2022-0007-0001). Available at: https://www.regulations.gov/document/FNS-2022-0007-0001. Accessed November 1, 2023

21. Farson Gray K, Balch-Crystal E, Giannarelli L, Johnson P. National- and state-level estimates of WIC eligibility and WIC program reach in 2019. Available at: https://fns-prod.azureedge.us/sites/default/files/resource-files/WICEligibles2019-Volume1-revised.pdf. Accessed November 1, 2023

22. United States Department of Agriculture Food and Nutrition Service. WIC and WIC FMNP informational memorandum: American Rescue Plan Act of 2021 (PL. 117-2), Program Modernization. Available at: https://fns-prod.azureedge.us/sites/default/files/resource-files/WICandFMNPInfoMemo-American-Rescue-Plan-Act-Pgm-Modernization.pdf.pdf. Accessed November 1, 2023

23. Gortmaker SL, Wang YC, Long MW, et al. Three interventions that reduce childhood obesity are projected to save more than they cost to implement. *Health Aff (Millwood).* 2015;34(11):1932–1939

24. Cradock AL, Barrett JL, Kenney EL, et al. Using cost-effectiveness analysis to prioritize policy and programmatic approaches to physical activity promotion and obesity prevention in childhood. *Prev Med.* 2017;95(suppl):S17–S27

25. Sharifi M, Franz C, Horan CM, et al. Cost-effectiveness of a clinical childhood obesity intervention. *Pediatrics.* 2017;140(5):e20162998

26. Kenney EL, Cradock AL, Long MW, et al. Cost effectiveness of water promotion strategies in schools for preventing childhood obesity and increasing water intake. *Obesity (Silver Spring).* 2019;27(12):2037–2045

27. United States Department of Agriculture Food and Nutrition Service. National- and state-level estimates of Special Supplemental Nutrition Program for Women, Infants, and Children (WIC) eligibles and program reach in 2014, and updated estimates for 2005–2013. Available at: https://fns-prod.azureedge.us/sites/default/files/ops/WICEligibles2014.pdf. Accessed November 20, 2022

28. United States Department of Agriculture Food and Nutrition Service. National- and state-level estimates of WIC eligibles and WIC program reach in 2015, final report: volume 1. Available at: https://fns-prod.azureedge.us/sites/default/files/ops/WICEligibles2015-Volume1.pdf. Accessed November 20, 2022

29. United States Department of Agriculture Food and Nutrition Service. National- and state-level estimates of WIC eligibility and WIC program reach in 2017, final report: volume 1. Available at: https://fns-prod.azureedge.us/sites/default/files/resource-files/WICEligibles2017-Volume1.pdf. Accessed November 20, 2022

30. United States Department of Agriculture Food and Nutrition Service. National- and state-level estimates of WIC eligibility and WIC program reach in 2016, final report: volume 1. Available at: https://fns-prod.azureedge.us/sites/default/files/resource-files/WICEligibles2016-Volume1.pdf. Accessed November 20, 2022

31. United States Department of Agriculture. WIC policy memorandum 2011-5: WIC nutrition risk criteria. Available at: https://fns-prod.azureedge.us/sites/default/files/2011-5-WICNutritionRiskCriteria.pdf. Accessed November 6, 2023

32. Drummond MF, Sculpher MJ, Claxton K, Stoddart GL, Torrance GW. *Methods for the Economic Evaluation of Health Care Programmes.* Oxford University Press; 2015

33. Gold MR, Siegel JE, Russell LB. *Cost-Effectiveness in Health and Medicine.* Oxford University Press; 1996

34. Gleason S, Morgan R, Bell L, Pooler J. Impact of the revised WIC food package on small WIC vendors: insight from a four-state evaluation. Available at: https://www.calwic.org/storage/FourStateWICFoodPackageEvaluation-Full_Report-20May11.pdf. Accessed November 1, 2023

35. National Academies of Sciences Engineering Medicine. Review of WIC food packages: improving balance and choice. Available at: https://nap.nationalacademies.org/catalog/23655/review-of-wic-food-packages-improving-balance-and-choice-final. Accessed November 1, 2023

36. U.S. Bureau of Labor Statistics. Employer costs for employee compensation – September 2014, USDL-14-2208. Available at: https://www.bls.gov/news.release/archives/ecec_12102014.pdf. Accessed October 13, 2022

37. U.S. Bureau of Labor Statistics. May 2019 national occupational employment and wage estimates. Available at: https://www.bls.gov/oes/2019/may/oes_nat.htm. Accessed October 13, 2022

38. Ward ZJ, Long MW, Resch SC, Giles CM, Cradock AL, Gortmaker SL. Simulation of growth trajectories of childhood obesity into adulthood. *N Engl J Med.* 2017;377(22):2145–2153

39. Ward ZJ, Bleich SN, Long MW, Gortmaker SL. Association of body mass index with health care expenditures in the United States by age and sex. *PLoS One.* 2021;16(3):e0247307

40. Kwon J, Kim SW, Ungar WJ, Tsiplova K, Madan J, Petrou S. A systematic review and meta-analysis of childhood health utilities. *Med Decis Making.* 2018;38(3):277–305

41. Shaw JW, Johnson JA, Coons SJ. US valuation of the EQ-5D health states: development and testing of the D1 valuation model. *Med Care.* 2005;43(3):203–220

42. Muennig P, Lubetkin E, Jia H, Franks P. Gender and the burden of disease attributable to obesity. *Am J Public Health.* 2006;96(9):1662–1668

43. Dupuis R, Block JP, Barrett JL, et al. Cost effectiveness of calorie labeling at large fast-food chains across the US [published online ahead of print August 14, 2023]. *Am J Prev Med.* doi: 10.1097/00005650-200503000-00003

44. Neumann PJ, Cohen JT, Weinstein MC. Updating cost-effectiveness—the curious resilience of the $50,000-per-QALY threshold. *N Engl J Med.* 2014;371(9):796–797

45. Vanness DJ, Lomas J, Ahn H. A health opportunity cost threshold for cost-effectiveness analysis in the United States. *Ann Intern Med.* 2021;174(1):25–32

46. Kline N, Zvavitch P, Wroblewska K, Worden M, Mwombela B, Thorn B. WIC participant and program characteristics 2020. Available at: https://fns-prod.azureedge.us/sites/default/files/resource-files/WICPC2020-1.pdf. Accessed November 2, 2022

47. Gago CM, Wynne JO, Moore MJ, et al. Caregiver perspectives on underutilization of WIC: a qualitative study. *Pediatrics*. 2022;149(2): e2021053889

48. Weber SJ, Wichelecki J, Chavez N, Bess S, Reese L, Odoms-Young A. Understanding the factors influencing low-income caregivers' perceived value of a federal nutrition programme, the Special Supplemental Nutrition Program for Women, Infants and Children (WIC). *Public Health Nutr*. 2019;22(6):1056–1065

49. Chauvenet C, De Marco M, Barnes C, Ammerman AS. WIC recipients in the retail environment: a qualitative study assessing customer experience and satisfaction. *J Acad Nutr Diet*. 2019;119(3):416–424.e2

50. Zimmer MC, Beaird J, Steeves EA. WIC participants' perspectives of facilitators and barriers to shopping with eWIC compared with paper vouchers. *J Nutr Educ Behav*. 2021;53(3):195–203

51. Vasan A, Kenyon CC, Feudtner C, Fiks AG, Venkataramani AS. Association of WIC participation and electronic benefits transfer implementation. *JAMA Pediatr*. 2021;175(6):609–616

52. United States Department of Agriculture Food and Nutrition Services. Child nutrition programs: COVID-19 waivers by state. Available at: https://www.fns.usda.gov/disaster/pandemic/covid-19/cn-waivers-flexibilities. Accessed November 1, 2023

53. Long MW, Polacsek M, Bruno P, et al. Cost-effectiveness analysis and stakeholder evaluation of 2 obesity prevention policies in Maine, US. *J Nutr Educ Behav*. 2019;51(10):1177–1187

54. Tiehen L, Frazão E. Where do WIC participants redeem their food benefits? An analysis of WIC food dollar redemption patterns by store type. Available at: https://www.ers.usda.gov/webdocs/publications/44073/57246_eib152.pdf?v=0. Accessed March 12, 2023

55. United States Department of Agriculture Food and Nutrition Service. 2013 WIC vendor management study. Available at: https://fns-prod.azureedge.us/sites/default/files/resource-files/2013WICVendor.pdf. Accessed March 12, 2023

56. Andreyeva T, Middleton AE, Long MW, Luedicke J, Schwartz MB. Food retailer practices, attitudes and beliefs about the supply of healthy foods. *Public Health Nutr*. 2011;14(6):1024–1031

Trends in Severe Obesity Among Children Aged 2 to 4 Years in WIC: 2010 to 2020

Lixia Zhao, PhD, David S. Freedman, PhD, Heidi M. Blanck, PhD, Sohyun Park, PhD

OBJECTIVES: To examine the prevalence and trends in severe obesity among 16.6 million children aged 2 to 4 years enrolled in the Special Supplemental Nutrition Program for Women, Infants, and Children (WIC) from 2010 to 2020.

METHODS: Severe obesity was defined as a sex-specific BMI for age $\geq$120% of the 95th percentile on the Centers for Disease Control and Prevention growth charts or BMI $\geq$35 kg/m^2. Joinpoint regression was used to identify when changes occurred in the overall trend. Logistic regression was used to compute the adjusted prevalence differences between years controlling for sex, age, and race and ethnicity.

RESULTS: The prevalence of severe obesity significantly decreased from 2.1% in 2010 to 1.8% in 2016 and then increased to 2.0% in 2020. From 2010 to 2016, the prevalence decreased significantly among all sociodemographic subgroups except for American Indian/Alaska Native (AI/AN) children. The largest decreases were among 4-year-olds, Asian/Pacific Islander and Hispanic children, and children from higher-income households. However, from 2016 to 2020, the prevalence increased significantly overall and among sociodemographic subgroups, except for AI/AN and non-Hispanic white children. The largest increases occurred in 4-year-olds and Hispanic children. Among 56 WIC agencies, the prevalence significantly declined in 17 agencies, and 1 agency (Mississippi) showed a significant increase from 2010 to 2016. In contrast, 21 agencies had significant increases, and only Alaska had a significant decrease from 2016 to 2020.

CONCLUSIONS: Although severe obesity prevalence in toddlers declined from 2010 to 2016, recent trends are upward. Early identification and access to evidence-based family healthy weight programs for at-risk children can support families and child health.

Division of Nutrition, Physical Activity, and Obesity, Centers for Disease Control and Prevention, Atlanta, Georgia

Dr Zhao conducted the data analyses, drafted the initial manuscript, revised the manuscript, and contributed to conceptualization of the study; Drs Freedman, Blanck, and Park contributed to the conceptualization, writing, reviewing, and editing of the manuscript; and all authors approved the final manuscript as submitted and agree to be accountable for all aspects of the work.

The findings and conclusions in this report are those of the authors and do not necessarily represent the official position of the Centers for Disease Control and Prevention.

DOI: https://doi.org/10.1542/peds.2023-062461

Accepted for publication Aug 15, 2023

Address correspondence to Lixia Zhao, PhD, Division of Nutrition, Physical Activity, and Obesity, National Center for Chronic Disease Prevention and Health Promotion, Centers for Disease Control and Prevention, 4770 Buford Highway, NE, Atlanta, GA 30341. E-mail: ynl3@cdc.gov

PEDIATRICS (ISSN Numbers: Print, 0031-4005; Online, 1098-4275).

WHAT'S KNOWN ON THIS SUBJECT: The prevalence of severe obesity among low-income children modestly declined from 2004 to 2014. However, little is known about (1) whether this declining trend has continued and (2) the state-level prevalence and trends in severe obesity.

WHAT THIS STUDY ADDS: The declining trends in severe obesity among 16.6 million low-income children between 2010 and 2016 have been reversed. The upward trends are concerning. Early identification and referral to family healthy weight programs for at-risk children can support healthy child growth.

> **To cite:** Zhao L, Freedman DS, Blanck HM, et al. Trends in Severe Obesity Among Children Aged 2 to 4 Years in WIC: 2010 to 2020. *Pediatrics.* 2024;153(1):e2023062461

ARTICLE

The prevalence of childhood obesity remains high in the United States; ~1 in 5 US children and adolescents have obesity.[1,2] The trends of childhood obesity have been well-documented by using the National Health and Nutrition Examination Survey (NHANES). Among youth aged 2 to 19 years, obesity prevalence has plateaued or slightly increased in the recent decades,[2-6] whereas the prevalence of severe obesity rose from 3.6% in 1999–2000 to 6.1% in 2017–2018.[5] In addition to these trends, recent cohort studies revealed substantial weight gain, particularly among children with excessive weight, during the early phase of the coronavirus disease 2019 (COVID-19) pandemic.[7,8] However, it is noteworthy that the accelerated weight gain during the early pandemic was largely attenuated later in the pandemic (January to November 2021).[9] These findings indicate a potential fluctuation in weight changes among children and the need for ongoing monitoring and interventions.

Children with severe obesity, compared with their peers with moderate obesity (BMI ≥95th percentile to <120% of the 95th percentile), are at a greater risk of various health complications, including cardiovascular disease, metabolic syndrome, type 2 diabetes, fatty liver disease, and premature death.[10-12] Despite these significant health implications, there has been limited attention given to understanding the prevalence of severe obesity among children aged 2 to 5 years, a critical age group for public health interventions.[13-15] Nevertheless, the authors of a few NHANES studies examined the prevalence and trends of severe obesity among children aged 2 to 5 years. One study revealed that the prevalence of severe obesity among this age group was 3.0% in 2009–2010, 1.7% in 2015–2016, and 2.9% in 2017–2018.[4] Hales and colleagues reported similar changes between 2009–2010 (2.7%) and 2015–2016 (1.8%).[3] Another study revealed that the prevalence of severe obesity was 2.2% in 2015–2018.[6] However, the 95% confidence intervals (CIs) for these estimates were wide, and no significant trends were observed over the study period. As a result of the small sample size and low cases of severe obesity, NHANES data provide limited ability to monitor trends among this age group, especially by sociodemographic characteristics.

Data from the Special Supplemental Nutrition Program for Women, Infants, and Children (WIC) Participant and Program Characteristics study have been used to monitor weight status among low-income children <5 years of age.[16-20] WIC is a federal assistance program that provides healthy foods, nutrition education, health care referrals, and other services to millions of low-income pregnant and postpartum women, as well as infants and children up to age 5, who are at nutritional risk.[21] In 2019, 20.4% of children in the United States received WIC benefits.[22] A previous study that examined trends in severe obesity among young children enrolled in WIC reported an increase from 1.80% in 2000 to 2.11%

in 2004, followed by a modest decline from 2.11% to 1.96% from 2004 to 2014.[23] However, it is unknown whether this declining trend has been sustained, and little is known about the prevalence and trends in severe obesity at the state level. Understanding the ongoing state-specific trends can help inform targeted intervention strategies for children at risk. In this study, with the latest data from WIC Participant and Program Characteristics (WIC-PC), we aimed to provide an updated prevalence of severe obesity among low-income children aged 2 to 4 years enrolled in WIC, and we examined trends in severe obesity by sex, age, race and ethnicity, household income, and by WIC State agency from 2010 to 2020.

METHODS

Data Sources and Study Population

The WIC-PC is a biennial census of participants certified to receive WIC benefits as of April of the reporting years (even years). WIC benefits include nutritious supplemental foods, nutrition education and counseling, and referrals to health care and social services, etc.[21] It is one of the largest federal nutrition programs, serving millions of people. The program helps maintain and improve the health of low-income pregnant, postpartum, and breastfeeding women, as well as infants and children up to age 5, who are at nutritional risk.[21] Enrollees must meet residential, nutritional risk, and income requirements to qualify for the benefits. Income eligibility is based on a household income of no more than 185% of the federal poverty income guidelines or participation in other federal programs, such as the Supplemental Nutrition Assistance Program, Temporary Assistance for Needy Families, or Medicaid.[24] The US Department of Agriculture's (USDA's) Food and Nutrition Service manages WIC at the federal level, and WIC is administered at the local level by state health departments or Indian tribal organizations in each state or territory. Children's weight and height (or length) are measured and collected by trained program staff during certification or recertification visits, and the data are used to calculate BMI. Weights were measured to the nearest one-quarter pound, and heights to the nearest one-eighth inch according to the Centers for Disease Control and Prevention (CDC) nutrition surveillance program standards.[25,26] The validity of these measurements was found to be sufficiently accurate.[27] This study did not need review by the Institutional Review Board of the CDC because we used deidentified secondary data.

The data for this study are from 6 WIC-PC censuses (2010 to 2020). The initial population included ~17.2 million children aged 2 to 4 years enrolled in WIC from 50 states, the District of Columbia, and 5 territories. We excluded 17 children whose weight and height were measured >1 year before the reporting year and 206 912 children whose sex, weight, height, or BMI were missing or biologically implausible based on the suggested CDC cutpoints.[28] We further excluded 308 091 children who were certified in March and April 2020 given data quality concerns due to the COVID-19 pandemic, which is ~15.8% of 2020 WIC participating children.[29] This yielded an analytical sample of 16 557 172 children ranging from 3 307 442 in 2010 to 1 646 747 in 2020.

Defining Severe Obesity

Severe obesity was defined as a sex-specific BMI for age ≥120% of the 95th percentile based on the CDC growth charts or a BMI ≥35 kg/m². Of the 4717 children in this analysis who had a BMI ≥35 kg/m², none were <120% of the 95th percentile.

Sociodemographic Characteristics

Sociodemographic variables included sex, age group (2, 3, or 4 years), race and ethnicity, and household income. Race and ethnicity are social constructs and were based on self-reports. USDA's WIC study team classified these self-reports into 5 mutually exclusive categories (American Indian/Alaska Native [AI/AN], Asian/Pacific Islander, Black, non-Hispanic [Black], Hispanic, or white, non-Hispanic [white]). Children with multiple race and ethnicity designations were not forced into a single category. Instead, a mapping approach developed by the USDA was employed to assign individuals to the appropriate category within the 5-category classification.[25] Children whose race or ethnicity was unknown were not included in analyses that specifically focused on (or adjusted for) race and ethnicity. Household income included income from all sources that were assessed at each WIC certification or recertification appointment. It was expressed as a percentage of the federal poverty level (% FPL) and categorized into <50% FPL, 50% to <100% FPL, 100% to <150% FPL, and ≥150% FPL.

Statistical Analyses

Descriptive analyses were conducted in SAS 9.4 (SAS Institute, Cary, NC) for the overall population, by sociodemographic characteristics and WIC state or territorial agency. The unadjusted prevalence of severe obesity and 95% CI were computed overall and for each subgroup. For trend analyses, we first used Joinpoint trend analysis software (National Cancer Institute, version 4.9.0, https://surveillance. cancer.gov/joinpoint) to identify possible knots in the overall trend in severe obesity prevalence from 2010 to 2020, and the software identified 2016 as the inflection year. Therefore, we focused on 2 periods, 2010 to 2016 and 2016 to 2020, to study the prevalence differences between years. We used logistic regression controlling for age in months, sex, and race and ethnicity to obtain the adjusted prevalence differences (APDs) during each period. We included race and

ethnicity as a confounding factor in the analysis, in addition to age and sex, because previous studies have revealed racial and ethnic disparities in severe obesity among young children.[15,23] The APDs were computed as 100 times the average marginal effect of year (2010 vs 2016 and 2016 vs 2020). The calculations were conducted in R with the "margins" package.[30,31] The APD was considered statistically significant if the 2-sided P value was <.05. A negative number of APD means that the adjusted prevalence in the latter year decreased compared with the earlier year.

RESULTS

The sociodemographic characteristics of children aged 2 to 4 years enrolled in WIC are shown in Table 1. The number of children included in this analysis was ~3.3 million in 2010, ~2.8 million in 2016, and ~1.6 million in 2020. The study population in 2010 had a slightly higher proportion of 4-year-olds than those in more recent years. The proportion of Black children increased from 18.7% in 2010% to 22.7% in 2020, whereas the proportion of Hispanic children decreased from 46.5% in 2010% to 43.3% in 2020. In addition, the proportion of children from families with household income <50% FPL increased from 2010 to 2020 (Table 1).

In all years, girls had slightly higher severe obesity prevalence than boys, the prevalence of severe obesity increased with age, and the highest prevalence was observed among 4-year-olds. Within racial and ethnic subgroups, AI/AN and Hispanic children had the highest prevalence. The prevalence of severe obesity was higher among children from families below the poverty level (<100% FPL) than children from families with relatively higher (100% to <150% FPL) or highest (≥150% FPL) household income (Table 2, Fig 1).

From 2010 to 2016, the overall prevalence of severe obesity decreased significantly by 0.19% points (95% CI [−0.21 to −0.16]; P < .001) after adjusting for age, sex, and race and ethnicity (Table 2). There were significant decreasing trends among all sociodemographic subgroups except for AI/AN children, for whom the adjusted prevalence decrease was not statistically significant (Table 2, Fig 1). Within the various subgroups, the largest adjusted prevalence decreases were observed among 4-year-olds (−0.32%, 95% CI [−0.38 to −0.27]), Asian/Pacific Islander (−0.32% [−0.41 to −0.23]), Hispanic children (−0.31% [−0.34 to −0.27]), and children from families with relative higher household income (100% to <150% FPL) (−0.27% [−0.32 to −0.22]; Table 2).

From 2016 to 2020, the prevalence of severe obesity increased significantly from 1.8% to 2.0% overall (APD, 0.23% [0.21 to 0.26], P < .001) and among most sociodemographic subgroups except for AI/AN and white children, for which the prevalence remained stable between 2016 and 2020 (Table 2, Fig 1). The adjusted prevalence increases were similar among boys and girls and among household

TABLE 1 Sociodemographic Characteristics of Children Aged 2 to 4 Years Enrolled in WIC Program in Selected Years, 2010 to 2020[a]

Characteristics	2010 n (%)	2016 n (%)	2020[b] n (%)
Total, n	3 307 442	2 818 594	1 646 747
Sex			
Male	1 676 395 (50.7)	1 431 197 (50.8)	837 069 (50.8)
Female	1 631 047 (49.3)	1 387 397 (49.2)	809 678 (49.2)
Age, y			
2	1 333 334 (40.3)	1 152 176 (40.9)	678 668 (41.2)
3	1 166 350 (35.3)	1 027 505 (36.5)	606 069 (36.8)
4	807 758 (24.4)	638 913 (22.7)	362 010 (22.0)
Race/ethnicity			
American Indian/Alaska Native	38 661 (1.2)	35 682 (1.3)	20 977 (1.3)
Asian/Pacific Islander	121 667 (3.7)	136 141 (4.8)	83 365 (5.1)
Black, non-Hispanic	618 580 (18.7)	594 060 (21.1)	373 567 (22.7)
Hispanic	1 536 644 (46.5)	1 274 650 (45.2)	712 904 (43.3)
White, non-Hispanic	966 673 (29.2)	776 843 (27.6)	455 005 (27.6)
Unknown	25 217 (0.8)	1218 (0.04)	929 (0.1)
Household income, % FPL			
<50	980 903 (29.7)	904 683 (32.1)	522 630 (31.7)
50 to <100	1 137 558 (34.4)	983 100 (34.9)	533 270 (32.4)
100 to <150	630 706 (19.1)	497 656 (17.7)	317 305 (19.3)
≥150	331 316 (10.0)	225 424 (8.0)	169 206 (10.3)
Unknown	226 959 (6.9)	207 731 (7.4)	104 336 (6.3)

[a] Included children who were enrolled in WIC from 50 states, the District of Columbia, and 5 US territories.
[b] Children with anthropometric data examined in March and April 2020 were excluded because of the COVID-19 pandemic.

income subgroups. The largest adjusted prevalence increases occurred among 4-year-olds (0.35% [0.28 to 0.42]) and Hispanic children (0.41% [0.36 to 0.46]; Table 2).

Table 3 reveals the crude prevalence and adjusted prevalence changes of severe obesity during the study period for the 56 WIC agencies, including 50 US states, the District of Columbia, and 5 territories. From 2010 to 2016, after adjusting for age, sex, and race and ethnicity, 14 states and 3 territories revealed significant decreases in the prevalence of severe obesity, and 1 state (Mississippi) showed a significant increase. The largest significant decrease among states was observed in Arizona (APD, −0.74% [−0.88 to −0.60]), and the largest decrease among territories was in the Northern Mariana Islands (APD, −1.99% [−2.78 to −1.20]). In contrast, from 2016 to 2020, the prevalence significantly increased in 20 states and Puerto Rico (APD, 0.30% [0.12 to 0.48]). Seven states had a significant increase of >0.3%, and the largest significant increase was in California (APD, 0.54% [0.45 to 0.62]). Alaska was the only WIC agency showing a significant decrease (APD, −0.59% [−1.18 to 0.0]) between 2016 and 2020.

DISCUSSION

We found a modest declining trends in severe obesity prevalence from 2010 to 2016, followed by a modestly increasing trend from 2016 to 2020 among low-income children aged 2 to 4 years enrolled in WIC. Although the magnitudes of the decline and the increase were small, the finding of a reversal in trends from decreasing to increasing is concerning, particularly if the upward trend continues. Our data reveal that the prevalence of severe obesity increased significantly from 2016 to 2020 overall and among all age, sex, household income groups, and race and ethnicity groups, except for American Indian/Alaska Native and non-Hispanic white children. Additionally, we found that 21 of 56 WIC agencies had a significant increase, and only Alaska had a significant decrease in severe obesity prevalence between 2016 and 2020. Our study revealed that 2.0% of low-income young children had severe obesity in 2020. A previous WIC-PC study revealed that the severe obesity prevalence increased from 2000 to 2004 and decreased from 2004 to 2014 among low-income children aged 2 to 4 years.[23] The decrease is similar to what we observed in our study.

A few earlier studies have revealed decreasing trends in obesity among WIC infants and young children from 2000 to 2016 or 2018, but none of these studies examined trends in severe obesity.[18-20] Multiple factors might have contributed to the declines, as noted in these studies. For example, the decreasing trends could be influenced by the revised 2009 WIC food packages that provided cash allowances for various healthy food options in addition to federal, state, and local obesity prevention initiatives and programs. The revised WIC food package includes extra cash allowances for fruits, vegetables, and whole grains,

TABLE 2 Trends in the Prevalence of Severe Obesity[a] Among Children Aged 2 to 4 Years Enrolled in WIC Program in Selected Years, 2010 to 2020

Characteristics	Crude Prevalence, % (95% CI)			APD,[b] % (95% CI)	
	2010	2016	2020[c]	2016 vs 2010	2020 vs 2016
Overall	2.12 (2.10 to 2.13)	1.84 (1.83 to 1.86)	2.03 (2.01 to 2.05)	−0.19 (−0.21 to −0.16)[d]	0.23 (0.21 to 0.26)[d]
Sex					
Male	2.06 (2.03 to 2.08)	1.75 (1.73 to 1.77)	1.95 (1.92 to 1.98)	−0.21 (−0.24 to −0.18)[d]	0.25 (0.21 to 0.28)[d]
Female	2.18 (2.16 to 2.20)	1.94 (1.92 to 1.96)	2.11 (2.08 to 2.15)	−0.16 (−0.19 to −0.13)[d]	0.22 (0.18 to 0.26)[d]
Age, y					
2	1.30 (1.28 to 1.32)	1.16 (1.14 to 1.18)	1.25 (1.23 to 1.28)	−0.10 (−0.13 to −0.07)[d]	0.11 (0.08 to 0.15)[d]
3	2.23 (2.20 to 2.26)	1.97 (1.95 to 2.00)	2.24 (2.20 to 2.27)	−0.22 (−0.26 to −0.18)[d]	0.28 (0.24 to 0.33)[d]
4	3.31 (3.27 to 3.35)	2.87 (2.83 to 2.91)	3.14 (3.09 to 3.20)	−0.32 (−0.38 to −0.27)[d]	0.35 (0.28 to 0.42)[d]
Race/ethnicity[e]					
American Indian/Alaska Native	2.66 (2.50 to 2.82)	2.41 (2.26 to 2.57)	2.36 (2.17 to 2.58)	−0.18 (−0.40 to 0.05)	−0.01 (−0.27 to 0.25)
Asian/Pacific Islander	1.51 (1.44 to 1.58)	1.14 (1.08 to 1.20)	1.43 (1.35 to 1.51)	−0.32 (−0.41 to −0.23)[d]	0.28 (0.19 to 0.38)[d]
Black, non-Hispanic	1.51 (1.48 to 1.54)	1.38 (1.35 to 1.41)	1.48 (1.44 to 1.52)	−0.09 (−0.13 to −0.05)[d]	0.13 (0.08 to 0.18)[d]
Hispanic	2.81 (2.78 to 2.83)	2.41 (2.38 to 2.44)	2.79 (2.76 to 2.83)	−0.31 (−0.34 to −0.27)[d]	0.41 (0.36 to 0.46)[d]
White, non-Hispanic	1.45 (1.42 to 1.47)	1.36 (1.34 to 1.39)	1.38 (1.35 to 1.42)	−0.05 (−0.08 to −0.01)[d]	0.03 (−0.01 to 0.07)
Household income, % FPL					
<50	2.18 (2.16 to 2.21)	1.90 (1.88 to 1.93)	2.11 (2.07 to 2.15)	−0.16 (−0.20 to −0.12)[d]	0.24 (0.19 to 0.29)[d]
50 to <100	2.27 (2.25 to 2.30)	1.97 (1.94 to 1.99)	2.19 (2.15 to 2.23)	−0.20 (−0.23 to −0.16)[d]	0.29 (0.24 to 0.34)[d]
100 to <150	2.02 (1.98 to 2.05)	1.66 (1.63 to 1.70)	1.88 (1.83 to 1.93)	−0.27 (−0.32 to −0.22)[d]	0.23 (0.18 to 0.29)[d]
≥150	1.66 (1.61 to 1.70)	1.45 (1.40 to 1.50)	1.72 (1.66 to 1.79)	−0.16 (−0.23 to −0.09)[d]	0.24 (0.16 to 0.32)[d]

[a] Defined as a BMI of 120% or more of the 95th percentile for age and sex on the CDC growth charts or BMI ≥35 kg/m^2.
[b] Represents 100 times the average marginal effect of year (2016 vs 2010, 2020 vs 2016) controlling for sex, age, and race/ethnicity. Children with missing information on race/ethnicity were excluded. A negative value indicates that the prevalence decreased.
[c] Children with anthropometric data examined in March and April 2020 were excluded because of the COVID-19 pandemic.
[d] Statistically significant difference at the 0.05 level based on logistic regression adjusting for age, sex, and race/ethnicity.
[e] Children with multiple race/ethnicity designations were assigned to the appropriate race/ethnicity category presented in the table.

reductions in milk, cheese, and juice allowances, restrictions on milk fat content, and incentives to encourage breastfeeding.[32] Several studies have revealed that these revisions improved the dietary intake habits of WIC participants, potentially contributing to the reduction in obesity prevalence among WIC children.[33–35] However, it is important to note that the effects of the revised food packages on the prevalence of obesity may vary by sex.[36,37] For instance, the food package changes appear to have limited benefits for girls, suggesting that other factors beyond the food packages may influence obesity trends. Additionally, the recent upward trends in severe obesity since 2016 are concerning, indicating that current population-level preventive efforts may not be fully effective. This highlights the need for the ongoing evaluation and refinement of obesity prevention strategies to address the persistent challenge of severe obesity among WIC children and identify additional interventions that can complement the impact of the revised food package.

In addition, we found significant increases in severe obesity among 21 of 56 WIC agencies from 2016 to 2020. The reasons for these increases remain unclear and are likely influenced by a complex interplay of various factors. These factors may include levels of state social resources to families (eg, earned income tax credit, wage supports, Medicaid, housing supports) and variations in funding to support local WIC agencies and clinics, as well as the implementation of the WIC benefits (such as breastfeeding support, provision of supplemental foods, and nutrition education and counseling). Additionally, state policy and environmental changes to improve the availability of healthier food and opportunities for physical activity in communities, alongside efforts to incorporate breastfeeding support, nutrition, and physical activity requirements, into early care and education programs,[38,39] may have played a role. However, further research is needed to understand the specific factors driving the increases in severe obesity across different states.

Although our study did not capture data during the COVID-19 pandemic, it is important to acknowledge the substantial impact of the pandemic on the daily routines of children and adolescents. The pandemic has introduced various challenges, including reduced opportunities for physical activity, increased sedentary behaviors, limited access to healthy food, and heightened stress levels within households.[40] These factors can have significant implications for weight gain, particularly among children with excessive weight, and may potentially influence future trend in severe obesity.[41]

An important avenue for addressing the problem of severe obesity for all children, including those with low

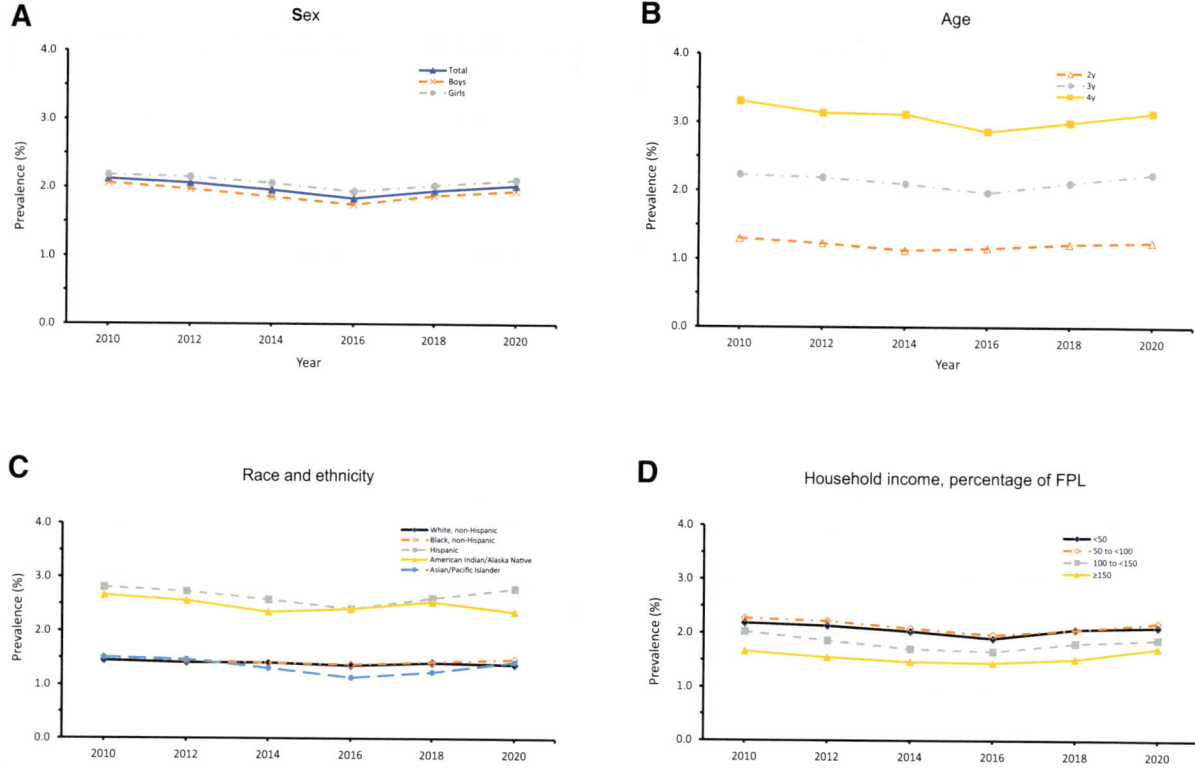

FIGURE 1

Trends in the prevalence of severe obesity among children aged 2 to 4 years enrolled in WIC from 2010 to 2020 by (A) sex, (B) age, (C) race and ethnicity, and (D) household income.

household incomes, is ensuring quality treatment. For young children aged 2 to 5 years who are obese, the American Academy of Pediatrics' new clinical practice guideline recommends intensive health behavior and lifestyle treatment (IHBLT), also called Family Healthy Weight Programs.[42,43] The most effective IHBLT interventions include 26 or more hours of intense, in-person, family-based multicomponent treatment from health care providers over a 3- to 12-month period. IHBLT includes coaching on nutrition, physical activity, and behavioral change support, such as parent modeling of healthy behaviors. Such intensive treatment is not universally available and needs training and support to deliver.[42] Collaborative and continued efforts involving multiple sectors, including state, local, communities, and clinicians, can help ensure that these family-centered intervention strategies are accessible for low-income young children with severe obesity.

The findings in this study are subject to several limitations that should be considered when interpreting the results. Firstly, the findings apply to low-income children enrolled in WIC, limiting the generalizability of the results to children from families of all income levels. Secondly, we did not include children participating in the tribal WIC programs. Therefore, the prevalence and trends

of severe obesity among AI/AN children may not be representative of all AI/AN children enrolled in WIC. Thirdly, although height and weight were measured by trained program staff following standardized protocols, potential variations in data collection practices across different WIC agencies could exist. Moreover, it is important to note that the number of children enrolled in the WIC program has steadily decreased since 2010,[44] and nearly 16% of records in 2020 were excluded from the analysis because of data quality issues related to the COVID-19 pandemic. Consequently, children's demographic characteristics in the sample may have changed throughout the study. We accounted for some of these changes in the trend analyses. However, residual confounding resulting from other factors, such as socioeconomic status, parental education level, and household composition, may remain.

CONCLUSIONS

Despite the declining trend of severe obesity among young children enrolled in the WIC program from 2010 to 2016, the small upward trend in severe obesity since 2016 is concerning. Given that children with higher BMI are at

TABLE 3 Prevalence of Severe Obesity[a] Among Children Aged 2 to 4 Years Enrolled in WIC Program, by US State or Territory, 2010 to 2020

WIC Agency	2010		2016		2020		2016 vs 2010	2020 vs 2016
	n	%[b] (95% CI)	n	%[b] (95% CI)	n	%[b] (95% CI)	APD,[c] % (95% CI)	APD,[c] % (95% CI)
State								
Alabama	45 743	2.12 (2.00 to 2.26)	42 671	2.25 (2.12 to 2.40)	29 284	2.10 (1.94 to 2.27)	0.10 (−0.09 to 0.29)	0.09 (−0.13, 0.31)
Alaska	10 108	2.6 (2.31 to 2.93)	5983	2.36 (2.00 to 2.77)	3390	1.74 (1.35 to 2.24)	−0.29 (−0.78 to 0.20)	−0.59 (−1.18 to 0.0)[d]
Arizona	72 933	2.07 (1.97 to 2.17)	58 054	1.29 (1.20 to 1.39)	40 182	1.41 (1.30 to 1.53)	−0.74 (−0.88 to −0.60)[d]	0.15 (0.0 to 0.29)
Arkansas	31 245	1.9 (1.76 to 2.06)	23 647	1.81 (1.64 to 1.98)	11 735	2.06 (1.82 to 2.34)	−0.07 (−0.30 to 0.16)	0.30 (−0.01 to 0.61)
California	583 008	2.73 (2.69 to 2.77)	495 095	2.26 (2.22 to 2.30)	202 526	2.77 (2.70 to 2.84)	−0.28 (−0.34 to −0.22)[d]	0.54 (0.45 to 0.62)[d]
Colorado	39 612	1.12 (1.02 to 1.22)	31 307	1.02 (0.92 to 1.14)	21 702	1.23 (1.10 to 1.39)	−0.10 (−0.25 to 0.05)	0.29 (0.10 to 0.48)[d]
Connecticut	22 988	2.32 (2.13 to 2.52)	18 748	1.84 (1.66 to 2.04)	13 271	2.19 (1.96 to 2.46)	−0.31 (−0.58 to −0.03)[d]	0.19 (−0.12 to 0.51)
Delaware	7650	2.81 (2.46 to 3.21)	6906	2.11 (1.8 to 2.48)	4610	2.32 (1.92 to 2.8)	−0.27 (−0.78 to 0.24)	0.19 (−0.36 to 0.73)
District of Columbia	5182	2.06 (1.71 to 2.49)	5181	1.41 (1.12 to 1.77)	3480	1.52 (1.17 to 1.99)	−0.45 (−0.95 to 0.05)	0.11 (−0.40 to 0.63)
Florida	194 924	1.83 (1.77 to 1.89)	193 749	1.61 (1.55 to 1.66)	125 469	1.74 (1.67 to 1.82)	−0.23 (−0.31 to −0.15)[d]	0.18 (0.08 to 0.27)[d]
Georgia	104 959	1.76 (1.68 to 1.84)	78 023	1.55 (1.46 to 1.63)	42 661	1.85 (1.73 to 1.98)	−0.23 (−0.35 to −0.11)[d]	0.40 (0.24 to 0.56)[d]
Hawaii	14 504	1.29 (1.12 to 1.49)	11 589	1.33 (1.14 to 1.55)	8441	1.55 (1.31 to 1.84)	0.03 (−0.25 to 0.31)	0.37 (0.02 to 0.72)[d]
Idaho	18 704	1.29 (1.14 to 1.47)	14 521	1.47 (1.29 to 1.68)	8859	1.47 (1.24 to 1.74)	0.16 (−0.09 to 0.41)	0.07 (−0.25 to 0.39)
Illinois	108 762	2.02 (1.94 to 2.10)	79 949	2.05 (1.96 to 2.15)	41 503	2.20 (2.07 to 2.35)	0.12 (−0.02 to 0.25)	0.22 (0.05 to 0.39)[d]
Indiana	63 220	2.07 (1.97 to 2.19)	55 955	1.54 (1.45 to 1.65)	35 126	1.65 (1.52 to 1.79)	−0.24 (−0.39 to −0.09)[d]	−0.06 (−0.23 to 0.10)
Iowa	29 481	2.01 (1.86 to 2.18)	24 427	1.99 (1.82 to 2.17)	14 447	1.88 (1.67 to 2.11)	0.02 (−0.22 to 0.26)	−0.12 (−0.40 to 0.16)
Kansas	30 458	1.69 (1.56 to 1.85)	24 306	1.52 (1.37 to 1.68)	15 555	1.64 (1.45 to 1.85)	−0.18 (−0.39 to 0.03)	0.22 (−0.04 to 0.47)
Kentucky	45 761	2.73 (2.58 to 2.88)	38 361	2.42 (2.28 to 2.58)	17 697	2.34 (2.13 to 2.57)	−0.30 (−0.52 to −0.09)[d]	−0.06 (−0.34 to 0.21)
Louisiana	48 145	1.85 (1.74 to 1.98)	37 527	1.76 (1.63 to 1.90)	21 090	1.95 (1.77 to 2.14)	−0.15 (−0.33 to 0.03)	0.26 (0.02 to 0.49)[d]
Maine	10 410	1.69 (1.46 to 1.96)	8233	1.63 (1.38 to 1.92)	4665	1.82 (1.48 to 2.25)	−0.07 (−0.44 to 0.30)	0.22 (−0.25 to 0.69)
Maryland	51 280	2.12 (2.00 to 2.25)	50 469	2.00 (1.88 to 2.12)	35 210	2.25 (2.10 to 2.41)	−0.03 (−0.21 to 0.14)	0.26 (0.06 to 0.46)[d]
Massachusetts	49 178	2.16 (2.03 to 2.29)	41 740	2.07 (1.94 to 2.22)	28 562	2.36 (2.19 to 2.54)	−0.13 (−0.32 to 0.06)	0.23 (0.01 to 0.45)[d]
Michigan	85 293	1.67 (1.59 to 1.76)	84 387	1.40 (1.32 to 1.48)	61 119	1.61 (1.51 to 1.71)	−0.12 (−0.23 to 0.0)	0.21 (0.08 to 0.34)[d]
Minnesota	57 529	1.30 (1.21 to 1.40)	47 219	1.45 (1.35 to 1.56)	27 074	1.30 (1.18 to 1.45)	0.11 (−0.03 to 0.26)	−0.08 (−0.25 to 0.09)
Mississippi	36 519	2.07 (1.93 to 2.22)	28 493	2.39 (2.22 to 2.57)	19 685	2.15 (1.96 to 2.36)	0.26 (0.03 to 0.49)[d]	−0.18 (−0.45 to 0.09)
Missouri	50 575	1.58 (1.48 to 1.69)	43 404	1.42 (1.32 to 1.54)	22 856	1.50 (1.35 to 1.67)	−0.15 (−0.31 to 0.0)	0.12 (−0.07 to 0.32)
Montana	7194	1.60 (1.33 to 1.92)	6647	1.43 (1.17 to 1.74)	3621	1.16 (0.86 to 1.56)	−0.22 (−0.62 to 0.19)	−0.22 (−0.68 to 0.23)
Nebraska	15 622	1.86 (1.66 to 2.09)	13 807	2.14 (1.91 to 2.39)	7376	1.84 (1.56 to 2.18)	0.24 (−0.08 to 0.56)	−0.26 (−0.65 to 0.13)
Nevada	25 855	2.02 (1.85 to 2.19)	24 493	1.70 (1.55 to 1.87)	15 790	1.64 (1.45 to 1.85)	−0.23 (−0.47 to 0.0)	0.07 (−0.19 to 0.33)
New Hampshire	7263	1.65 (1.38 to 1.97)	6042	1.77 (1.47 to 2.14)	4402	2.02 (1.65 to 2.48)	0.08 (−0.36 to 0.52)	0.31 (−0.23 to 0.84)
New Jersey	59 000	2.45 (2.33 to 2.58)	53 917	2.09 (1.97 to 2.21)	42 528	2.28 (2.15 to 2.43)	−0.40 (−0.58 to −0.23)[d]	0.39 (0.20 to 0.58)[d]
New Mexico	21 968	1.86 (1.69 to 2.05)	18 619	1.57 (1.40 to 1.76)	11 781	1.98 (1.74 to 2.25)	−0.27 (−0.52 to −0.01)[d]	0.33 (0.02 to 0.63)[d]
New York	186 760	2.10 (2.03 to 2.16)	182 401	1.66 (1.60 to 1.72)	103 959	1.95 (1.87 to 2.04)	−0.27 (−0.36 to −0.19)[d]	0.19 (0.09 to 0.29)[d]
North Carolina	89 798	1.85 (1.77 to 1.94)	97 286	1.83 (1.74 to 1.91)	57 101	1.91 (1.8 to 2.03)	0.0 (−0.12 to 0.13)	0.17 (0.03 to 0.31)[d]
North Dakota	5484	1.53 (1.24 to 1.89)	4723	1.69 (1.36 to 2.10)	3072	1.89 (1.46 to 2.43)	0.14 (−0.35 to 0.64)	0.26 (−0.35 to 0.87)
Ohio	102 803	1.62 (1.55 to 1.70)	74 753	1.45 (1.37 to 1.54)	35 864	1.61 (1.49 to 1.75)	−0.17 (−0.28 to −0.05)[d]	0.18 (0.02 to 0.33)[d]
Oklahoma	37 849	1.75 (1.62 to 1.88)	34 486	1.68 (1.55 to 1.83)	19 665	1.64 (1.47 to 1.83)	−0.07 (−0.26 to 0.12)	−0.04 (−0.27 to 0.18)
Oregon	43 209	1.73 (1.61 to 1.85)	34 485	1.77 (1.63 to 1.91)	21 315	1.97 (1.79 to 2.17)	0.06 (−0.13 to 0.24)	0.27 (0.04 to 0.51)[d]
Pennsylvania	96 762	1.65 (1.57 to 1.73)	80 202	1.56 (1.48 to 1.65)	55 283	1.71 (1.61 to 1.82)	−0.02 (−0.14 to 0.1)	0.05 (−0.09 to 0.19)
Rhode Island	10 783	2.28 (2.02 to 2.58)	6984	1.93 (1.64 to 2.28)	4938	2.37 (1.98 to 2.83)	−0.36 (−0.79 to 0.07)	0.41 (−0.12 to 0.95)
South Carolina	39 785	1.65 (1.53 to 1.78)	32 399	1.56 (1.43 to 1.70)	16 461	1.75 (1.56 to 1.96)	0.04 (−0.14 to 0.23)	0.20 (−0.04 to 0.44)
South Dakota	7884	1.84 (1.57 to 2.16)	6771	1.76 (1.47 to 2.10)	4194	1.74 (1.39 to 2.18)	−0.14 (−0.58 to 0.29)	−0.11 (−0.61 to 0.39)
Tennessee	57 153	2.12 (2.01 to 2.24)	51 157	2.01 (1.89 to 2.13)	30 061	2.09 (1.93 to 2.25)	−0.14 (−0.31 to 0.03)	0.20 (0.0 to 0.41)
Texas	361 823	2.33 (2.29 to 2.38)	268 787	2.02 (1.97 to 2.07)	180 615	2.40 (2.33 to 2.47)	−0.14 (−0.21 to −0.06)[d]	0.45 (0.36 to 0.54)[d]
Utah	26 045	1.22 (1.09 to 1.36)	21 599	0.97 (0.85 to 1.11)	11 707	1.17 (0.99 to 1.38)	−0.24 (−0.43 to −0.06)[d]	0.25 (0.01 to 0.49)[d]
Vermont	6964	1.71 (1.43 to 2.04)	5254	1.79 (1.46 to 2.18)	3904	1.74 (1.38 to 2.2)	0.06 (−0.41 to 0.54)	−0.04 (−0.59 to 0.50)
Virginia	48 920	2.72 (2.58 to 2.87)	47 376	1.99 (1.86 to 2.12)	28 038	2.16 (2.00 to 2.34)	−0.55 (−0.74 to −0.36)[d]	0.16 (−0.05 to 0.37)
Washington	78 336	1.81 (1.72 to 1.90)	69 870	1.74 (1.65 to 1.84)	43 618	1.90 (1.78 to 2.03)	−0.09 (−0.22 to 0.05)	0.38 (0.22 to 0.55)[d]
West Virginia	17 669	2.33 (2.12 to 2.56)	14 222	2.52 (2.27 to 2.79)	7598	2.34 (2.03 to 2.71)	0.15 (−0.19 to 0.49)	−0.12 (−0.55 to 0.31)
Wisconsin	48 511	1.79 (1.68 to 1.92)	37 116	1.79 (1.66 to 1.93)	26 177	1.90 (1.74 to 2.08)	0.04 (−0.14 to 0.22)	0.26 (0.04 to 0.47)[d]

TABLE 3 Continued

WIC Agency	2010		2016		2020		2016 vs 2010	2020 vs 2016
	n	%[b] (95% CI)	n	%[b] (95% CI)	n	%[b] (95% CI)	APD,[c] % (95% CI)	APD,[c] % (95% CI)
Wyoming	4413	0.95 (0.70 to 1.28)	3458	1.33 (1.00 to 1.77)	2007	1.74 (1.26 to 2.42)	0.34 (−0.13 to 0.82)	0.45 (−0.24 to 1.14)
Territory								
American Samoa	3221	1.55 (1.18 to 2.04)	2824	1.10 (0.77 to 1.55)	1421	1.76 (1.19 to 2.58)	−0.45 (−1.02 to 0.13)	0.62 (−0.16 to 1.39)
Guam	3248	1.45 (1.09 to 1.92)	2710	0.70 (0.45 to 1.09)	2234	0.81 (0.51 to 1.27)	−0.76 (−1.28 to −0.24)[d]	0.11 (−0.38 to 0.59)
Northern Mariana Islands	2157	2.60 (2.00 to 3.36)	1418	0.63 (0.33 to 1.20)	1095	0.82 (0.43 to 1.55)	−1.99 (−2.78 to −1.20)[d]	0.16 (−0.52 to 0.84)
Puerto Rico	70 699	3.09 (2.97 to 3.22)	63 251	1.90 (1.80 to 2.01)	40 056	2.14 (2.00 to 2.29)	−1.17 (−1.33 to −1.00)[d]	0.30 (0.12 to 0.48)[d]
Virgin Islands	2093	1.72 (1.24 to 2.37)	1593	1.76 (1.22 to 2.53)	667	1.65 (0.92 to 2.93)	0.03 (−0.82 to 0.88)	−0.09 (−1.25 to 1.08)

[a] Defined as a BMI of 120% or more of the 95th percentile for age and sex on the CDC growth charts or BMI ≥35 kg/m².
[b] Crude prevalence of severe obesity.
[c] Represents 100 times the average marginal effect of year (2016 vs 2010, 2020 vs 2016) controlling for sex, age, and race/ethnicity. Children with missing information on race/ethnicity were excluded. A negative value indicates that the adjusted prevalence decreased.
[d] Statistically significant difference at the 0.05 level based on logistic regression adjusting for age, sex, and race/ethnicity.

greater risk of future health consequences, continued understanding of the ongoing state trends of obesity, especially severe obesity among young children, is warranted. Ensuring that children and families from low-income households have access to early clinical detection, and referrals to effective and sustainable family-based interventions, could help promote healthy child growth.

ACKNOWLEDGMENTS

We thank Amanda Reat (USDA) for the critical review of the article. We also acknowledge the staff from USDA Food and Nutrition Service for providing WIC-PC data.

ABBREVIATIONS

AI/AN: American Indian/Alaska Native
APD: adjusted prevalence difference
CDC: Centers for Disease Control and Prevention
CI: confidence interval
COVID-19: coronavirus disease 2019
FPL: federal poverty level
IHBLT: intensive behavior and lifestyle treatment
NHANES: National Health and Nutrition Examination Survey
USDA: US Department of Agriculture
WIC: Special Supplemental Nutrition Program for Women, Infants, and Children
WIC-PC: WIC Participant and Program Characteristics

FUNDING: No external funding.

CONFLICT OF INTEREST DISCLOSURES: The authors have indicated they have no potential conflicts of interest relevant to this article to disclose.

COMPANION PAPER: A companion to this article can be found online at www.pediatrics.org/cgi/doi/10.1542/peds.2023-063799.

REFERENCES

1. National Center for Health Statistics. NHANES 2017–March 2020 prepandemic data files. Available at: https://www.cdc.gov/nchs/data/nhsr/nhsr158-508.pdf. Accessed February 17, 2023

2. Hu K, Staiano AE. Trends in obesity prevalence among children and adolescents aged 2 to 19 years in the US from 2011 to 2020. *JAMA Pediatr.* 2022;176(10):1037–1039

3. Hales CM, Fryar CD, Carroll MD, et al. Trends in obesity and severe obesity prevalence in US youth and adults by sex and age, 2007–2008 to 2015–2016. *JAMA.* 2018;319(16):1723–1725

4. Tsoi MF, Li HL, Feng Q, et al. Prevalence of childhood obesity in the United States in 1999-2018: a 20-year analysis. *Obes Facts.* 2022;15(4):560–569

5. QuickStats: prevalence of obesity* and severe obesity† among persons aged 2–19 years - national health and nutrition examination survey, 1999–2000 through 2017–2018. *MMWR Morb Mortal Wkly Rep.* 2020;69(13):390

6. Ogden CL, Fryar CD, Martin CB, et al. Trends in obesity prevalence by race and Hispanic origin-1999–2000 to 2017–2018. *JAMA.* 2020;324(12):1208–1210

7. Woolford SJ, Sidell M, Li X, et al. Changes in body mass index among children and adolescents during the COVID-19 pandemic. *JAMA.* 2021;326(14):1434–1436

8. Lange SJ, Kompaniyets L, Freedman DS, et al; DNP3. Longitudinal trends in body mass index before and during the COVID-19 pandemic among persons aged 2–19 years - United States, 2018–2020. *MMWR Morb Mortal Wkly Rep.* 2021;70(37):1278–1283

9. Pierce SL, Kompaniyets L, Freedman DS, et al. Children's rates of BMI change during pre-pandemic and two COVID-19 pandemic periods, IQVIA Ambulatory Electronic Medical Record, January 2018 through November 2021. *Obesity (Silver Spring).* 2023;31(3):693–698

10. Kelly AS, Barlow SE, Rao G, et al; American Heart Association Atherosclerosis, Hypertension, and Obesity in the Young Committee of the Council on Cardiovascular Disease in the Young, Council on Nutrition, Physical Activity and Metabolism, and Council on Clinical Cardiology. Severe obesity in children and adolescents: identification, associated health risks, and treatment approaches: a scientific statement from the American Heart Association. *Circulation.* 2013;128(15):1689–1712

11. Bass R, Eneli I. Severe childhood obesity: an under-recognised and growing health problem. *Postgrad Med J.* 2015;91(1081): 639–645

12. Calcaterra V, Klersy C, Muratori T, et al. Prevalence of metabolic syndrome (MS) in children and adolescents with varying degrees of obesity. *Clin Endocrinol (Oxf).* 2008;68(6):868–872

13. Porter RM, Tindall A, Gaffka BJ, et al. A review of modifiable risk factors for severe obesity in children ages 5 and under. *Child Obes.* 2018;14(7):468–476

14. Mirza N, Phan TL, Tester J, et al. A narrative review of medical and genetic risk factors among children age 5 and younger with severe obesity. *Child Obes.* 2018;14(7):443–452

15. Tester JM, Phan TT, Tucker JM, et al. Characteristics of children 2 to 5 years of age with severe obesity. *Pediatrics.* 2018; 141(3):e20173228

16. Pan L, Freedman DS, Sharma AJ, et al. Trends in obesity among participants aged 2–4 years in the Special Supplemental Nutrition Program for Women, Infants, and Children - United States, 2000–2014. *MMWR Morb Mortal Wkly Rep.* 2016;65(45):1256–1260

17. Freedman DS, Sharma AJ, Hamner HC, et al. Trends in weight-for-length among infants in WIC From 2000 to 2014. *Pediatrics.* 2017;139(1):e20162034

18. Pan L, Freedman DS, Park S, et al. Changes in obesity among US children aged 2 through 4 years enrolled in WIC during 2010-2016. *JAMA.* 2019;321(23):2364–2366

19. Pan L, Blanck HM, Park S, et al. State-specific prevalence of obesity among children aged 2–4 years enrolled in the Special Supplemental Nutrition Program for Women, Infants, and Children - United States, 2010-2016. *MMWR Morb Mortal Wkly Rep.* 2019;68(46):1057–1061

20. Pan L, Blanck HM, Galuska DA, et al. Changes in high weight-for-length among infants enrolled in Special Supplemental Nutrition Program for Women, Infants, and Children during 2010–2018. *Child Obes.* 2021;17(6):408–419

21. USDA Food and Nutrition Services. The Special Supplemental Nutrition Program for Women, Infants and Children (WIC). Available at: https://www.fns.usda.gov/wic/about-wic. Accessed February 17, 2023

22. Farson Gray K, Balch-Crystal E, Giannarelli L, Johnson P; U.S. Department of Agriculture Food and Nutrition Service. National- and state-level estimates of WIC eligibility and WIC program reach in 2019. Available at: https://fns-prod.azureedge.us/sites/default/files/resource-files/WICEligibles2019-Volume1-revised.pdf. Accessed April 28, 2023

23. Pan L, Park S, Slayton R, et al. Trends in severe obesity among children aged 2 to 4 years enrolled in Special Supplemental Nutrition Program for Women, Infants, and Children From 2000 to 2014. *JAMA Pediatr.* 2018;172(3):232–238

24. USDA Food and Nutrition Services. WIC eligibility requirements. Available at: https://www.fns.usda.gov/wic/wic-eligibility-requirements. Accessed February 17, 2023

25. US Department of Agriculture. National sample file for public use codebook: WIC participant and program characteristics 2018. Available at: https://data.nal.usda.gov/dataset/wic-participant-and-program-characteristics-2018/resource/e5bf8469-d6de-48c0-99e0-0fc2efa254d8. Accessed June 6, 2023

26. Minnesota Department of Health. WIC anthropometrics manual 2022. Available at: https://www.health.state.mn.us/docs/people/wic/localagency/training/nutrition/nst/anthro.pdf. Accessed June 6, 2023

27. Crespi CM, Alfonso VH, Whaley SE, Wang MC. Validity of child anthropometric measurements in the Special Supplemental Nutrition Program for Women, Infants, and Children. *Pediatr Res.* 2012;71(3):286–292

28. Centers for Disease Control and Prevention (CDC). The SAS Program for CDC growth charts that includes the extended BMI calculations. Available at: https://www.cdc.gov/nccdphp/dnpao/growthcharts/resources/sas.htm. Accessed February 17, 2023

29. USDA Food and Nutrition Services. WIC participant and program characteristics 2020 final report. Available at: https://fns-prod.azureedge.us/sites/default/files/resource-files/WICPC2020-1.pdf. Accessed February 17, 2023

30. Leeper TJ; CRAN. Margins: marginal effects for model objects. R package version 0.3.26. Available at: https://rdrr.io/cran/margins/. Accessed November 8, 2022

31. R Core Team; R Foundation for Statistical Computing. R: a language and environment for statistical computing. Available at: https://www.R-project.org/. Accessed November 8, 2022

32. USDA Food and Nutrition Services. Special Supplemental Nutrition Program for Women, Infants and Children (WIC): revisions in the WIC food packages, 2009. Available at: https://www.federalregister.gov/documents/2009/12/31/E9-30991/special-supplemental-nutrition-program-for-women-infants-and-children-wic-revisions-in-the-wic-food. Accessed June 6, 2023

33. Daepp MIG, Gortmaker SL, Wang YC, et al. WIC food package changes: trends in childhood obesity prevalence. *Pediatrics.* 2019;143(5):e20182841

34. Schultz DJ, Byker Shanks C, Houghtaling B. The impact of the 2009 Special Supplemental Nutrition Program for Women,

Infants, and Children food package revisions on participants: a systematic review. *J Acad Nutr Diet.* 2015;115(11):1832–1846

35. Andreyeva T, Tripp AS. The healthfulness of food and beverage purchases after the federal food package revisions: the case of two New England states. *Prev Med.* 2016;91:204–210

36. Chaparro MP, Anderson CE, Crespi CM, et al. The effect of the 2009 WIC food package change on childhood obesity varies by gender and initial weight status in Los Angeles County. *Pediatr Obes.* 2019;14(9):e12526

37. Chaparro MP, Crespi CM, Anderson CE, et al. The 2009 Special Supplemental Nutrition Program for Women, Infants, and Children (WIC) food package change and children's growth trajectories and obesity in Los Angeles County. *Am J Clin Nutr.* 2019;109(5):1414–1421

38. Centers for Disease Control and Prevention (CDC). Priority obesity strategy: early care and education (ECE) policies and activities. Available at: https://www.cdc.gov/obesity/strategies/priority-obesity-strategy.html. Accessed February 24, 2023

39. Pelletier JE, Schreiber LRN, Laska MN. Minimum stocking requirements for retailers in the Special Supplemental Nutrition Program for Women, Infants, and Children: disparities across US states. *Am J Public Health.* 2017;107(7):1171–1174

40. Browne NT, Snethen JA, Greenberg CS, et al. When pandemics collide: the impact of COVID-19 on childhood obesity. *J Pediatr Nurs.* 2021;56:90–98

41. Cena H, Fiechtner L, Vincenti A, et al. COVID-19 pandemic as risk factors for excessive weight gain in pediatrics: the role of changes in nutrition behavior. A narrative review. *Nutrients.* 2021;13(12):4255

42. Hampl SE, Hassink SG, Skinner AC, et al. Clinical practice guideline for the evaluation and treatment of children and adolescents with obesity. *Pediatrics.* 2023;151(2):e2022060640

43. Centers for Disease Control and Prevention (CDC). Family healthy weight programs. Available at: https://www.cdc.gov/obesity/strategies/family-healthy-weight-programs.html. Accessed March 22, 2023

44. USDA Food and Nutrition Services. WIC participant and program characteristics 2020 - charts. Available at: https://www.fns.usda.gov/wic/participant-program-characteristics-2020-charts. Accessed February 24, 2023

Universal Free School Meals Policy and Childhood Obesity

Anna M. Localio, MPH,[a] Melissa A. Knox, PhD,[b] Anirban Basu, PhD, MS,[a,c] Tom Lindman, MPP,[d]
Lina Pinero Walkinshaw, MPH,[a] Jessica C. Jones-Smith, PhD, MPH, RD[a,e]

BACKGROUND AND OBJECTIVES: The Community Eligibility Provision (CEP), a universal free school meals policy, increases school meal participation by allowing schools in low-income areas to provide free breakfast and lunch to all students; however, its impact on obesity remains uncertain. The objective of this study is to estimate the association of CEP with child obesity.

METHODS: School obesity prevalence was calculated using BMI measurements collected annually between 2013 and 2019 from students in California public schools in grades 5, 7, and 9. To estimate the association of CEP with obesity, we used a difference-in-differences approach for staggered policy adoption with an outcome regression model conditional on covariates, weighted by student population size.

RESULTS: The analysis included 3531 CEP-eligible schools using school-level obesity prevalence calculated from 3 546 803 BMI measurements. At baseline, on average, 72% of students identified as Hispanic, 11% identified as white, 7% identified as Black, and 80% were eligible for free or reduced-price meals. Baseline obesity prevalence was 25%. Schools that participated in CEP were associated with a 0.60-percentage-point net decrease in obesity prevalence after policy adoption (95% confidence interval: −1.07 to −0.14 percentage points, $P = .01$) compared with eligible, nonparticipating schools, corresponding with a 2.4% relative reduction, given baseline prevalence. Meals served increased during this period in CEP-participating schools only.

CONCLUSIONS: In a balanced sample of California schools, CEP participation was associated with a modest net decrease in obesity prevalence compared with eligible, nonparticipating schools. These findings add to the growing literature revealing potential benefits of universal free school meals for children's well-being.

Departments of [a]Health Systems and Population Health, [b]Economics, [c]Pharmacy, [e]Epidemiology and [d]Evans School of Public Policy and Governance, University of Washington, Seattle, Washington

Ms Localio contributed to study design, cleaned and managed data, conducted the initial data analyses, contributed to data interpretation, and drafted the manuscript; Drs Knox and Basu conceptualized and designed the study and contributed to data analysis and interpretation; Mr Lindman contributed to the study design and contributed to data analysis and interpretation; Ms Walkinshaw coordinated data acquisition, managed the project, and assisted in data cleaning and management; Dr Jones-Smith conceptualized and designed the study, acquired study funding, coordinated and supervised data acquisition, and contributed to data analysis and interpretation; and all authors critically reviewed and revised the manuscript, approved the final manuscript as submitted, and agree to be accountable for all aspects of the work.

DOI: https://doi.org/10.1542/peds.2023-063749

Accepted for publication Jan 23, 2024

Address correspondence to Anna M. Localio, MPH, Department of Health Systems and Population Health, University of Washington, 3980 15th Ave NE, Seattle, WA 98195. E-mail: alocalio@uw.edu

WHAT'S KNOWN ON THIS SUBJECT: The Healthy, Hunger-Free Kids Act improved the nutritional quality of school meals, which are healthier than alternatives. CEP increases school meal participation by providing free meals to all students; however, its impact on obesity remains uncertain.

WHAT THIS STUDY ADDS: In low-income California schools between 2013 and 2019, participation in CEP was associated with a relative decrease in obesity prevalence compared with eligible, nonparticipating schools, suggesting that universal free school meals policies may be effective for addressing childhood obesity.

To cite: Localio AM, Knox MA, Basu A, et al. Universal Free School Meals Policy and Childhood Obesity. Pediatrics. 2024;153(4):e2023063749

ARTICLE

Childhood obesity is a pressing public health concern for which solutions remain elusive. Obesity often tracks into adulthood[1] and increases the risk of chronic conditions and premature death.[2] Because obesity disproportionately impacts racially and ethnically minoritized and low-income children,[3] effective population-level obesity-reduction strategies must address social determinants of health.[4,5] Universal free school meals (UFM) policies represent one potential approach.

The Community Eligibility Provision (CEP) is a federal UFM policy authorized by the 2010 Healthy, Hunger-Free Kids Act (HHFKA). CEP operates through the National School Lunch Program and School Breakfast Program, which provide free and reduced-price meals to qualifying students. Schools that adopt CEP offer free meals to all students, saving schools the administrative burden of processing meal applications. Participating schools receive federal reimbursement based on the identified student percentage (ISP), which is calculated by using the percentage of students directly certified to receive free meals without an application, such as through participation in a means-tested safety net program, multiplied by 1.6 to approximate additional certification via application.[6] CEP became an option for high-poverty schools nationwide in 2014. By 2023, >40% of US public schools were participating, reaching nearly 20 million children.[6]

CEP expands access to and reduces the stigma of receiving free meals,[7] thus increasing school meal participation.[8–11] Increased school meal participation may reduce obesity because school meals are more nutritious than meals obtained elsewhere.[12–16] This may be particularly true for low-income children, for whom several income-stratified analyses reveal greater positive associations of nutritional quality and school meal participation relative to those observed in higher-income students.[13,17,18] In addition to authorizing CEP, the HHFKA improved nutrition standards for school meals, resulting in improved nutritional quality among school meal participants.[15,18–21] CEP also relaxes budget constraints for low-income families. Students receiving free breakfast and lunch save approximately $4.70 per day ($850 per year) compared with paying full price.[22] This allows families to purchase more nutritious groceries and spend less overall,[23] potentially increasing disposable income. Evidence also suggests that UFM policies improve food insecurity[15,23] and child academic performance.[8,11,15,24] Although CEP has the potential to reduce obesity, its impact remains uncertain. Preliminary evidence suggests that UFM policies may be associated with obesity reduction;[10,24–26] however, more rigorous research is needed. To add to this small body of literature, with this study, we seek to evaluate the association of CEP with child obesity.

METHODS

Because we hypothesize that CEP reduces obesity by increasing participation in school meals, we first conducted a simple, unadjusted, difference-in-differences analysis of the change in free, reduced-price, full-price, and total meals served per child per year, comparing schools that adopted CEP in school year 2018 to 2019 with eligible, nonparticipating schools. The California Department of Education (CDE) provided meals served counts from 2017 to 2019 (the only years available during the study period).

For our primary analysis of the association of CEP with obesity prevalence, we used a difference-in-differences design for staggered policy adoption.[27] The design was repeated cross-sectional at the child level and longitudinal at the school level, comparing schools that participated in CEP with eligible schools that did not participate between 2013 and 2019. As secondary analyses, we examined the association of CEP with normal weight and overweight prevalence. The University of Washington Institutional Review Board determined the research exempt from oversight.

Primary Outcome

School-level obesity prevalence from school years 2013−14 through 2018−19 came from California's physical fitness testing program which collects BMI each spring from fifth-, seventh-, and ninth-grade students.[28] Although neither individual nor aggregate continuous BMI measurements are publicly available, they report categorical aggregate measures of students with obesity, defined as BMI greater than or equal to the 95th percentile for age and sex according to the Centers for Disease Control and Prevention growth charts.[28,29]

Secondary Outcomes

We examined obesity as our primary outcome because it is most clearly associated with future risk of disease.[1,30–32] As secondary outcomes, we assessed change in normal weight (here defined as BMI below the 85th percentile because CDE did not report a separate underweight category) and overweight (BMI at or above the 85th percentile but below the 95th percentile) prevalence.

Exposure

Treatment was defined as school participation in CEP, reported annually by CDE and the National Center for Education Statistics.

Covariates

Cross-sectional studies have revealed CEP adoption to be positively associated with ISP and the percentage of Hispanic and Black students and potentially associated with school size, school level, and rurality.[33,34] Accordingly, we controlled for pretreatment school-level characteristics: percentage of students eligible for free and reduced-price meals (approximating ISP which was not available at baseline [2013–14]), percentage of fifth-grade students (of fifth, seventh, and ninth-grade students measured) because some schools group grades differently, percentage of students identifying as Hispanic because they comprise the majority of the sample, and participation in US Department of Agriculture (USDA) Provisions 2 and 3 (described in the Supplemental Information). School covariate data came from CDE and the National Center for Education Statistics. We also included county-level rurality (from the National Center for Health Statistics), unemployment rate (from the Bureau of Labor Statistics), and percentage of adults 25 and older with a bachelor's degree or higher (from the American Community Survey), which could impact policy adoption and obesity outcomes beyond school-level subsidized meal eligibility. The models were weighted by school population size. As a sensitivity analysis, we replaced unemployment and education variables with a composite measure of socioeconomic status.[35]

Exclusion Criteria

Figure 1 depicts school exclusion criteria. Beginning with 9841 public schools participating in California's physical fitness testing program, we excluded 1904 schools that did not report obesity outcomes in all 6 study years, 3744 schools that were ineligible for CEP (ISP <40%) to create comparable treatment and control groups, and 19 schools that switched from participating to not participating in CEP because our analytic approach required treated schools to remain treated. Schools reporting improbable outcomes were excluded from our sample; these included 433 schools reporting zero students with obesity. Obesity prevalence had a near-normal distribution, except for a disproportionate number of zeros. In these schools, obesity prevalence in the years before and after zero was often high. The majority of these schools also reported zero overweight prevalence. The high prevalence of obesity in US children[3] makes this large spike at zero improbable and was considered a reporting error. Additionally, we excluded 210 schools reporting a >25-percentage-point (pp) change in obesity prevalence between years, which was beyond the first (−23 pp) and 99th (23 pp) percentiles of the distribution. This was deemed a change too large between years to be plausible and likely a reporting error. To check that our results were robust to how we defined outliers, we conducted sensitivity analyses, changing this cutoff to 20 and 30 pp.

Statistical Analysis

In our primary analysis, we estimated the association of CEP with obesity prevalence by using a difference-

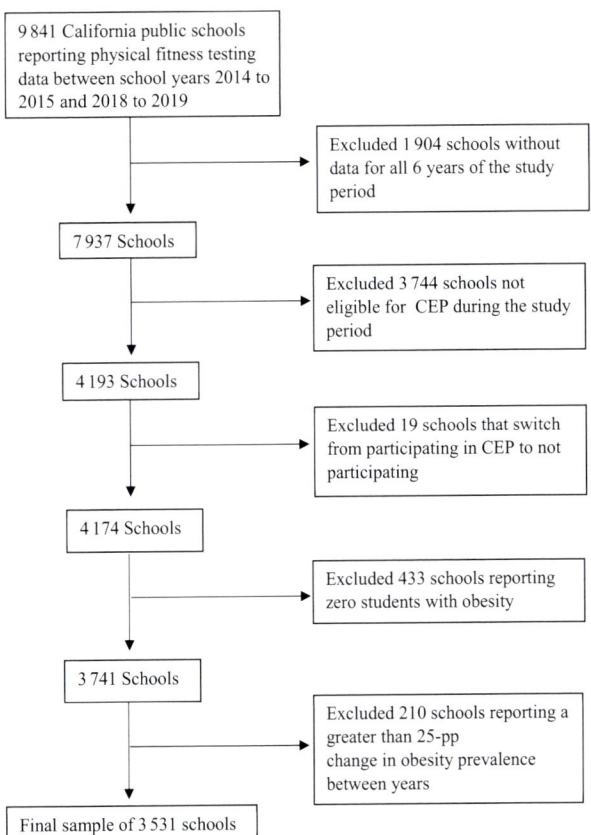

FIGURE 1
Flowchart of California public schools excluded from analysis.

in-differences approach, which accounts for heterogeneous treatment effects due to staggered policy adoption.[27] This approach leverages the same mechanism as a traditional difference-in-differences design (comparing treated and untreated groups before and after policy implementation) but does so for each cohort of schools newly participating in CEP (eg, schools newly participating in school year 2014–15, 2015–16, etc), comparing each year of participation to 1 year before policy adoption (eg, for the 2014–15 cohort, a separate treatment effect is estimated for school year 2013–14 vs 2014–15, 2013–14 vs 2015–16, 2013–14 vs 2016–17, 2013–14 vs 2017–18, and 2013–14 vs 2018–19). Our primary approach used an "outcome regression" model based on ordinary least squares, conditional on covariates, as described by Callaway, Sant'Anna, Heckman, and colleagues[27,36,37] (Supplemental Information). This avoids the potential biases of two-way fixed effects models (including fixed effects for time and unit in a linear regression model).[38–40] This difference-in-differences approach relies on a conditional parallel trends assumption: baseline outcomes do not need to be the same for both groups; however, trends in the outcome before policy adoption should be similar to provide evidence that the parallel trends assumption post-policy is reasonable. Accordingly, we assess pretreatment trends in the outcome. Additional assumptions are described in the Supplemental Information.

We performed several additional sensitivity analyses. First, to assess the robustness of parallel pretrends, in the preperiod we designated the reference year as that before policy adoption. This is in contrast to our main analysis, which provides a short-term, year-over-year comparison in the pre-policy period.[27] Second, we changed our comparison group to include not-yet-treated schools in addition to eligible, never-treated schools. Third, we used a doubly robust model that combines the outcome regression model from our primary analysis with inverse probability weighting, which yields valid results even if 1 of the 2 models is misspecified but can produce larger standard errors.[42,60] Lastly, we repeated our main analysis, dropping all schools that participated in Provisions 2 or 3 during the study period (see the Supplemental Information). We used a P value of <.1 as a threshold for statistical significance, consistent with other studies on CEP.[8,10,11,43] For the analyses, we used xthdidregress in Stata/MP 18.0.[41] The Supplemental Information includes code to produce estimates and figures.

STUDY RESULTS

The balanced sample included 3531 CEP-eligible schools between school years 2013−14 and 2018−19. Aggregate obesity data came from 3 546 803 BMI measurements from students in grades 5, 7, and 9. Table 1 reveals baseline school and county demographics overall and by the year in which the schools initiated CEP. Nonparticipating schools and those that adopted CEP in later years had higher average percentages of white and non-economically disadvantaged students. At baseline, on average, schools were composed of 72% students identifying as Hispanic, 11% identifying as white, 7% identifying as Black, and 5% identifying as Asian. On average, 80% of students were eligible for free or reduced-price lunch. Supplemental Table 4 reveals the baseline characteristics of CEP-eligible schools included in versus excluded from our analysis. The characteristics were not meaningfully different between the 2 groups, except for the percentage of fifth graders, which was higher among excluded schools. Supplemental Fig 5 reveals the percentage of schools that adopted CEP in our sample by district and year. Figure 2 reveals unadjusted trends in obesity prevalence by cohort (year in which schools began participating in CEP), weighted by school population size. The mean baseline obesity prevalence

TABLE 1 Baseline School and County Demographic Characteristics by Year Schools Adopted the CEP

	Overall	Year Schools Began Participating in CEP					
		Never	2014−15	2015−16	2016−17	2017−18	2018−19
	$n = 3531$	$n = 1618$	$n = 127$	$n = 426$	$n = 264$	$n = 128$	$n = 968$
School characteristics							
Sex							
Male	51%	51%	51%	51%	51%	51%	51%
Race and ethnicity							
Hispanic	72%	69%	73%	85%	71%	62%	73%
White	11%	13%	8%	3%	9%	13%	13%
Black	7%	7%	7%	7%	8%	12%	7%
Asian	5%	6%	9%	2%	7%	7%	3%
2 or more races	2%	2%	1%	0.4%	2%	2%	1%
Filipino	2%	2%	0.3%	1%	2%	2%	1%
American Indian	1%	1%	1%	0.4%	1%	1%	1%
Pacific Islander	1%	1%	0.4%	0.1%	0.4%	1%	0.4%
Economic status[a]							
Disadvantaged	82%	79%	93%	96%	89%	71%	80%
Not disadvantaged	13%	16%	6%	3%	8%	20%	15%
No economic information	5%	5%	1%	1%	3%	10%	5%
Eligible for free or reduced-price meals	80%	77%	86%	85%	86%	80%	81%
Grade level							
Percentage of students in fifth grade	52%	49%	66%	61%	55%	50%	51%
County characteristics							
Percentage unemployed	10%	10%	12%	11%	9%	11%	11%
Percentage bachelor's degree or higher	26%	27%	22%	27%	29%	24%	23%
Rurality[b]	1.8	1.7	1.9	1.5	1.8	2.2	2.0

Percentages weighted by school population size. All schools were untreated in the first study year (2013−14).
[a] Economically disadvantaged defined as neither student's parents received a high school diploma and/or student is eligible for free or reduced-price meals.
[b] Mean rurality on a scale from 1 to 6, with 6 indicating most rural.

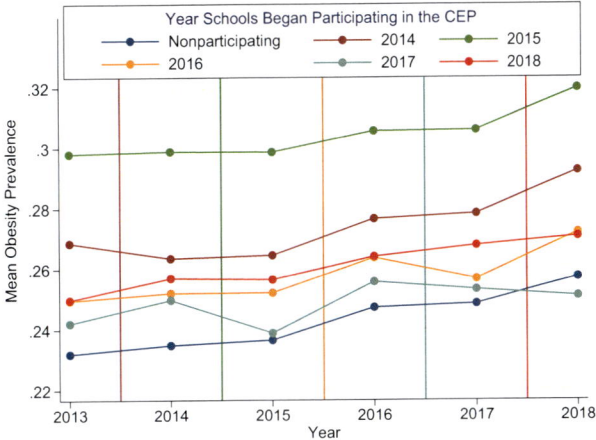

FIGURE 2

Unadjusted trends in obesity prevalence over time by the year in which schools began participating in CEP. Sample includes 3531 CEP-eligible schools between school years 2013–14 and 2018–19. All schools were untreated in the 2013–14 school year. Schools are grouped by the year they began participating in CEP. Color-coded vertical lines correspond to the first year that each group adopted CEP. The mean obesity prevalence is weighted by school population size.

was 25% overall. Table 2 reveals the unadjusted difference-in-differences in free, reduced-price, full-price, and total meals served in school years 2017–18 and 2018–19, comparing schools that began participating in CEP in 2018–19 with eligible nonparticipating schools. Total meals served increased by an average of 13.4 meals per student per year (95% confidence interval [CI]: 5.7 to 21.2), free meals increased by 44.8 meals (95% CI: 37.8 to 51.8), full-price meals decreased by 11.3 meals (95% CI: −12.9 to −9.7), and reduced-price meals decreased by 20.1 meals (95% CI −21.0 to −19.2).

Table 3 and Figs 3 and 4 display results from our adjusted difference-in-differences model. Table 3 reveals the overall average treatment effect estimate, indicating that schools that participated in CEP experienced a 0.60-pp net reduction in obesity prevalence after policy adoption compared with eligible nonparticipating schools, conditional on covariates (95% CI: −1.07 to −0.14 pp, $P = .01$), corresponding to a 2.40% relative reduction, given baseline obesity prevalence (95% CI: −4.28% to −0.56%). Table 3 and Fig 3 display average treatment effects aggregated by

cohort. Although all posttreatment cohort effects were negative, effects were largest for later-treated cohorts. Table 3 and Fig 4 reveal dynamic treatment effects (indexed by time relative to CEP adoption). The joint test that all pretreatment effects are zero was not statistically significant ($P = .55$), indicating parallel pre-policy trends, which lends support to the parallel trends assumption. In other words, despite differences in average baseline obesity prevalence, the differences in trends in obesity prevalence for CEP-participating versus eligible, nonparticipating schools were not different from zero. All dynamic treatment effect estimates were negative but only statistically significant for the first 2 years of CEP participation.

We observed no significant association of CEP with overweight prevalence and a relative increase in normal weight prevalence associated with CEP (0.58 pp, 95% CI: 0.08 to 1.08; Supplemental Table 5 and Supplemental Figs 6–9). Our primary results were not substantively changed when replacing county-level education and unemployment measures as covariates with a Social Deprivation Index,[35] changing the cutoff for excluding outlier schools, or changing the reference year, comparison group, estimation technique, and sample inclusion criteria (Supplemental Tables 6 and 7 and Supplemental Figs 10–22). Pre-policy trends were not significant in any of our sensitivity analyses, supporting the parallel trends and no anticipation assumptions, with the exception of the analysis which dropped schools that participated in Provisions 2 or 3 during the study period (Supplemental Fig 22). However, this analysis dropped a substantial portion of our sample (36%), including 915 schools that switched from participating in Provisions 2 or 3 to CEP between 2013 and 2019.

DISCUSSION

Among 3531 low-income California public schools, those that implemented universal free meals through CEP experienced an average net reduction in obesity prevalence of 2.4% compared with eligible, nonparticipating schools. The strengths of our study include its use of a balanced sample of schools and a comparison group of eligible nonparticipating schools. In addition, we used a novel difference-in-differences approach for staggered policy adoption,

TABLE 2 Difference-in-Differences in Free, Reduced-Price, Full-Price, and Total Meals Served per Student per Year, 2017 to 2019

Mean Meals Served per Student per Year	CEP Schools ($n = 965$)			Non-CEP Schools ($n = 1571$)			Difference-in-Differences (95% CI)
	2017–18	2018–19	Difference	2017–18	2018–19	Difference	
Free	159.9	201.0	41.1	138.1	134.4	−3.7	44.8 (37.8 to 51.8)
Reduced-price	19.3	0	−19.3	21.1	21.9	0.8	−20.1 (−21.0 to −19.2)
Full-price	20.2	10.2	−10.0	21.2	22.5	1.3	−11.3 (−12.9 to −9.7)
Total	199.4	211.1	11.7	180.4	178.8	−1.6	13.4 (5.7 to 21.2)

Meals served data from a subset of 2536 schools that adopted the CEP in the 2018–19 school year or were eligible for but did not participate in CEP during the study period 2013 to 2019.

TABLE 3 Aggregate Post-Policy Treatment Effect Estimates of School Participation in the CEP on Obesity Prevalence

	Estimate (pp)	95% CI
Overall	−0.60*	(−1.07 to −0.14)
Cohort (y of policy adoption)		
2014 − 2015	−0.41	(−1.60 to 0.78)
2015 − 2016	−0.62	(−1.55 to 0.30)
2016 − 2017	−0.38	(−1.20 to 0.43)
2017 − 2018	−0.97	(−2.16 to 0.21)
2018 − 2019	−0.78*	(−1.39 to −0.16)
Duration of policy exposure, y		
1	−0.49*	(−0.90 to −0.08)
2	−0.95**	(−1.59 to −0.30)
3	−0.50	(−1.26 to 0.25)
4	−0.69	(−1.66 to 0.28)
5	−0.09	(−1.67 to 1.48)

Sample includes 3531 schools eligible for the CEP during the study period 2013 to 2019. Treatment effects were estimated using the Callaway/Sant'Anna difference-in-differences outcome regression estimator,[27] weighted by school size and conditional on covariates.
*$P < .05$
**$P < .01$

allowing treatment effects to vary over time.[27,38] By conditioning on covariates, we accounted for covariate-specific trends.[27]

Examining treatment effects by year of CEP adoption, we found that although effects were negative for all cohorts, they were largest for later-treated cohorts (school years 2017–18 and 2018–19). In computing dynamic treatment effects by years of policy exposure, the strongest associations were observed in the first 2 years of policy adoption, with weaker negative associations in the

third and fourth years of adoption. These findings are consistent because later-adopting cohorts contribute to estimates in the first and second years of policy adoption. For instance, schools adopting CEP in the 2017–18 school year were only observed for 2 years post-policy, so they contributed to the first- and second-year post-policy estimates but not the third-, fourth-, or fifth-year estimates. Alternatively, these findings could indicate a reduction in the policy's effectiveness over time. The authors of future research should explore the sustainability of CEP's effects.

In our sample, later-treated cohorts had, on average, fewer students already eligible for free or reduced-price meals before CEP adoption. In these schools, CEP may result in a larger proportion of children newly participating in school meals, which is a plausible mechanism for the observed relative reduction in obesity, as evidence reveals that school meals are healthier than alternatives,[13,14,17,44] particularly after stricter nutrition standards introduced by the HHFKA resulted in improved nutritional quality.[15,18,19] Newly participating children may substitute up to half of their diet during the school year with more nutritious meals, potentially saving money for families.[23] This is supported by the observed increase in meals served in 2018–19 CEP-adopting schools. We are not aware of changes in physical activity or other curriculum requirements in California schools during this time that coincide with the adoption of CEP (and are not a direct result of CEP) that could contribute to the observed effect.

Our results build on findings from other researchers. Kenney et al found that the timing of the HHFKA was associated with a reduction in obesity among low-income children in a nationally representative sample.[25] In this

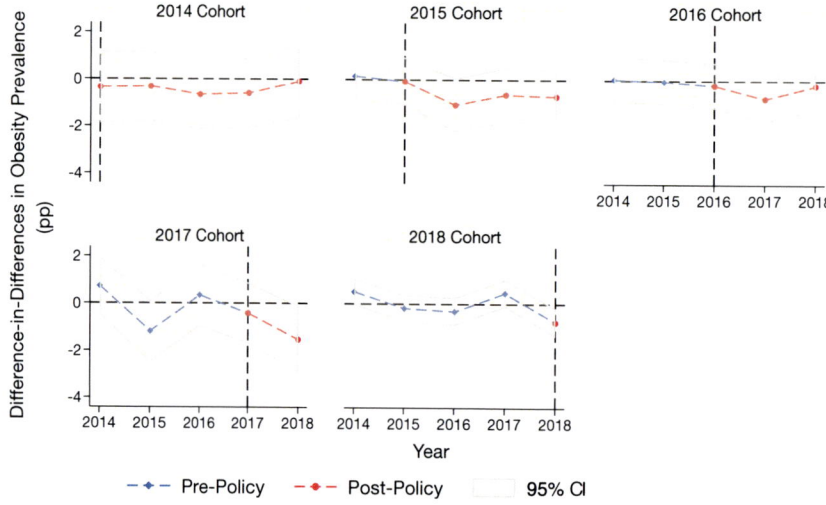

FIGURE 3

Cohort treatment effects of participation in CEP on obesity prevalence. Difference-in-differences estimates are from the Callaway/Sant'Anna outcome regression estimator.[27,36,37] Estimates are grouped by the year schools adopted CEP, conditional on covariates. The reference group is eligible, nonparticipating schools, and the reference year is 1 year before policy adoption.

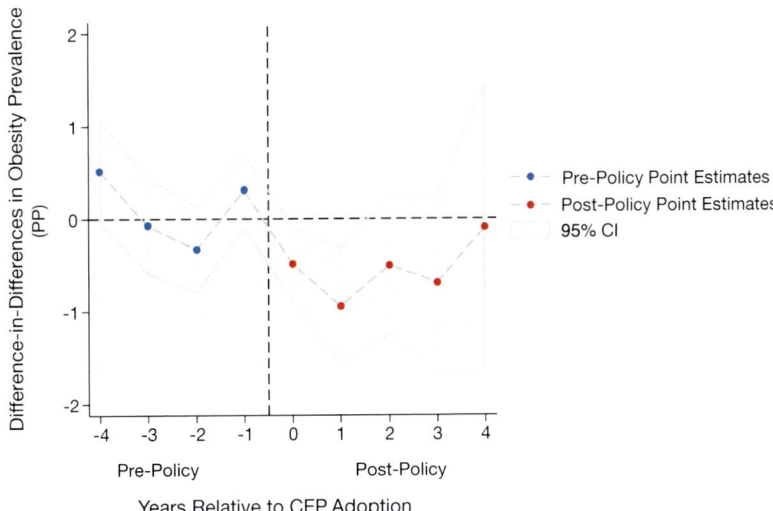

FIGURE 4
Dynamic treatment effects of participation in CEP on obesity prevalence. Pre- and posttreatment difference-in-differences estimates are from the Callaway/ Sant'Anna outcome regression estimator.[27,36,37] Estimates are aggregated relative to the year schools adopted CEP (time = 0). The panel of schools is balanced in calendar time, not event time.

study, however, the authors did not examine CEP specifically, nor did they have a control group.[25] The authors of another study found that BMI increases associated with school meal participation among low-income students attenuated after the HHFKA's nutrition standards took effect.[26] The authors of this study also did not examine CEP specifically and lacked a comparison group.[26] Rothbart and colleagues found that obesity decreased among seventh and 10th graders, but not younger students, in New York state school districts.[10] Schwartz and Rothbart found that, in New York City middle schools, UFM was associated with reduced obesity among children from households at >185% of the federal poverty level.[24] In a nationally representative sample of elementary schoolchildren, Andreyeva and Sun did not find an effect of CEP on obesity but observed a reduced probability of overweight among students from households at <200% of the federal poverty level.[8] Internationally, the authors of several studies have found associations of UFM with reduced obesity.[45–47]

In our study, we observed a reduction in obesity prevalence among CEP-participating schools relative to nonparticipating schools; however, prevalence increased over time for CEP and non-CEP schools. Although UFM policies may slow rising childhood obesity rates, they alone will not be sufficient to reverse trends and should be considered in conjunction with other obesity-reduction strategies. Although the observed effect size is modest, few population-level interventions have been successful at reducing obesity prevalence, particularly among lower-income populations;[48,49]

therefore, even small improvements are noteworthy. With this research, we add to a growing body of literature revealing the potential benefits of UFM to child well-being, including increasing participation in school meals,[8–11] improving diet quality,[15,18–20] reducing food insecurity,[15] and improving academic outcomes.[8,11,15,24] The coronavirus disease 2019 pandemic prompted the USDA to issue temporary waivers between 2020 and 2022 allowing schools nationwide to provide UFM.[50] Beginning in 2022, California expanded UFM to all public schools.[51] The authors of future research should explore whether such universal expansions impact health.

Data obtained from CDE were aggregated at the school level rather than the child level. Although California has a large and diverse population, these data are not nationally representative; the majority of students identified as Hispanic, which is representative of low-income children in California. The effects of CEP may vary by geographic region. For example, Davis et al found that CEP was associated with an increase in BMI and the probability of overweight (but not obesity) in 1 Atlanta school district.[52] Data are from students in grades 5, 7, and 9 and are not generalizable to younger students. Additionally, data were collected and reported by schools, not necessarily for research; however, we attempted to minimize the perceived erroneous outcome measures. Evidence reveals that teacher-measured BMI is highly accurate,[53,54] suggesting that the observed outliers were due to reporting rather than measurement error, adding support to the validity of nonoutlier measurements.

CONCLUSIONS

In a balanced sample of low-income, predominantly Hispanic California schools, participating in CEP was associated with a modest net reduction in obesity prevalence compared with eligible, nonparticipating schools. These findings add to the growing literature revealing the potential benefits of UFM for child well-being. Such policies represent a promising strategy for addressing childhood obesity.

ABBREVIATIONS

CDE: California Department of Education
CEP: Community Eligibility Provision
CI: confidence interval
HHFKA: Healthy, Hunger-Free Kids Act
ISP: identified student percentage
pp: percentage point
UFM: universal free school meals
USDA: United States Department of Agriculture

PEDIATRICS (ISSN Numbers: Print, 0031-4005; Online, 1098-4275).

Copyright © 2024 by the American Academy of Pediatrics

FUNDING: Funded by the National Institutes of Health (NIH). All phases of this study were supported by the Eunice Kennedy Shriver National Institute of Child Health & Development of the NIH under award number R01HD105666. The NIH had no role in the design and conduct of this study. The content is solely the responsibility of the authors and does not necessarily represent the official views of the National Institutes of Health.

CONFLICT OF INTEREST DISCLOSURES: The authors have indicated they have no potential conflicts of interest relevant to this article to disclose.

REFERENCES

1. Simmonds M, Llewellyn A, Owen CG, Woolacott N. Predicting adult obesity from childhood obesity: a systematic review and meta-analysis. *Obes Rev.* 2016;17(2):95–107

2. Hruby A, Manson JE, Qi L, et al. Determinants and consequences of obesity. *Am J Public Health.* 2016;106(9):1656–1662

3. Stierman B, Afful J, Carroll MD, et al; National Center for Health Statistics. National health and nutrition examination survey 2017–March 2020 prepandemic data files development of files and prevalence estimates for selected health outcomes. *Nat Health Stat Reports.* 2021;158:1–20

4. Dietz WH. We need a new approach to prevent obesity in low-income minority populations. *Pediatrics.* 2019;143(6):e20190839

5. Kumanyika SK. A framework for increasing equity impact in obesity prevention. *Am J Public Health.* 2019;109(10):1350–1357

6. Food Research & Action Center. Community eligibility: the key to hunger-free schools, school year 2022–2023. Available at: https://frac.org/wp-content/uploads/cep-report-2023.pdf. Accessed December 8, 2023

7. Bhatia R, Jones P, Reicker Z. Competitive foods, discrimination, and participation in the National School Lunch Program. *Am J Public Health.* 2011;101(8):1380–1386

8. Andreyeva T, Sun X. Universal school meals in the US: what can we learn from the community eligibility provision? *Nutrients.* 2021;13(8):2634

9. Tan ML, Laraia B, Madsen KA, et al. Community eligibility provision and school meal participation among student subgroups. *J Sch Health.* 2020;90(10):802–811

10. Rothbart MW, Schwartz AE, Gutierrez E. Paying for free lunch: the impact of CEP universal free meals on revenues, spending, and student health. *Ed Finance Policy.* 2023;18(4):708–737

11. Ruffini K. Universal access to free school meals and student achievement: evidence from the community eligibility provision. *J Hum Resour.* 2022;57(3):776–820

12. Liu J, Micha R, Li Y, Mozaffarian D. Trends in food sources and diet quality among US children and adults, 2003-2018. *JAMA Netw Open.* 2021;4(4):e215262

13. Vernarelli JA, O'Brien B. A vote for school lunches: school lunches provide superior nutrient quality than lunches obtained from other sources in a nationally representative sample of US children. *Nutrients.* 2017;9(9):924

14. Au LE, Rosen NJ, Fenton K, et al. Eating school lunch is associated with higher diet quality among elementary school students. *J Acad Nutr Diet.* 2016;116(11):1817–1824

15. Cohen JFW, Hecht AA, McLoughlin GM, et al. Universal school meals and associations with student participation, attendance, academic performance, diet quality, food security, and body mass index: a systematic review. *Nutrients.* 2021;13(3):911

16. Au LE, Gurzo K, Gosliner W, et al. Eating school meals daily is associated with healthier dietary intakes: the healthy communities study. *J Acad Nutr Diet.* 2018;118(8):1474–1481.e1

17. Hanson KL, Olson CM. School meals participation and weekday dietary quality were associated after controlling for weekend eating among U. S. school children aged 6 to 17 Years. 2013;143(5):714–721

18. Kinderknecht K, Harris C, Jones-Smith J. Association of the healthy, hunger-free kids act with dietary quality among children in the US national school lunch program. *JAMA.* 2020;324(4):359–368

19. Johnson DB, Podrabsky M, Rocha A, Otten JJ. Effect of the Healthy Hunger-Free Kids Act on the nutritional quality of meals selected by students and school lunch participation rates. *JAMA Pediatr.* 2016;170(1):e153918

20. Dietz WH. Better diet quality in the Healthy Hunger-Free Kids Act and WIC package reduced childhood obesity. *Pediatrics*. 2021; 147(4):e2020032375

21. Food and Nutrition Service, USDA. Nutrition standards in the national school lunch and school breakfast programs. Final rule. *Fed Regist*. 2012;77(17):4088–4167

22. School Nutrition Association. 2023 school nutrition trends report. Available at: https://schoolnutrition.org/wp-content/uploads/2023/01/2023-School-Nutrition-Trends-Report.pdf. Accessed March 2, 2023

23. Marcus M, Yewell KG. The effect of free school meals on household food purchases: evidence from the community eligibility provision. *J Health Econ*. 2022;84:102646

24. Schwartz AE, Rothbart MW. Let them eat lunch: the impact of universal free meals on student performance. *J Policy Anal Manage*. 2019;39(2):376–410

25. Kenney EL, Barrett JL, Bleich SN, et al. Impact of the Healthy, Hunger-Free Kids Act on obesity trends. *Health Aff (Millwood)*. 2020; 39(7):1122–1129

26. Richardson AS, Weden MM, Cabreros I, Datar A. Association of the Healthy, Hunger-Free Kids Act of 2010 with body mass trajectories of children in low-income families. *JAMA Netw Open*. 2022;5(5):e2210480

27. Callaway B, Sant'Anna P. Difference-in-differences with multiple time periods. *J Econom*. 2021;225:200–230

28. California Department of Education. Physical fitness testing (PFT). Available at: https://www.cde.ca.gov/ta/tg/pf/. Accessed February 8, 2023

29. Centers for Disease Control and Prevention, National Center for Health Statistics. CDC growth charts: United States. Available at: www.cdc.gov/growthcharts/. Accessed February 7, 2024

30. Gordon-Larsen P, The NS, Adair LS. Longitudinal trends in obesity in the United States from adolescence to the third decade of life. *Obesity (Silver Spring)*. 2010;18(9):1801–1804

31. Rundle AG, Factor-Litvak P, Suglia SF, et al. Tracking of obesity in childhood into adulthood: effects on body mass index and fat mass index at age 50. *Child Obes*. 2020;16(3):226–233

32. Flegal KM, Kit BK, Orpana H, Graubard BI. Association of all-cause mortality with overweight and obesity using standard body mass index categories: a systematic review and meta-analysis. *JAMA*. 2013;309(1):71–82

33. Turner L, Guthrie JF, Ralston K. Community eligibility and other provisions for universal free meals at school: impact on student breakfast and lunch participation in California public schools. *Transl Behav Med*. 2019;9(5):931–941

34. Hecht AA, Stuart EA, Pollack Porter KM. Factors associated with universal free school meal provision adoption among US public schools. *J Acad Nutr Diet*. 2022;122(1):49–63

35. Robert Graham Center. Social deprivation index (SDI). Available at: https://www.graham-center.org/maps-data-tools/social-deprivation-index.html. Accessed October 23, 2023

36. Heckman JJ, Ichimura H, Todd PE. Matching as an econometric evaluation estimator: evidence from evaluating a job training programme. *Rev Econ Stud*. 1997;64(4):605–654

37. Heckman J, Ichimura H, Smith J, Todd P. Characterizing selection bias using experimental data. *Econometrica*. 1998;66(5):1017

38. Goodman-Bacon A. Difference-in-differences with variation in treatment timing. *J Econom*. 2021;225(2):254–277

39. Baker AC, Larcker DF, Wang CCY. How much should we trust staggered difference-in-differences estimates? *J Financ Econ*. 2022; 144(2):370–395

40. Sun L, Abraham S. Estimating dynamic treatment effects in event studies with heterogeneous treatment effects. *J Econom*. 2021; 225(2):175–199

41. StataCorp. Stata statistical software: release 18. Available at: https://www.stata.com/support/faqs/resources/citing-software-documentation-faqs/. Accessed February 7, 2024

42. Tan Z. Bounded, efficient and doubly robust estimation with inverse weighting. *Biometrika*. 2010;97(3):661–682

43. Wasserstein RL, Lazar NA. The ASA statement on *p*-values: context, process, and purpose. *Am Stat*. 2016;70(2):129–133

44. Johnston CA, Moreno JP, El-Mubasher A, Woehler D. School lunches and lunches brought from home: a comparative analysis. *Child Obes*. 2012;8(4):364–368

45. Caro JC. Scaled-up nutrition services for child development: evidence from the chilean school meals program. *Am J Health Econ*. 2023;9(4):649–673

46. Bethmann D, Cho JI. The impacts of free school lunch policies on adolescent BMI and mental health: evidence from a natural experiment in South Korea. *SSM Popul Health*. 2022;18:101072

47. Holford A, Rabe B. Going universal. The impact of free school lunches on child body weight outcomes. *Journal of Public Economics Plus*. 2022;3:100016

48. Kumanyika SK. Advancing health equity efforts to reduce obesity: changing the course. *Annu Rev Nutr*. 2022;42(1):453–480

49. Roberto CA, Swinburn B, Hawkes C, et al. Patchy progress on obesity prevention: emerging examples, entrenched barriers, and new thinking. *Lancet*. 2015;385(9985):2400–2409

50. Food Research and Action Center. Large school district report operating school nutrition programs during the pandemic. Available at: https://frac.org/wp-content/uploads/large-school-district-report-2022.pdf. Accessed March 2, 2023

51. California Department of Education. California universal meals. Available at: https://www.cde.ca.gov/ls/nu/sn/cauniversalmeals.asp. Accessed February 7, 2024

52. Davis W, Kreisman D, Musaddiq T. The effect of universal free school meals on child BMI. *Edu Finance Policy*. 2023:1–31

53. Thompson HR, Linchey JK, King B, et al. Accuracy of school staff-measured height and weight used for body mass index screening and reporting. *J Sch Health*. 2019;89(8):629–635

54. Morrow Jr JR, Martin SB, Jackson AW. Reliability and validity of the FITNESSGRAM: quality of teacher-collected health-related fitness surveillance data. *Res Q Exerc Sport*. 2010;81(3 Suppl):S24–S30

Food Insecurity and Childhood Obesity: A Systematic Review

Christine St. Pierre, MPH, RDN,[a] Michele Ver Ploeg, PhD,[a] William H. Dietz, MD, PhD,[a,b] Sydney Pryor, MPH,[a] Chioniso S. Jakazi, MPH,[a] Elizabeth Layman, MPH,[a] Deborah Noymer, RDN,[a] Tessa Coughtrey-Davenport, MPH,[a] Jennifer M. Sacheck, PhD [a]

abstract

BACKGROUND AND OBJECTIVES: Addressing food insecurity while promoting healthy body weights among children is a major public health challenge. Our objective is to examine longitudinal associations between food insecurity and obesity in US children aged 1 to 19 years.

METHODS: Sources for this research include PubMed, CINAHL, and Scopus databases (January 2000 to February 2022). We included English language studies that examined food insecurity as a predictor of obesity or increased weight gain. We excluded studies outside the United States and those that only considered the unadjusted relationship between food security and obesity. Characteristics extracted included study design, demographics, methods of food security assessment, and anthropometric outcomes.

RESULTS: Literature searches identified 2272 articles; 13 met our inclusion criteria. Five studies investigated the relationship between food insecurity and obesity directly, whereas 12 examined its relationship with body mass index or body mass index z-score. Three studies assessed multiple outcomes. Overall, evidence of associations between food insecurity and obesity was mixed. There is evidence for possible associations between food insecurity and obesity or greater weight gain in early childhood, for girls, and for children experiencing food insecurity at multiple time points. Heterogeneity in study methods limited comparison across studies.

CONCLUSIONS: Evidence is stronger for associations between food insecurity and obesity among specific subgroups than for children overall. Deeper understanding of the nuances of this relationship is critically needed to effectively intervene against childhood obesity.

[a]Milken Institute School of Public Health, and [b]Sumner M. Redstone Center for Prevention and Wellness, The George Washington University, Washington, District of Columbia

Ms St. Pierre and Dr Ver Ploeg conceptualized and designed the study, coordinated and supervised data collection, drafted the initial manuscript, and reviewed and revised the manuscript; Drs Dietz and Sacheck conceptualized and designed the study and critically reviewed the manuscript for important intellectual content; Ms Pryor, Ms Jakazi, Ms Layman, Ms Noymer, and Ms Coughtrey-Davenport collected data, conducted the initial analyses, and reviewed and revised the manuscript; and all authors approved the final manuscript as submitted and agree to be accountable for all aspects of the work.

DOI: https://doi.org/10.1542/peds.2021-055571

Accepted for publication Apr 15, 2022

Address correspondence to Christine St. Pierre, MPH, RDN, Department of Exercise and Nutrition Sciences, Milken Institute School of Public Health, The George Washington University, 950 New Hampshire Ave NW, Washington, DC 20052. E-mail: cstpierre@gwu.edu

PEDIATRICS (ISSN Numbers: Print, 0031-4005; Online, 1098-4275).

FUNDING: This research was supported by Healthy Eating Research, a national program of the Robert Wood Johnson Foundation.

CONFLICT OF INTEREST DISCLOSURES: The authors have indicated they have no conflicts of interest to disclose.

To cite: St. Pierre C, Ver Ploeg M, Dietz WH, et al. Food Insecurity and Childhood Obesity: A Systematic Review. *Pediatrics*. 2022;150(1):e2021055571

REVIEW ARTICLE

The United States faces 2 important public health challenges in reducing childhood obesity while ensuring that children and their families have enough nutritious food for an active, healthy life. From 2017 to 2018, ~20% of US children aged 2 to 19 were estimated to have obesity, a prevalence level that has increased by nearly 40% over the past 20 years.[1] In 2020, the first year of the COVID-19 pandemic, food insecurity among US households with children was 14.8%, an increase over the 2019 level of 13.6% and a reversal of the declining trend observed over the previous decade.[2]

Childhood obesity and food insecurity are more prevalent in lower-income households,[2,3] suggesting a potentially simultaneous occurrence of both under- and over-nutrition. Despite almost 3 decades since these dual problems were first observed,[4] no consensus exists about the underlying mechanisms of their relationship. The increases in food insecurity[2,5] and accelerated weight gain[6-8] observed among children during the COVID-19 pandemic indicate that greater understanding of how these 2 issues interact is of great importance for child health, particularly in terms of associations between food insecurity episodes and weight status over the long term.

In this systematic review, we examined longitudinal associations between food insecurity and obesity in US children aged 1 to 19 years. The review summarizes the overall evidence, then discusses differences in the evidence according to relevant demographics and the experience of multiple food insecurity episodes.

METHODS AND LITERATURE SEARCH

This review was conducted in accordance with the Preferred Reporting Items for Systematic Reviews and Meta-Analysis. Searches were performed in December 2020 in PubMed, CINHAL, and Scopus databases and restricted to English language studies published between January 1, 2000, and November 30, 2020. Studies published before 2000 were excluded to maximize homogeneity in food security and child weight status assessment tools. Results were uploaded to the Covidence systematic review tool (Covidence, Melbourne, Australia) for screening.

Studies eligible for inclusion were those with participants who were infants or children in the United States from 1 to 19 years of age; that assessed food security or insufficiency at the household or child level; compared outcomes by food security status; and examined obesity or body mass index (BMI) as the primary outcome of interest (see full search strategy Supplemental Table 3). Included studies were limited to those conducted in the United States to reduce heterogeneity in the food security assessment tools employed. Studies were excluded if they only reported unadjusted relationships between food security and obesity, or if the study population was limited to only youth with overweight or obesity at baseline. Studies with less than 30 participants, the traditional minimum in statistics for a reliable confidence interval, were also excluded. Title and abstract screening, full-text screening and data extraction were performed by 2 independent reviewers; conflicts were resolved by consultation between researchers. Database searches were re-run in September 2021 and February 2022, and results were hand-searched to add

relevant studies published between December 2020 and February 2022.

Study quality was assessed using the National Institutes of Health (NIH) quality assessment tool for observational cohort and cross-sectional studies (NIH, Bethesda, Maryland). Although quality assessment tools for clinical trials are well established, there is no consensus on the best methods to assess the quality of observational nutrition studies.[9] We selected the NIH tool because it could be applied consistently to all included studies. Two researchers applied the assessment tool independently. Disagreements were resolved via discussion among the research team.

RESULTS

The database search yielded 2272 studies after duplicates were removed. Following title and abstract review, 91 papers were retained for full-text screening. Forty-two were excluded for 1 of the following: methods (no adjusted estimate of the relationship between food security and anthropometrics); outcome (did not assess likelihood of obesity or a continuous BMI-related outcome); population (participants over 19 years old); or location (outside the United States). A total of 41 studies met the inclusion criteria after the initial screening, 4 studies were subsequently added following the search and screening process in September 2021, and no additional studies meeting the inclusion criteria were identified in the February 2022 search (Fig 1).

A total of 45 papers were originally included for data extraction. Data on sample size, demographic characteristics of study participants, nutrition assistance program participation (when available), food security assessment methods,

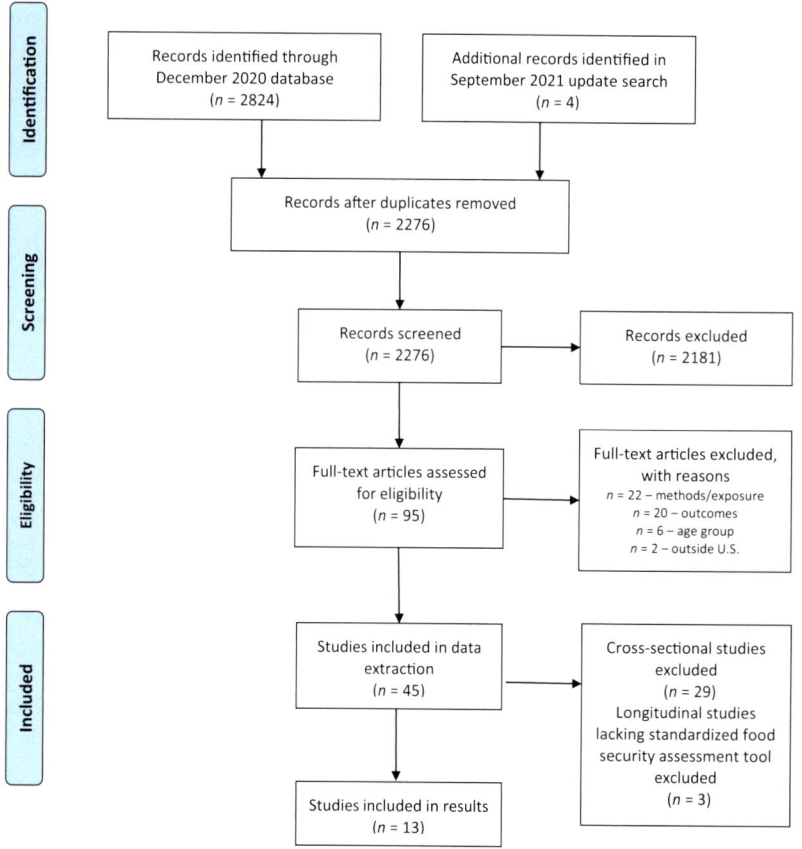

FIGURE 1

Preferred Reporting Items for Systematic Reviews and Meta-Analysis flow diagram detailing review search process. PRISMA statement distributed under the terms of the Creative Commons Attribution License. Original source: Mohr D, Liberati A, Tetzlaff J, Altmann DC, the PRISMA Group. Preferred reporting items for systematic reviews and meta-analysis: the PRISMA statement. *PLoS Med.* 2009;6(7);e1000098.[37]

outcomes measured, method of analysis, covariates included in analysis, adjusted results, and tests for interaction with any subsequent stratified results, were extracted using a piloted, standardized extraction spreadsheet. Although both longitudinal and cross-sectional studies were initially included, only the longitudinal studies ($n = 16$) were ultimately retained for evidence analysis because of their overall higher study quality and ability to provide insight into potential relationships between food insecurity and obesity over time.

In the quality analysis, all longitudinal studies were rated "good" or "fair" (Supplemental Table 4). Thirteen studies[10–22] used either the "gold standard" USDA 18-item Household Food Security Survey Module or a shorter subset derived directly from the full module to assess food security, whereas 3 studies used single-item measures. These 3 studies were excluded from the overall results synthesis because they lacked a standardized food security assessment instrument.

In the final 13 studies, variation in outcomes measured, food security categorization (eg, binary vs

multilevel and categorical versus continuous), and analysis methods prevented us from conducting a meta-analysis. We instead present the results according to the 3 different outcomes analyzed in the included studies. Our primary interest was examining the relationship between food insecurity and obesity. We focused on obesity rather than both overweight and obesity because obesity has a greater sensitivity and specificity for identifying excess body fat and carries a higher risk for adverse health outcomes.[23] To examine potential differences in trajectories of BMI growth, we also synthesized the evidence for associations between food insecurity and changes in BMI and BMI z-score. Both variables present interpretation challenges as longitudinal outcomes. BMI changes are not indexed to age and sex-specific references in studies and may not account for the normative dip in BMI that occurs in early childhood.[24] BMI z-score changes are smaller at higher levels of adiposity and do not adequately reflect large changes in weight and adiposity.[25] Despite these limitations, the growth trajectories identified in these analyses can illuminate associations between food insecurity and excess weight gain in children. When included studies measured multiple outcomes, we included the findings in each of the applicable syntheses. Table 1 summarizes the characteristics of all included studies.

Food Insecurity and Obesity

Five studies examined the association between food insecurity and obesity.[12,14,19–21] Among a cohort of participants in the Special Supplemental Nutrition Program for Women, Infants, and Children (WIC) in Massachusetts, an association was found between low food security

TABLE 1 Characteristics of Included Studies

Source	Number	Location or Cohort	Age Range	Race and Ethnicity	Food Security Assessment Tool	Food Security Level of Assessment	Food Security Categories for Analysis	Covariates Included in Final Model	Outcome(s) Assessed	Main Analysis Findings for Food Insecurity Independent Variable	Tests for Interactions and Findings
Benjamin-Neelon et al[10] (2020)	666	Nurture study: birth cohort of women and their infants from 2 clinics in the southeastern United States. Mothers enrolled during pregnancy, children followed from 1–12 mo	Mothers enrolled during pregnancy, children followed from 1–12 mo	14.9% White, 68.6% Black, 14.9% non-White, and non-Black or more than 1 race	USDA 18-item HFSSM, but over the past 30 d at each assessment instead of over the past 12 mo	Household; assessed at infant age 3, 6, 9, an d 12 mo	(1) High food security, (2) marginal food security, (3) low food security, and (4) very low food security	Infant race, sex, birth weight for gestational age z-score, breastfeeding, maternal age, race, education, and prepregnancy BMI; number of children in household, Supplemental Nutrition Assistance Program (SNAP) participation, and WIC participation	BMI z-score using WHO reference data	Very low food security associated with increased BMI z-score	Food insecurity x SNAP: null; food insecurity x WIC: null
Bhargava et al[11] (2008)	7635	ECLS-K (national)	Followed from first through fifth grade, mean age in first grade: 73 mo	9% Black, 16% Hispanic model only controlled for non-Hispanic Black race or Hispanic ethnicity; authors also reported the following demographics: 65% White and 4% Asian	USDA 18-item HFSSM	Household; assessed at first, third, and fifth grades	Continuous variable for aggregate number of affirmative responses (higher score, greater food insecurity)	Child race (binary variables for Black and Hispanic), age (quadratic; not included in BMI z-score model), parental education, number of siblings, health of respondent limited activities (Y/N), emotional wellbeing of respondent, minutes per day TV time, hours per week nonparental care, physical exercise (days per week with > 20 min), and household income lagged dependent variable	BMI, BMI z-score	Null in both models	None reported
Bronte-Tinkew et al[12] (2007)	8693	ECLS-birth cohort (national)	Followed from 9 to 24 mo, age range	Specific proportions in analysis sample not reported and	USDA 18-item Household Food Security Survey	Household; assessed at 9-mo wave	(1) High and marginal, (2) low, and (3) very low	Child age, child sex, family structure, parental education, mother's age at	Obesity status at 24 mo (wt-for-length)	Direct relationship: null; mediated relationship:	None reported

TABLE 1 Continued

Source	Number	Location or Cohort	Age Range	Race and Ethnicity	Food Security Assessment Tool	Food Security Level of Assessment	Food Security Categories for Analysis	Covariates Included in Final Model	Outcome(s) Assessed	Main Analysis Findings for Food Insecurity Independent Variable	Tests for Interactions and Findings
			was 6 to 22 mo for the 9-mo wave; 16 to 38 mo for 24-mo wave	race not included as covariate	Module (HFSSM)			birth, appropriate number of well-baby visits, smoking in household, maternal employment status, household SNAP participation, WIC participation, and household poverty index ratio; mediators: maternal depression, parenting practices, and infant feeding practices		food insecurity associated with poorer positive parenting practices, good positive parenting practices associated with good infant feeding practices, and good infant feeding practices associated with decreased odds of obesity	
Burke et al[15] (2016)	15 827	ECLS-K (national)	Followed from K through eighth grade	Boys, at fall K: 60.5% White, 12.6% Black, 16.7% Hispanic, 10.2% non-White, non-Black, and non-Hispanic; Girls, at fall K: 59.5% White, 13.3% Black, 17.3% Hispanic, 9.9% non-White, non-Black and non-Hispanic	USDA 18-item HFSSM	Household; assessed at fall K, spring K, spring third, spring fifth, and spring eighth	(1) Food secure (high and marginal) and (2) food insecure (low and very low)	Child age, height (quadratic), birth weight, race and ethnicity, health insurance coverage, parental perception of child exercise level (same as, more, or less than other children), school lunch receipt, number of parents in household, urbanicity, region of the United States, SNAP participation, total household size, and socioeconomic status	BMI growth from K to eighth grade using data from fall kindergarten, spring kindergarten, spring third grade, spring fifth grade, and spring eighth grade	Growth curve models stratified by sex: for girls, lower BMI in K and higher BMI in eighth grade for those from food insecure households	Food security status x year: for girls, BMI growth from K to eighth grade was greater for those from food insecure households

TABLE 1 Continued

Source	Number	Location or Cohort	Age Range	Race and Ethnicity	Food Security Assessment Tool	Food Security Level of Assessment	Food Security Categories for Analysis	Covariates Included in Final Model	Outcome(s) Assessed	Main Analysis Findings for Food Insecurity Independent Variable	Tests for Interactions and Findings
Gamba et al[14] (2021)	204	CHAMACOS, Salinas, CA	Mothers enrolled during pregnancy, followed children from age 5 to 12 y for this analysis	100% Hispanic (mothers)	USDA 6-item Short Form	Household; assessed at child ages 5, 7, 9, and 10.5	(1) Fully food secure and (2) marginal food security or food insecure, also examined status over multiple time points	Child sex, birth weight (low to normal versus high), early life food insecurity, hours per day TV time, hours per day playing outside, puberty status (prepubescent or pubescent); maternal age (range), marital status, prepregnancy BMI, parity, proportion of life spent in the United States, education level and household income (above or below FPL)	Change in obesity status across age intervals: 5 to 7 y, 7 to 9 y, 9 to 10.5 y, 10.5 to 12 y, change in BMI z-score and BMI over specific age intervals: 5 to 7 y, 7 to 9 y, 9 to 10.5 y, 10.5 to 12 y and change in BMI z-score and BMI across 2 intervals and 3 intervals	Null findings for associations between food insecurity and obesity in all models. Food insecurity at age 9 associated with a decrease in BMI z-score from 9 to 10.5 y, to food security status across 2 intervals, food insecurity across 2 time points associated with decrease in BMI z-score, change from food secure to food insecure across 2 time points associated with decreases in both BMI z-score and BMI	None reported in obesity analysis, for BMI z-score and BMI: Food insecurity x maternal prepregnancy BMI: null, food insecurity x child sex: null
Jackson et al[15] (2017)	128	Generating rural options for wt (GROW)-healthy kids and communities: sample from	Elementary students followed over 1 y, mean age 8.0 ± 1.9 y	89.2% White and 10.8% non-White	2-item Hunger Vital Signs food security screening tool	Household; assessed at baseline	(1) Not at risk for food insecurity and (2) at risk for food insecurity	Child BMI z-score at baseline, participation in GROW intervention, (main analysis was crosssectional)	Change in BMI z-score from baseline to 1-y follow-up	Null	None reported

TABLE 1 Continued

Source	Number	Location or Cohort	Age Range	Race and Ethnicity	Food Security Assessment Tool	Food Security Level of Assessment	Food Security Categories for Analysis	Covariates Included in Final Model	Outcome(s) Assessed	Main Analysis Findings for Food Insecurity Independent Variable	Tests for Interactions and Findings
		rural communities in 3 Oregon counties	at baseline				(affirmative to either item)				
Jansen et al[16] (2017)	501	Growing Healthy Study: preschoolers in Head Start programs in urban and rural Michigan	Followed over 6 mo (fall to spring of 1 school year) mean age 4.4 ± 0.6 y at baseline	60.3% White, 28.7% Black, 6.6% Hispanic, 4.4% non-White, non-Black, and non-Hispanic	USDA 18-item HFSSM	Household; assessed at baseline and follow-up	(1) Food secure (high and marginal) and (2) food insecure (low and very low), created measure using the 2 categories and 2 time points for 4 different food security categories in analysis	Caregiver race and ethnicity, education level, and household income to needs ratio	Change in BMI z-score	Models stratified by child sex: for girls, greater increase in BMI z-score for those whose households became food insecure over the interval	None reported
Jyoti et al[17] (2005)	11 460	ECLS-K (national)	Followed from spring of K to spring of third grade, mean age in spring of K 6.2 y	62.1% White, 11.4% Black, 16.6% Hispanic, 10.0% non-White, non-Black, and non-Hispanic or more than 1 race	USDA 18-item HFSSM	Household; assessed at K and third grade	(1) Food secure (high) and (2) food insecure (marginal, low, and very low), created measure using the 2 categories and 2 time points for 4 different food security categories in analysis	Child sex, age, birth weight (low or not), race and ethnicity, disability (yes or no), initial height, change in height, BMI in kindergarten, health insurance coverage, exercise frequency (days per week), home language (English or other), household income, number of parents in household, household size, mother's age, father's age, parent marital status, mother's age at first birth, parent employment, parent	Change in BMI from K–3rd grade	When controlling for only kindergarten BMI, food insecurity in kindergarten associated with increased third grade BMI, null when additional covariates are added; food insecurity over time, and food insecurity at both time points	Food insecurity x sex: increased BMI gain for girls when experienced food insecurity in K; increased BMI gain for girls if food insecure at both time points

TABLE 1 Continued

Source	Number	Location or Cohort	Age Range	Race and Ethnicity	Food Security Assessment Tool	Food Security Level of Assessment	Food Security Categories for Analysis	Covariates Included in Final Model	Outcome(s) Assessed	Main Analysis Findings for Food Insecurity Independent Variable	Tests for Interactions and Findings
								highest education level, childcare arrangements, number of siblings, parent self-assessment of depression, region of residence, urbanicity, and neighborhood safety rating		associated with increased BMI gain	
Kamdar et al[18] (2019)	137	Cohort recruited from self-identified Hispanic parent-child dyads enrolled in Head Start in Houston, Texas	Followed children for 18 mo, mean age 4.8 y at baseline and 6.3 y at follow-up	100% Hispanic (parent)	5-item, self-administered paper version of USDA 6-item Short Form	Household; assessed at baseline	(1) Food secure (high and marginal) and (2) food insecure (low and very low), interval-level scale score used in analysis	Child BMI z-score at baseline, maternal English acculturation, maternal BMI mediators: parental feeding demandingness, parental feeding responsiveness, and child diet quality at follow-up	BMI z-score	Null (both direct and indirect effects)	Food insecurity x maternal English acculturation: null
Lee et al[19] (2018)	8167	ECLS-K:2011 (national	Followed from spring of K to spring of third grade, mean age in fall of K: 5.6 y	55.9% White, 9.1% Black, 25.6% Hispanic, 0.9% AI and AN, 4.5% Asian or PI, 4.0% Multiracial or unreported	USDA 18-item HFSS	Household; assessed at K and first grad	(1) Food secure (high and marginal) and (2) food insecure (low and very low, separate analyses for status in kindergarten and status in first grade	Sex, race and ethnicity, income quintile, and parental level of education	Odds of obesity in third grade, BMI z-score in third grade	Null, food insecurity in first grade associated with higher BMI z-score in third grade	Food insecurity x WIC participation: null, food insecurity x WIC participation: null
Metallinos-Katsaras et al[20] (2012)	28 353	WIC participants, Massachusetts	Retrospective cohort, followed from first WIC infancy visit to	41.4% White, 20.6% Black, 31.6% Hispanic, and 6.5% Asian	4-item subscale of USDA 18-item HFSSM	Household: assessed at infant visit and child visit	(1) Food secure, (2) food insecure without hunger (older term for low food	Child sex, race and ethnicity, birth weight, age at the last WIC visit, maternal age, education, prepregnancy wt	Odds of obesity at child visit (underweight children excluded), BMI z-score	Food insecurity without hunger at both time points associated with	Food security status in infancy x maternal prepregnancy wt status: if mothers were

TABLE 1 Continued

Source	Number	Location or Cohort	Age Range	Race and Ethnicity	Food Security Assessment Tool	Food Security Level of Assessment	Food Security Categories for Analysis	Covariates Included in Final Model	Outcome(s) Assessed	Main Analysis Findings for Food Insecurity Independent Variable	Tests for Interactions and Findings
			last WIC child visit (2–5 y), mean age at child visit: 36.9 ± 9.7 mo				security), and (3) food insecure with hunger (older term for very low food security), created time-integrated measure using 3 categories and 2 time points for 9 different food security categories in analysis	status, and household size		increased and odds of obesity relative to food secure at both time points, no difference in BMI z-score for either food insecure group relative to food security in infancy, food insecurity without hunger in infancy associated with higher BMI z-score at child visit relative to food insecurity with hunger in infancy	either underweight or overweight or with obesity, positive association between food insecurity without hunger at both time points and odds of child obesity relative to food secure at both time points; if mothers were overweight or with obesity, positive association between food insecurity without hunger in infancy and BMI z-score at child visit, relative to food security in infancy
Rose and Bodor[21] (2006)	12 890	ECLS-K (national)	Followed from spring of K to spring of first grade, mean age in spring	58.8% White, 15.5% Black, 18.6% Hispanic, 2.7% Asian, 4.4% non-White, non-Black, non-Hispanic, and non-Asian	USDA 18-item HFSSM	Household: assessed at K	(1) Food secure (high and marginal) and (2) food insecure (with and without hunger, ie, low and very low	Child age, sex, race and ethnicity, interaction between sex and race and ethnicity, birth weight, (dummy variables for low or high); household poverty index ratio, maternal education, urbanization, region	Odds of obesity in first grade, odds of high wt gain between K and first (high wt gain defined as a BMI gain in the top 15%	Null, food insecurity in K associated with lower odds of high wt gain from K to first grade	None reported for longitudinal analyses

TABLE 1 Continued

Source	Number	Location or Cohort	Age Range	Race and Ethnicity	Food Security Assessment Tool	Food Security Level of Assessment	Food Security Categories for Analysis	Covariates Included in Final Model	Outcome(s) Assessed	Main Analysis Findings for Food Insecurity Independent Variable	Tests for Interactions and Findings
			of K: 74.4 mo				low food security)	of the country, frequency of family meals, parent perception of child's physical activity (relative to other children), and TV time (> 2 h per day or not)	distribution for age and sex)		
Zhu et al[22] (2020)	6368	ECLS-K (national)	Followed from K-8th grade	Food secure in K: 69.7% White, 7.5% Black, 14.1% Hispanic, 8.6% Asian or non-White, non-Black and non-Hispanic; food insecure in K: 39.1% White, 12.4% Black, 34.1% Hispanic, 14.4% Asian or non-White, non-Black and non-Hispanic, race and ethnicity reported by food security status in kindergarten; significant difference in demographics between food secure and food insecure groups (P < .001)	USDA 18-item HFSSM	Household: assessed at K, third, fifth, and eighth grades	(1) Food secure (high and marginal) and (2) food insecure (low and very low)	Child sex, race and ethnicity, birth weight (low, normal, or high), health insurance status, household poverty (at and above or below FPL), parental depression, maternal nativity (born in U.S. or no), maternal education level	BMI z-score at third, fifth, and eighth grades	Food insecurity in fifth grade associated with higher BMI z-score in eighth grade	Interaction between food security status at adjacent time points: null food security by race and ethnicity: null, food security by household poverty: null, food security by sex: null

Only analyses meeting our inclusion criteria are presented in the table; studies may have analyzed other outcomes that did not fit our criteria

Only analyses meeting our inclusion criteria are presented in the table; studies may have analyzed other outcomes that did not fit our criteria (worried about food but no disruption to eating patterns, as opposed to very low food security, which also includes disruption of eating patterns) when present in both infancy and preschool and greater odds of obesity in preschool.[20] This relationship was also moderated by maternal prepregnancy weight status, with greater odds of obesity for children in households with low food security at both time points and whose mothers were either overweight, had obesity, or were underweight prepregnancy. An analysis of the Early Childhood Longitudinal Study (ECLS) birth cohort using structural equation modeling found no direct association between food insecurity and obesity, but in mediation analysis, food insecurity affected parenting and infant feeding behaviors, which ultimately affected weight.[12] The 3 remaining studies found no significant associations between food insecurity and obesity; 2 used data from the ECLS-K[21] and ECLS-K: 2011[19] cohorts, and the third used findings from a cohort of Hispanic mothers and their children in California (CHAMACOS).[14]

Food Insecurity and BMI

Four studies analyzed the relationship between food insecurity and changes in BMI over time. Of the 2 studies using ECLS-K data, 1 found a greater increase in BMI among children whose households were food insecure at 2 time points,[17] and both found higher BMI increases for girls from food insecure households but not for boys.[13,17] In a third study using ECLS-K data, the authors reported no significant associations but did not test for interactions by sex or consider food insecurity at multiple time points.[11] The CHAMACOS study found lower BMI gains among children whose households changed from highly food secure to

marginally food secure or food insecure across 2 time points.[14]

Food Insecurity and BMI z-Score

Nine studies investigated associations between food insecurity and changes in BMI z-score. The ECLS-K: 2011 study found an association between food insecurity in first grade and an increased BMI z-score in third grade, but no association between kindergarten food insecurity and third grade BMI z-score.[19] Likewise, a fourth ECLS-K study found an association between fifth grade food insecurity and a higher eighth grade BMI z-score but no significant associations when food insecurity occurred in younger grades.[22] In a Head Start preschool cohort, an association was found between food insecurity and increased BMI z-score for girls, but participants were only followed for an average of 6 months.[16] A birth cohort following infants through 12 months found an association between very low food security and a higher BMI z-score,[10] whereas the WIC cohort found no association in the main analysis but an association between food insecurity in infancy and an increased BMI z-score in early childhood if the mother was overweight or had obesity prepregnancy.[20] In the CHAMACOS cohort, food insecurity at age 9 was associated with a decrease in BMI z-score from ages 9 to 10.5, and food insecurity across 2 time points or changing from food secure to food insecure were also associated with decreased BMI z-score.[14] The remaining 3 studies found no significant associations.[11,15,18]

Results Synthesis

The studies are categorized by outcome and findings in Table 2. An association between food insecurity and obesity was found only in early childhood,[20] whereas 6 additional studies found evidence of associations between food insecurity

and increases in BMI or BMI z-score in limited age groups or sex-specific analyses.[10,13,16,17,19,22] One study of an exclusively Hispanic population found evidence of an association between food insecurity and decreases in BMI z-score or BMI, limited to a specific age group or changes in food security status.[14] Although all studies assessed food security based on standardized US Department of Agriculture assessment tools, comparison is challenging because of differences in food security categorization. Most studies categorized participants as either food secure (high or marginal food security according to survey responses) or food insecure (low or very low food security). However, 2 studies combined marginal food security with low and very low food security,[14,17] 3 studies used more than 2 categories for food security status,[10,12,20] and 1 used a continuous variable.[11] Studies also differed in the covariates used in their analyses. Child age, sex, race or ethnicity, household income, and parent or maternal education were consistently included as control variables, but other predictors of obesity, such as physical activity level, child birth weight, and maternal BMI, were included in no more than half of the studies. The variations in both the food security variable and covariates may help explain the mixed results observed across studies.

DISCUSSION

Our findings corroborate the previously published literature, indicating that potential relationships between food insecurity and childhood obesity and child weight changes are complex. Although the evidence did not allow us to draw broad conclusions about the relationship between food insecurity and obesity in children, we were nevertheless able to gain deeper insight and identify

TABLE 2 Findings by Outcome

Outcome	Number of Studies[a]	Increase	Decrease	No Association
Odds of obesity	5	Metallinos-Katsaras et al[20] (2012) (WIC)		Bronte-Tinkew et al[12] (2007) (ECLS-B), Gamba et al[14] (2021) (CHAMACOS), Lee et al[19] (2018) (ECLS-K:2011), Rose and Bodor[21] (2006) (ECLS-K)
Changes in BMI	4	Burke et al[13] (2016) (ECLS -K), Jyoti et al[17] (2005) (ECLS-K)	Gamba et al[14] (2021) (CHAMACOS)	Bhargava et ak[11] (2008) (ECLS-K)
Changes in BMI z-score	9	Benjamin-Neelon et al[10] (2020) (birth cohort), Jansen et al[16] (2017) (Head Start), Lee et al[19] (2018) (ECLS-K:2011), Metallinos-Katsaras et al[20] (2012) (WIC), Zhu et al[22] (2020) (ECLS-K)	Gamba et al[14] (2021) (CHAMACOS)	Bhargava et al[11] (2008) (ECLS-K), Jackson et al[15] (2017) (elementary, rural), Kamdar et al[18] (2019) (Head Start, Hispanic)

[a]The number of studies does not sum to 13 because some studies investigated multiple outcomes.

directions for further research by synthesizing results according to age, sex, and multiple experiences of food insecurity.

We observed associations between food insecurity and increases in BMI or BMI z-score among infants,[10] preschoolers,[16,20] elementary students,[17,19] and middle school students.[13,22] Although 5 of the studies with evidence of higher BMIs among food insecure youth were highly powered cohorts with large samples,[13,17,19,20,22] findings were limited to specific age ranges or subgroups within the sample, with the exception of the preschool study.[20] In the localized CHAMACOS cohort, food insecurity was associated with decreased BMI z-scores during mid- to late elementary years.[14] Thus, the mixed evidence is in agreement with the 2015 Dietary Guidelines Advisory Committee (DGAC) conclusion that limited evidence supports an association between food insecurity and higher anthropometric measurements in early childhood.[26] It is also particularly noteworthy that none of the studies followed children

beyond eighth grade. Eight of the 13 studies in our review were published after the 2015 DGAC identified the need for additional study of food insecurity and weight changes into the adolescent years,[26] but none provided evidence of potential associations beyond middle school.

Three of the studies in the review presented results stratified by child sex, and all found an association between food insecurity and increased BMI or BMI z-score for girls but not for boys.[13,16,17] Three additional studies tested for interaction by sex but found no associations.[14,20,22] Associations between food insecurity and higher BMI for preschool girls have also been found cross-sectionally.[27,28] Potential explanations for this association in girls but not in boys could include differential parent feeding practices by gender,[29] or different responses to stress, including the experience of food insecurity.[17] Lack of testing for interaction by sex in many studies could also be masking associations

in 1 of the groups, even if a relationship is not found in the overall population.[27] Following youth into adolescence and early adulthood could also help clarify differences in the interactions between food insecurity and weight by sex, particularly given recent evidence among adults that food insecurity was more prevalent among women with greater adiposity.[30]

Several of the longitudinal studies in the review categorized food security across multiple time points to examine how changes in food security status or multiple episodes of food insecurity were related to obesity and BMI.[13,14,16,17,20] In 3 large studies, food insecurity at multiple time points was associated with obesity or greater BMI growth relative to food security at all time points,[13,17,20] and 1 preschool study found that for girls, higher BMI z-scores were associated with the household changing from food secure to food insecure over the course of 1 school year.[16] One smaller study found an association with decreased BMI z-scores when food insecurity occurred at multiple time points or when households transitioned from food security to food insecurity,[14] but more evidence points to a potential cumulative positive effect of multiple experiences of food insecurity on weight gain, an effect also observed by the 2015 DGAC.[26] The effects of the duration and episodic nature of food insecurity may be of particular relevance to the increase in childhood obesity that has occurred during the COVID-19 pandemic.[6,7]

Potential differences by age range, sex, and the unknown effects of fluctuations in food security status over time indicate that a systems or structural modeling approach may provide better insight into how food insecurity and child weight status are related to one another through indirect channels. Household stress may play an important mediating role in the relationship between food insecurity and weight outcomes. One longitudinal study with a small sample size found an association between food insecurity and increased BMI when high stress was present at the child level,[31] and multiple studies have examined how interactions between maternal stress and food insecurity may affect child weight status.[32–35] Two of the studies included in this review included structural models that accounted for parental feeding practices,[12,18] and another structural model includes child dietary intake and both child and parent physical activity levels.[36] Further research can build on such models to better understand the complex mechanisms that affect the relationship between food insecurity and child weight status. Irrespective of any future conclusive evidence on the relationship mechanisms between food insecurity and childhood obesity, however, effective interventions against child food insecurity should be a public health priority to promote the physical, emotional, and cognitive wellbeing of children and parents.

Limitations

Although limiting our analysis to longitudinal studies strengthens the evidence relative to cross-sectional findings, following low-income populations over long periods is a challenging endeavor. The ECLS-K studies did not remain nationally representative over the follow-up periods, and 1 of them specifically noted that participants excluded because of missing data were more likely to be of lower socioeconomic status.[19] Recent evidence indicates that racial or ethnic disparities in childhood obesity have increased since the COVID-19 pandemic,[6] but our ability to explore potential differences by race or ethnicity in the food insecurity-childhood obesity relationship was limited by lack of testing for interaction by race or ethnicity. Two of the 3 studies that followed youth into puberty omitted any discussion of pubertal status, despite connections between puberty and anthropometric measurements that could have affected study findings. Differences in covariates, most notably omission of control variables for physical activity in most studies and for dietary quality in all studies, may contribute to the inconsistent findings. Finally, we were limited in our ability to assess the relationship between food insecurity and obesity by the diverse outcomes measured in the included studies. A greater proportion of studies used continuous BMI outcomes relative to weight categories. Although these studies showed changes in BMI trajectories, it was not apparent whether these changes indicated movement across weight categories.

CONCLUSIONS

We observed mixed evidence of associations between food insecurity and childhood obesity, but the mechanisms of their relationship remain difficult to ascertain. This review highlights the importance of understanding the many nuances of how food insecurity and childhood obesity interact with one another, which is even more critical as we have observed increased child food insecurity and widening disparities in the prevalence of obesity amid the COVID-19 pandemic. Ongoing and future studies need to consider interactions between food insecurity and salient demographics and the broader context of the household environment to enable us to meet the dual challenges of reducing childhood obesity and ensuring food security for all families.

ACKNOWLEDGMENTS

We thank the anonymous reviewers for their thoughtful and insightful feedback on this paper.

ABBREVIATIONS

BMI: body mass index
DGAC: Dietary Guidelines Advisory Committee
ECLS: Early Childhood Longitudinal Study
NIH: National Institutes of Health
SNAP: Supplemental Nutrition Assistance Program
WIC: Special Supplemental Nutrition Program for Women, Infants, and Children

REFERENCES

1. Fryar CD, Carroll MD, Afful J; Centers for Disease Control and Prevention; National Center for Health Statistics. Prevalence of overweight, obesity, and severe obesity among adults aged 20 and over: United States, 1960–1962 through 2017–2018. Available at: https://www.cdc.gov/nchs/data/hestat/obesity-adult-17-18/obesity-adult.htm. Accessed August 10, 2021

2. Coleman-Jensen A, Rabbitt MP, Gregory CA, Singh A; United States Department of Agriculture. Household food security in the United States in 2020. USDA economic research service report number 298. 2021. Available at: https://www.ers.usda.gov/publications/pub-details/?pubid=102075. Accessed September 21, 2021

3. Ogden CL, Carroll MD, Fakhouri TH, et al. Prevalence of obesity among youths by household income and education level of head of household—United States 2011–2014. *MMWR Morb Mortal Wkly Rep.* 2018;67(6):186–189

4. Dietz WH. Does hunger cause obesity? *Pediatrics.* 1995;95(5):766–767

5. Adams EL, Caccavale LJ, Smith D, Bean MK. Food insecurity, the home

food environment, and parent feeding practices in the era of COVID-19. *Obesity (Silver Spring)*. 2020;28(11):2056–2063

6. Jenssen BP, Kelly MK, Powell M, Bouchelle Z, Mayne SL, Fiks AG. COVID-19 and changes in child obesity. *Pediatrics*. 2021;147(5):e2021050123

7. Lange SJ, Kompaniyets L, Freedman DS, et al; DNP3. Longitudinal trends in body mass index before and during the COVID-19 pandemic among persons aged 2-19 years - United States, 2018-2020. *MMWR Morb Mortal Wkly Rep*. 2021;70(37):1278–1283

8. Weaver RG, Hunt ET, Armstrong B, et al. COVID-19 leads to accelerated increases in children's BMI z-score gain: an interrupted time-series study. *Am J Prev Med*. 2021;61(4):e161–e169

9. Tobias DK, Wittenbecher C, Hu FB. Grading nutrition evidence: where to go from here? *Am J Clin Nutr*. 2021;113(6): 1385–1387

10. Benjamin-Neelon SE, Allen C, Neelon B. Household food security and infant adiposity. *Pediatrics*. 2020;146(3): e20193725

11. Bhargava A, Jolliffe D, Howard LL. Socio-economic, behavioural and environmental factors predicted body weights and household food insecurity scores in the early childhood longitudinal study-kindergarten. *Br J Nutr*. 2008;100(2):438–444

12. Bronte-Tinkew J, Zaslow M, Capps R, Horowitz A, McNamara M. Food insecurity works through depression, parenting, and infant feeding to influence overweight and health in toddlers. *J Nutr*. 2007;137(9):2160–2165

13. Burke MP, Frongillo EA, Jones SJ, Bell BB, Hartline-Grafton H. Household food insecurity is associated with greater growth in body mass index among female children from kindergarten through eighth grade. *J Hunger Environ Nutr*. 2016;11(2):227–241

14. Gamba RJ, Eskenazi B, Madsen K, Hubbard A, Harley K, Laraia BA. Changing from a highly food secure household to a marginal or food insecure household is associated with decreased weight and body mass index z-scores among Latino children from CHAMACOS. *Pediatr Obes*. 2021;16(7):e12762

15. Jackson JA, Smit E, Branscum A, et al. The family home environment, food insecurity, and body mass index in rural children. *Health Educ Behav*. 2017;44(4):648–657

16. Jansen EC, Kasper N, Lumeng JC, et al. Changes in household food insecurity are related to changes in BMI and diet quality among Michigan Head Start preschoolers in a sex-specific manner. *Soc Sci Med*. 2017;181:168–176

17. Jyoti DF, Frongillo EA, Jones SJ. Food insecurity affects school children's academic performance, weight gain, and social skills. *J Nutr*. 2005;135(12): 2831–2839

18. Kamdar N, Hughes SO, Chan W, Power TG, Meininger J. Indirect effects of food insecurity on body mass index through feeding style and dietary quality among low-income Hispanic preschoolers. *J Nutr Educ Behav*. 2019;51(7): 876–884

19. Lee AM, Scharf RJ, DeBoer MD. Association between kindergarten and first-grade food insecurity and weight status in US children. *Nutrition*. 2018;51-52:1–5

20. Metallinos-Katsaras E, Must A, Gorman K. A longitudinal study of food insecurity on obesity in preschool children. *J Acad Nutr Diet*. 2012;112(12): 1949–1958

21. Rose D, Bodor JN. Household food insecurity and overweight status in young school children: results from the early childhood longitudinal study. *Pediatrics*. 2006;117(2):464–473

22. Zhu Y, Mangini LD, Hayward MD, Forman MR. Food insecurity and the extremes of childhood weight: defining windows of vulnerability. *Int J Epidemiol*. 2020; 49(2):519–527

23. Freedman DS, Sherry B. The validity of BMI as an indicator of body fatness and risk among children. *Pediatrics*. 2009;124(Suppl 1):S23–S34

24. Jabakhanji SB, Boland F, Ward M, Biesma R. Body mass index changes in early childhood. *J Pediatr*. 2018;202: 106–114

25. Cole TJ, Faith MS, Pietrobelli A, Heo M. What is the best measure of adiposity change in growing children: BMI, BMI %, BMI z-score or BMI centile? *Eur J Clin Nutr*. 2005;59(3):419–425

26. 2015 Dietary Guidelines Advisory Committee. Systematic reviews of the individual diet and physical activity behavior change subcommittee. Available at: https://nesr.usda.gov/individual-diet-and-physical-activity-behavior-change-subcommittee. Accessed January 24, 2022

27. Metallinos-Katsaras E, Sherry B, Kallio J. Food insecurity is associated with overweight in children younger than 5 years of age. *J Am Diet Assoc*. 2009;109(10):1790–1794

28. Speirs KE, Fiese BH; STRONG Kids Research Team. The relationship between food insecurity and BMI for preschool children. *Matern Child Health J*. 2016;20(4):925–933

29. Faith MS, Scanlon KS, Birch LL, Francis LA, Sherry B. Parent-child feeding strategies and their relationships to child eating and weight status. *Obes Res*. 2004;12(11): 1711–1722

30. Myers CA, Mire EF, Katzmarzyk PT. Trends in adiposity and food insecurity among US adults. *JAMA Netw Open*. 2020;3(8):e2012767

31. Distel LML, Egbert AH, Bohnert AM, Santiago CD. Chronic stress and food insecurity: examining key environmental family factors related to body mass index among low-income Mexican-origin youth. *Fam Community Health*. 2019;42(3):213–220

32. Gundersen C, Lohman BJ, Garasky S, Stewart S, Eisenmann J. Food security, maternal stressors, and overweight among low-income US children: results from the national health and nutrition examination survey (1999-2002). *Pediatrics*. 2008;122(3):e529–e540

33. Lohman BJ, Stewart S, Gundersen C, Garasky S, Eisenmann JC. Adolescent overweight and obesity: links to food insecurity and individual, maternal, and family stressors. *J Adolesc Health*. 2009;45(3):230–237

34. McClain AC, Evans GW, Dickin KL. Maternal stress moderates the relationship of food insufficiency with body mass index trajectories from childhood to early adulthood among U.S. rural youth. *Child Obes*. 2021;17(4):263–271

35. Eagleton SG, Na M, Savage JS. Food insecurity is associated with higher food responsiveness in low-income children: the moderating role of parent stress and family functioning. *Pediatr Obes.* 2022;(1):e12837

36. Huang H, Wan Mohamed Radzi CWJB, Salarzadeh Jenatabadi H. Family environment and childhood obesity: a new framework with structural equation modeling. *Int J Environ Res Public Health.* 2017;14(2):181

37. Moher D, Liberati A, Tetzlaff J, Altman DG, The PRIMSA Group. Preferred reporting items for systematic reviews and Meta-analyses: the PRISMA statement. *PLoS Med.* 2009;6(7):e1000097

Food Insecurity and Cardiometabolic Markers: Results From the Study of Latino Youth

Luis E. Maldonado, PhD,[a,b,c] Daniela Sotres-Alvarez, DrPH,[d] Josiemer Mattei, PhD,[e] Krista M. Perreira, PhD,[f] Amanda C. McClain, PhD,[g] Linda C. Gallo, PhD,[h] Carmen R. Isasi, MD, PhD,[i] Sandra S. Albrecht, PhD[j]

abstract

OBJECTIVES: Hispanic/Latino youth bear a disproportionate burden of food insecurity and poor metabolic outcomes, but research linking the two in this diverse population is lacking. We evaluated whether lower household and child food security (FS) were adversely associated with a metabolic syndrome (MetS) composite variable and clinically measured cardiometabolic markers: waist circumference, fasting plasma glucose, triglycerides, high-density lipoprotein cholesterol, and systolic and diastolic blood pressure.

METHODS: This cross-sectional study included 1325 Hispanic/Latino youth aged 8 to 16 years from the Hispanic Community Children's Health Study/Study of Latino Youth, a study of offspring of adults enrolled in the Hispanic Community Health Survey/Study of Latinos. Multivariable regression analyses were used to assess relationships between household FS (high, marginal, low, very low) and child FS (high, marginal, low/very low) status, separately, and our dependent variables, adjusting for participant age, sex, site, parental education, and poverty-income ratio.

RESULTS: For both FS measures, youth in the lowest FS category had significantly lower high-density lipoprotein cholesterol than those with high FS (household FS: −3.17, 95% confidence interval [CI]: −5.65 to −0.70, child FS: −1.81, 95% CI: −3.54 to −0.09). Low/very low versus high child FS was associated with greater fasting plasma glucose (β = 1.37, 95% CI: 0.08 to 2.65), triglycerides (β = 8.68, 95% CI: 1.75 to 15.61), and MetS expected log counts (β = 2.12, 95% CI: 0.02 to 0.45).

CONCLUSIONS: Lower FS is associated with unfavorable MetS-relevant cardiometabolic markers in Hispanic/Latino youth. These findings also support the use of a child-level versus a household-level measure to capture the health implications of food insecurity in this population.

Full article can be found online at www.pediatrics.org/cgi/doi/10.1542/peds.2021-053781

[a]Carolina Population Center, [b]Departments of Nutrition, and [d]Biostatistics, Gillings School of Global Public Health, and [f]Social Medicine, University of North Carolina, Chapel Hill, North Carolina; [c]Department of Population and Public Health Sciences, Keck School of Medicine, University of Southern California, Los Angeles, California; [e]Department of Nutrition, Harvard T.H. Chan School of Public Health, Boston, Massachusetts; [g]School of Exercise and Nutritional Sciences, and [h]Department of Psychology, San Diego State University, San Diego, California; [i]Department of Epidemiology & Population Health, Albert Einstein College of Medicine, Bronx, New York; and [j]Department of Epidemiology, Mailman School of Public Health, Columbia University, New York City, New York

Dr Maldonado reviewed the literature, developed the study design, analyzed and interpreted the data, and wrote the manuscript; Dr Albrecht contributed to the study design, interpreted the data, and critically revised and edited the manuscript; Drs Sotres-Alvarez, Mattei, Perreira, McClain, Gallo, and Isasi assisted in data interpretation and reviewed and edited the manuscript; and all authors approved the final manuscript as submitted and agree to be accountable for all aspects of the work.

DOI: https://doi.org/10.1542/peds.2021-053781

Accepted for publication Jan 26, 2022

WHAT'S KNOWN ON THIS SUBJECT: Early appearance of components of the metabolic syndrome and a high prevalence of low food security have been documented among US Hispanic/Latino youth. However, it is unknown if the two are associated in this population.

WHAT THIS STUDY ADDS: This study is among the first to document adverse associations between household and child food security measures with cardiometabolic markers among Hispanic/Latino youth. It also supports using the child-level versus the household-level measure to capture the health implications of food insecurity in this population.

To cite: Maldonado LE, Sotres-Alvarez D, Mattei J, et al. Food Insecurity and Cardiometabolic Markers: Results From the Study of Latino Youth. *Pediatrics.* 2022;149(4):e2021053781

ARTICLE

Food insecurity (FI) is characterized by limited or uncertain access to nutritionally adequate and safe foods or the ability to obtain such foods in socially acceptable ways.[1,2] FI has been associated with reduced quality of food, disrupted eating patterns,[3] and high levels of stress,[4,5] all of which can adversely affect health.[4,6] Despite abundant food availability in higher-income countries like the United States, FI affects ~14% of households with youth,[7] a disproportionate number of whom are Hispanics/Latinos.[8–10] In fact, 2012 to 2014 data from the Hispanic Community Children's Health Study/Study of Latino Youth (SOL Youth), a random sample of Hispanic/Latino youth from 4 large US cities, demonstrated 42% of Hispanic/Latino households with youth reported some level of FI in the previous year[10]; meanwhile, 11% reported the highest form of FI, which involves the uneasy/painful sensation of hunger.[2]

In adults, FI has been consistently associated with several cardiometabolic diseases, including type 2 diabetes,[11–17] obesity,[18–20] hypertension and hyperlipidemia,[14] and other metabolic sequelae,[21] but little is known about FI's role on physical health in youth. Among Hispanic/Latino youth, the scarce FI literature is mixed and largely centers on overweight/obesity.[10,22–24] The few studies evaluating links between FI and other cardiometabolic markers (CMMs) in youth were mostly specific to non-Hispanic White individuals and revealed null findings.[16,25] Despite the concurrent disproportionate burden of FI,[10] insulin resistance (IR), and the metabolic syndrome (MetS)[8,10,26–29] among Hispanic/Latino youth, no study, to our knowledge has evaluated FI's role in MetS and MetS-relevant CMMs in this population.

The health implications of FI may also vary by parental place of birth. Although previous work suggests that healthier diets and strong social and familial ties among foreign-born Hispanic/Latino parents may help protect their children from adopting less healthy US behaviors,[30] FI may undermine the protection of these factors.[31] Thus, we expect associations with MetS and MetS-relevant CMMs to be more pronounced among youth with foreign-born Hispanic/Latino parents or caregivers. Lastly, although food assistance (eg, Supplemental Assistance Nutrition Program [SNAP]) may serve as a potential buffer against poor diet quality and obesity in adults,[32] research is needed to better understand whether receiving any food assistance helps minimize the adverse health implications of FI among Hispanic/Latino youth.

Taken together, FI may have health implications for Hispanic/Latino youth. Therefore, this study's primary aim was to evaluate associations of household and child FI measures with MetS and MetS-relevant CMMs: waist circumference (WC), fasting plasma glucose (FG), high-density lipoprotein cholesterol (HDL-C), triglycerides (TGs), and systolic blood pressure (SBP) and diastolic blood pressure (DBP) measures. Our secondary aim was to investigate whether associations differed by parental place of birth and receipt of any food assistance in the previous year.

METHODS

Study Population

Data came from SOL Youth, a study of Hispanic/Latino youth aged 8 to 16 years recruited between 2012 and 2014 from the Bronx, New York, Chicago, Illinois, Miami, Florida, and San Diego, California. Detailed information about the study design

and objectives can be found elsewhere.[33,34] Briefly, SOL Youth is an ancillary study that enrolled children and adolescents living with the adults enrolled in the Hispanic Community Health Study/Study of Latinos (HCHS/SOL). HCHS/SOL is a prospective cohort study of US Hispanic/Latino adults of diverse origin recruited through a 2-stage area probability sampling design from the same 4 communities. Study design and procedures of HCHS/SOL have also been previously documented.[35,36] A total of 1466 youth (82% of eligible) were enrolled. Youth were instructed to fast for 10 hours before the baseline clinic visit (2012–2014), which included in-person interviews (in English or Spanish) of youth participants and their accompanying parent or caregiver and a blood draw. Institutions participating in SOL Youth received study approval from their respective institutional review boards. Written informed consent and assent were obtained from participating parents or caregivers and their youth, respectively.

Household and Child Food Insecurity

Most FI studies in youth have used a household versus a child FI measure, but the latter may better reflect FI in the youth as available food in food-insecure households may be prioritized for them. Thus, a child- versus household-level FI measure may show stronger associations.[37] Household and child FI was measured by using the United States Department of Agriculture 18-item Household Food Security Survey Module, a well-validated questionnaire which asks parents or caregivers about food security (FS) status over the past 12 months in the household (10 items) and for the youth (8 items).[2] On the basis of the number of affirmative responses for each set of questions, household and child FS measures were generated, each with 4 United States Department of Agriculture standard categories across the range of severity: household FS (high [0], marginal [1–2], low [3–7], and very low [8–18]) and child FS (high [0], marginal [1], low [2–4], and very low [3–8]). Lower FS categories are often collapsed into a single category to represent FI, but growing evidence suggests marginal, low, and very low FS are distinctly influential to diet and health.[4] Because of very few observations in the lowest child FS category, however, we combined low and very low child FS categories.

MetS-Relevant CMMs and MetS Composite Score

FG, TGs, and HDL-C were assessed by using fasting ($\geq$ 10-hour) blood samples taken from each participant and processed overnight at the University of Minnesota. FG was measured on a Modular P Chemistry Analyzer by using a hexokinase enzymatic method (Roche Diagnostics, Indianapolis, IN), serum insulin on an Elecsys 2010 Analyzer by using a sandwich immunoassay method (Rocha Diagnostics Corp.), serum TGs with a glycerol blanking enzymatic method (Roche Diagnostics), and HDL-C with a direct magnesium/dextran sulfate method.[38] After a 5-minute rest, 3 seated blood pressure measures were recorded from each participant by trained personnel using a standard sphygmomanometer and then averaged. WC was also measured 3 times and averaged per participant by using standard protocol.[39] On the basis of a modified child version of the adult-specific guidelines (Adult Treatment Panel III) on cholesterol management issued by the National Cholesterol Education Program,[40] we created a composite MetS score variable for CMMs constituting MetS.[41–43] For instance, youth

received a score of 1 for each CMM criteria met: abdominal adiposity (WC $\geq$ 90th age- and sex-specific percentiles),[44] FG ($\geq$ 100 mg/dL),[45] TGs ($\geq$ 150 mg/dL),[45] HDL-C ($\leq$ 40 mg/dL),[45] SBP or DBP ($\geq$ 90th age-, sex-, and height-specific percentiles),[46] ranging between 0 and 5.

Covariates and Modifiers

Data collected from SOL Youth participants included sex (female or male) and age (years). Information collected from accompanying parents/caregivers included income (lowest and highest reported income categories were <$10 000 and >$100 000, respectively), parental education (less than high school, high school or equivalent, and more than high school), parental place of birth (US-born including born in Puerto Rico and foreign-born), site (Bronx, NY, Chicago, IL, Miami, FL, and San Diego, CA), and receipt of any food assistance in the previous 12 months (yes or no), including SNAP, Women, Infants, and Children (WIC), or National School Lunch Program for free or reduced school meals. We calculated the poverty-income ratio by determining the median income for a given reported income range and dividing by the state-specific federal poverty guidelines for the year in which data collection took place.[47,48]

Statistical Analysis

Of the 1466 youth enrolled, 140 participants had missing data on at least 1 MetS-relevant CMM ($n = 87$) or relevant covariates ($n = 53$). Our final analytic sample included 1325 SOL Youth participants. All analyses were weighted and accounted for the study's complex design by using Stata software, version 14.1 (StataCorp LLC, College Station, TX). Because of skewness in the CMM variables, we reported median and interquartile ranges in descriptive analyses and log-transformed all

CMMs in regression analyses. We tested differences in sociodemographic and CMM variables across household and child FS categories by using t tests and Mann-Whitney U (Wilcoxon rank sum) tests for continuous variables and Pearson χ^2 tests for categorical variables. We used multivariable linear regression to estimate associations between household and child FS measures separately and each of the MetS-relevant CMMs (WC, FG, TGs, SBP, DBP, and HDL-C), adjusting for each participant's sex, age, site, parental education, parental place of birth, and poverty-income ratio. To examine associations with the MetS score variable, we employed multivariable Poisson regression, adjusting for the same covariates. In a set of separate models, we also evaluated adjusted interactions between each of the FS measures and parental place of birth, testing the appropriate interaction terms (FS measures × parental place of birth). In these same models, we additionally adjusted for receipt of any food assistance, as participants may also be living with members of the household who are undocumented and, therefore, ineligible for government food assistance (eg, SNAP). In another set of models, we tested an adjusted interaction term between each FS measure and receipt of any food assistance in the previous year adjusting for the aforementioned covariates. All geometric mean estimates derived from linear regression analyses were back-transformed to their original scales to improve interpretation.[49] We considered statistical significance at $P < .05$ and for interactions at $P < .10$.

RESULTS

Table 1 shows MetS-relevant CMMs and sociodemographic characteristics by household and child FS measures. In general,

TABLE 1 CMMs and Sociodemographic Characteristics by Household and Child FS Status in the SOL Youth ($n = 1325$)

Characteristics	Household Food Security Status				Child Food Security Status		
	High ($n = 554$)	Marginal ($n = 220$)	Low ($n = 393$)	Very Low ($n = 158$)	High ($n = 740$)	Marginal ($n = 143$)	Low/Very Low ($n = 442$)
MetS-relevant CMMs[a]							
WC (cm)	75 (66–85)	72 (64–82)	76 (69–85)	78 (69–87)	74 (66–85)	73 (67–81)	77 (69–87)**
FG (mg/dL)	91 (87–95)	92 (88–96)	92 (88–96)	92 (89–96)	91 (87–95)	92 (87–96)	92 (89–96)
TGs (mg/dL)	66 (48–91)	68 (45–92)	71 (53–96)**	74 (53–103)**	67 (48–91)	68 (51–98)	72 (53–100)**
HDL-C (mg/dL)	52 (45–60)	50 (45–59)	50 (44–58)*	49 (42–55)**	52 (45–60)	52 (44–56)	49 (43–57)**
SBP (mm Hg)	105 (98–111)	104 (97–110)	105 (97–113)	106 (98–113)	105 (98–111)	105 (98–113)	106 (98–113)
DBP (mm Hg)	60 (56–66)	61 (56–65)	60 (56–66)	60 (56–65)	60 (56–65)	61 (56–66)	60 (56–65)
MetS score criteria,[b] n (%)							
Abdominal obesity (≥ 90th percentile)	138 (25.8)	52 (21.1)	108 (23.1)	46 (30.2)	184 (25)	33 (17.3)	27 (26.9)
FG (≥ 100 mg/dL)	52 (8.7)	30 (10.9)	45 (10.2)	21 (12.7)	69 (8.7)	23 (10.8)	56 (12.4)
TGs (≥150 mg/dL)	33 (6.7)	13 (8.1)	29 (7.9)	19 (11.2)	44 (6.3)	7 (7.3)	43 (10.4)
HDL-C (≤40 mg/dL)	80 (11.8)	26 (11.4)	59 (13.5)	32 (20.9)*	101 (11.1)	18 (10.2)	78 (18.0)**
SBP or DBP (≥90th percentile)	25 (5.1)	3 (1.8)	25 (8.3)	9 (6.7)	28 (4.3)	7 (7.8)	27 (7.6)
MetS (score)[a]	1 (1–2)	1 (1–2)	1 (1–2)	1 (1–2)	1 (1–2)	1 (1–1)	1 (1–2)
Sociodemographics, n (%)							
Child age, y	12.2 (2.6)	11.7 (2.7)	12.4 (2.5)	12.3 (2.6)	12.1 (2.6)	11.9 (2.5)	12.4 (2.6)
Female	271 (49)	104 (44.7)	207 (49.3)	79 (51)	365 (49.2)	70 (45.1)	226 (49.1)
Site, n (%)							
Bronx	142 (31.2)	64 (35.5)	116 (40.1)	66 (51.9)**	204 (34)	50 (41.9)	134 (40)
Chicago	116 (13.4)	57 (17.5)	103 (14.2)	35 (14.6)	163 (14.1)	31 (12.6)	117 (15.6)
Miami	103 (14.2)	48 (16.6)	64 (11.2)	29 (15.1)	143 (14.7)	18 (7.1)*	83 (14.4)
San Diego	193 (41.2)	51 (30.4)	110 (34.6)	28 (18.5)**	230 (37.3)	44 (38.4)	108 (30)
Parental education, n (%)							
< High school	175 (28.3)	69 (36.3)	180 (47.2)**	90 (58.2)**	230 (29.2)	58 (46.0)*	226 (52.2)**
High school or equivalent	152 (31.8)	73 (30.6)	118 (28.6)	30 (18.9)*	221 (32.4)	37 (22.7)	115 (26.1)
> High school	227 (39.9)	78 (33.1)	95 (24.2)**	38 (23.0)**	289 (38.4)	48 (31.3)	101 (21.7)**
US-born parent/caregiver, n (%)[c]	103 (17.6)	50 (24.9)	64 (20.5)	43 (31.6)*	146 (19.2)	48 (40.4)**	66 (17.6)
Food assistance in previous year, n (%)[d]	417 (76.6)	188 (87.7)*	346 (87.8)**	144 (88.3)**	577 (79.3)	123 (84.3)	395 (89.0)**
Poverty-income ratio[a,e]	1.3 (0.8–2.3)	0.8 (0.5–1.3)**	0.8 (0.6–1.2)**	0.6 (0.3–0.9)**	1.2 (0.6–1.8)	1.0 (0.7–1.4)*	0.8 (0.5–1.2)**

The SI conversion factors from mg/dL to mmol/L are as follows: multiply FG values by 0.0555, TG values by 0.0113, and HDL-C values by 0.0259 Values are means or percentages unless otherwise specified. All analyses were weighted for survey design, and. sample sizes are unweighted.

[a] Median and interquartile ranges reported for variables with nonnormal distributions. Mann-Whitney U (Wilcoxon rank sum) was used to test median differences.

[b] MetS score for meeting each of the following criteria: abdominal adiposity (WC ≥ 90th age- and sex-specific percentiles), FG (≥ 100 mg/dL), TGs (≥ 150 mg/dL), HDL-C (≤ 40 mg/dL), SBP or DBP (≥ 90th age-, sex-, and height-specific percentiles).

[c] US-born includes Puerto Rico.

[d] Receipt of food assistance in the previous 12 months includes SNAP, WIC, or National School Lunch Program for free or reduced school meals.

[e] We calculated poverty–income ratio by first determining the median income for a given reported income range and dividing by the state- and year-specific (based on recruitment year of the study) federal poverty guidelines specific to family size and issued by the US Department of Health and Human Services.

*$P < .05$ and **$P < .01$ for comparisons between the indicated FS category and the high FS category of each FS measure.

several CMMs were less favorable with lower FS. For instance, the lowest household and child FS categories had the highest median levels of WC (in cm) and TGs (in mg/dL), and the lowest median levels of HDL-C (in mg/dL). The proportions of youth meeting each of the MetS criteria also tended to be highest among individuals in the lowest categories of FS. In terms of sociodemographic characteristics, lower FS showed lower parental education, a greater proportion of youth receiving any food assistance in the previous year, and lower

poverty income ratio, although there was little difference by age and sex.

Table 2 presents adjusted differences of MetS-relevant CMMs and MetS scores by household and child FS measures. For both FS measures, Hispanic/Latino youth in the lowest versus high FS category had significantly lower HDL-C (household: −3.17, 95% CI: −5.65 to −0.70; child: −1.81, 95% CI: −3.54 to −0.09). However, only the child FS measure was associated with other MetS-relevant CMMs. Compared with youth with high

child FS, individuals with low/very low child FS had greater FG (1.37, 95% CI: 0.08 to 2.65), TGs (8.68, 95% CI: 1.75 to 15.61), and MetS expected log counts (2.12, 95% CI: 0.02 to 0.45).

We found statistically significant interactions between each of the 2 FS measures and parental place of birth for TGs only (P interactions: household = 0.05 and child = 0.008). To ease interpretation, Fig 1 shows multivariable TG mean differences by household and child FS stratified by parental place of birth (see

TABLE 2 Adjusted Back-Transformed Geometric Mean MetS CMM Differences and MetS Expected Log Count Differences by Household and Child FS Status in the SOL Youth (n = 1325)

Cardiometabolic Markers	Household Food Security Status			Child Food Security Status	
	Marginal (n = 220)	Low (n = 393)	Very Low (n = 158)	Marginal (n = 143)	Low/Very Low (n = 442)
WC (cm)[a]	−2.28 (−4.89 to 0.32)	−0.59 (−2.57 to 1.38)	1.49 (−1.02 to 4.01)	−1.24 (−3.67 to 1.20)	0.63 (−1.12 to 2.37)
FG (mg/dL)[a]	0.47 (−1.05 to 1.99)	0.81 (−0.69 to 2.32)	1.22 (−0.42 to 2.85)	−0.13 (−2.17 to 1.91)	1.37 (0.08 to 2.65)
TGs (mg/dL)[a]	1.85 (−9.82 to 13.51)	6.35 (−0.99 to 13.68)	10.26 (−0.15 to 20.67)	2.10 (−8.60 to 12.81)	8.68 (1.75 to 15.61)
HDL-C (mg/dL)[a]	−0.93 (−3.16 to 1.31)	−0.93 (−3.02 to 1.16)	−3.17 (−5.65 to −0.70)	−0.63 (−3.07 to 1.80)	−1.81 (−3.54 to −0.09)
SBP (mm Hg)[a]	−1.06 (−2.78 to 0.67)	0.29 (−1.52 to 2.11)	2.06 (−0.03 to 4.16)	0.63 (−1.65 to 2.90)	0.92 (−0.74 to 2.58)
DBP (mm Hg)[a]	0.46 (−0.90 to 1.83)	0.42 (−0.92 to 1.76)	1.13 (−0.58 to 2.84)	1.23 (−0.73 to 3.19)	0.32 (−0.90 to 1.53)
MetS risk count (score)[b]	−0.42 (−0.47 to 0.30)	0.07 (−0.22 to 0.24)	1.88 (−0.01 to 0.59)	−0.35 (−0.33 to 0.23)	2.12 (0.02 to 0.45)

The SI conversion factors from mg/dL to mmol/L are as follows: multiply FG values by 0.0555, TG values by 0.0113, and HDL-C values by 0.0259. Estimates are back-transformed geometric mean differences (95% CIs) and expected log count differences (for MetS score) comparing lowest to high FS status categories by household and child measures. Data are from interviewer-administered questionnaires and clinical examinations. All models were weighted for survey design and adjusted for age (years), sex (male or female), site (Bronx, NY, Chicago, IL, San Diego, CA, and Miami, FL), parental place of birth (US-born, including Puerto Rico and foreign-born), parental education (less than high school, high school or equivalent, and more than high school), and poverty-income ratio (continuous).

[a] Geometric mean estimates were back-transformed to their original scales and modeled by using linear regression.

[b] MetS score for meeting the following criteria: abdominal adiposity (WC ≥ 90th age- and sex-specific percentiles), FG (≥ 100 mg/dL), TGs (≥ 150 mg/dL), HDL-C (≤ 40 mg/dL), SBP or DBP (≥ 90th age-, sex-, and height-specific percentiles); modeled using Poisson regression.

Supplemental Table 3 for full findings). Among youth with foreign-born parents or caregivers, being in the lowest FS category was associated with significantly greater levels of TGs (household FS: 15.56, 95% CI: 1.63 to 29.48, child FS: 10.83 95% CI: 2.55 to 19.11) compared with the highest FS category. Findings were null among youth with US-born parents or caregivers. There were also no significant interactions for the remaining MetS-relevant CMMs.

We also found statistically significant interactions between each of the 2 FS measures and receipt of any food assistance in the previous year in models of TG (P interactions: household FS = 0.03 and child FS = 0.005) and HDL-C (P interactions: household FS = 0.01 and child FS = 0.04) (Fig 2; see Supplemental Table 4 for full findings). Only among participants whose families did not receive any food assistance in the previous year, being in the lowest versus high FS categories was associated with significantly greater TGs (household FS: 36.12, 95% CI: 14.23 to 58.01; child FS: 18.79, 95% CI: 5.40 to 32.17), and significantly lower

HDL-C (household FS: −10.17, 95% CI: −16.64 to −3.71; child FS: −6.99, 95% CI: −12.19 to −1.79). We also found statistically significant interactions for the child FS measure (but not household FS) in models of WC (P interaction = 0.008) and MetS score (P interaction = 0.009). Compared with youth with high child FS, those in the lowest child FS category had significantly higher WC (4.92, 95% CI: 0.15 to 9.69) and a higher MetS expected log count (0.75, 95% CI: 0.31 to 1.19), but only among youth whose families did not receive any food assistance in the previous year.

DISCUSSION

Our study is among the first to document adverse associations between household and child FS measures with a MetS score variable and several MetS-relevant CMMs among US Hispanic/Latino youth. In addition, findings suggest that the health implications of FI may be greater among youth with foreign-born parents or caregivers and whose families did not receive any food assistance in the previous year.

Unlike the current study, 2 studies using nationally representative data among adolescents found no associations between FS measures and relevant CMMs (FG, TGs, and HDL-C).[16,25] One reason for these discrepancies may have to do with the populations under study. Although Hispanic/Latino youth (mostly of Mexican origin) were included in these studies, they were aggregated with other racial or ethnic groups, potentially attenuating associations. Moreover, interactions with race or ethnicity and other important sociodemographic characteristics were not evaluated in these studies.

Relatedly, our findings suggest greater health implications of FI among Hispanic/Latino youth with foreign-born parents or caregivers and among those who did not receive any food assistance in the past year. The differential patterns by parental place of birth, in particular, are consistent with previous work related to mental health in HCHS/SOL Youth.[10] In these data, greater FI was associated with higher anxiety scores among youth with foreign-born parents or caregivers.[10] Meanwhile, compared

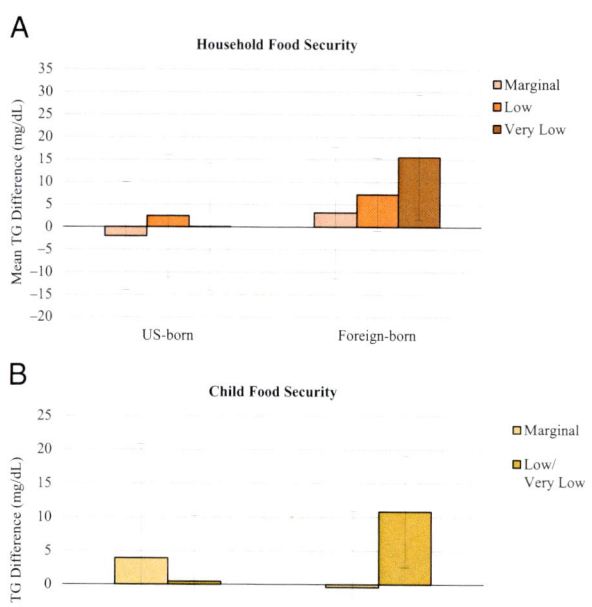

FIGURE 1

Adjusted-mean differences in TGs by (A) household and (B) child FS stratified by parental place of birth in the SOL Youth (*n* = 1325). Estimates are back-transformed adjusted-geometric-mean TG differences (95% CIs) from linear regression models comparing lower versus high household and child FS measures stratified by parental place of birth (US-born, including Puerto Rico and foreign-born). CIs not including zero indicate significant pairwise comparisons between lower FS and high FS (referent; not shown) at *P* < .05. Data are from interviewer-administered questionnaires and clinical examinations. Household FS: high (*n* = 554), marginal (*n* = 220), low (*n* = 393), very low (*n* = 158), child FS: high (*n* = 740), marginal (*n* = 143), low/very low (*n* = 442). All models were weighted for survey design and adjusted for participant's age (years), sex (male or female), site (Bronx, NY, Chicago, IL, San Diego, CA, and Miami, FL), parental education (less than high school, high school or equivalent, and more than high school), parental place of birth (US-born, including Puerto Rico and foreign-born), poverty–income ratio (continuous), and receipt of any food assistance in the previous year (yes or no). *P* interactions: household FS = 0.06 and child FS = 0.010.

with those with US-born parents or caregivers, youth with foreign-born parents or caregivers have been shown to experience several acculturative (eg, adjusting to US norms or family dynamics) and economic (eg, low-income status or parental unemployment) chronic stressors (in addition to FI),[30,31] which contribute to poor mental and physical health outcomes. Another study found similar findings for self-reported health status among youth with foreign-born parents or caregivers, showing a lower

probability of reporting very good health among children and adolescents of immigrants facing FI compared with their food-secure peers.[31] The combination of these factors may amplify the adverse health consequences of FI for youth in these families. These chronic stressors may also undermine the health-protective role of sociocultural (eg, strong family and social support networks, optimism, and resilience) and behavioral (eg, healthy eating) factors[30,46] that may otherwise contribute to a health

advantage among Hispanic/Latino youth with foreign-born parents/caregivers.

Youth with foreign-born parents or caregivers may also be living with members of the household who are undocumented and, therefore, ineligible for government food assistance (eg, SNAP), further worsening the impact of FI.[50,51] In our study, low levels of FS were adversely associated with MetS score, WC, TGs, and HDL-C to a greater extent for youth whose families did not receive any food assistance in the previous year than among those that did. However, even after adjusting for food assistance in interaction models with parental place of birth, the same adverse associations remained for youth with foreign-born parents or caregivers. Future research should more directly evaluate whether expansion and increased uptake of food assistance programs and other interventions among immigrant families can limit the adverse health consequences of FI in Hispanic/Latino youth.

Our study evaluated associations with 2 different FS measures and indicated that a child versus a household FS measure may better capture the role of FI in youth's health. For instance, although household and child FS status detected associations with HDL-C, only the child FS measure also detected associations with FG, TGs, and the MetS score. This could be because a child measure may be more sensitive for detecting FI in this population compared with a broader household measure. In a context of low household-level FS, older family members may prioritize food resources for younger family members, protecting them against some of the negative health consequences.[2,37] In contrast, a child

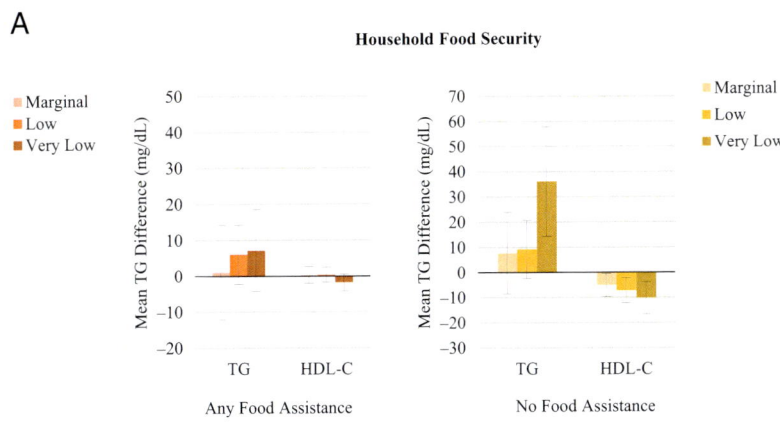

A

Household Food Security

Any Food Assistance

No Food Assistance

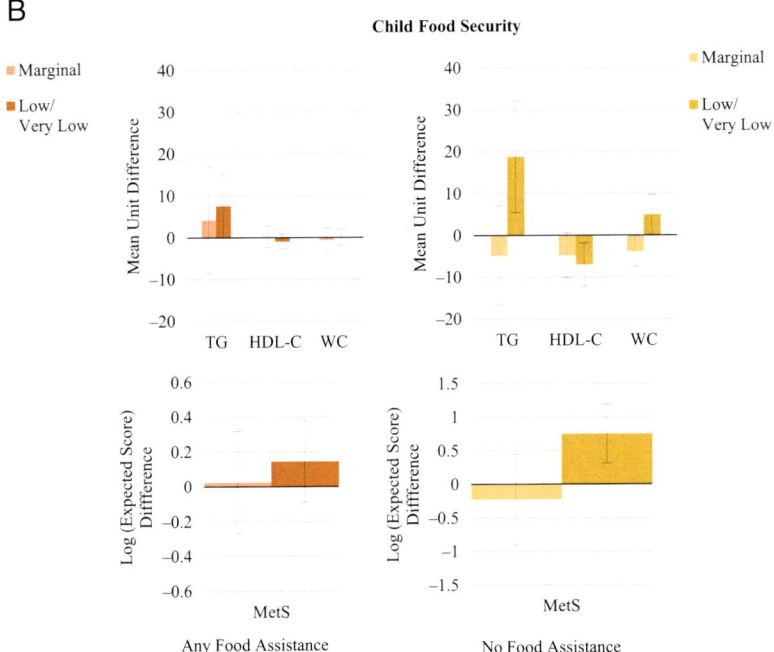

B

Child Food Security

Any Food Assistance

No Food Assistance

FIGURE 2

Adjusted-mean differences in MetS-relevant CMMs by (A) household and (B) child FS stratified by receipt of any food assistance in the previous year in the SOLYouth (n = 1325). Estimates are back-transformed adjusted geometric mean unit differences (95% CIs) comparing lower-versus-high FS by household and child FS measures stratified by receipt of any food assistance (SNAP, WIC, or National School Lunch Program for free/reduced school meals) in the previous year. CIs not including zero indicate significant pairwise comparisons between lower FS and high FS (referent; not shown) at P < .05. Data are from interviewer-administered questionnaires and clinical examinations. Household FS: high (n = 554), marginal (n = 220), low (n = 393), very low (n = 158), child FS: high (n = 740), marginal (n = 143), low/very low (n = 442). All models were weighted for survey design and adjusted for participant's age (years), sex (male or female), site (Bronx, NY, Chicago, IL, San Diego, CA, and Miami, FL), parental education (less than high school, high school or equivalent, and more than high school), parental place of birth (US-born, including Puerto Rico and foreign-born), and poverty–income ratio (continuous). TGs (in mg/dL), WC (in cm), and HDL-C (in mg/dL) were modeled by using linear regression whereas MetS score was modeled by using Poisson regression. MetS was calculated by summing the number of counts for each of the following criteria: abdominal adiposity (WC ≥ 90th age- and sex-specific percentiles), FG (≥ 100 mg/dL), TGs (≥ 150 mg/dL), HDL-C (≤ 40 mg/dL), SBP or DBP (≥ 90th age-, sex-, and height-specific percentiles). Household FS P interactions: TG = 0.04, HDL-C = 0.01, child FS P interactions: TG = 0.004, WC = 0.008, HDL-C = 0.03, MetS score = 0.009.

FS measure is more likely to capture food availability for these specific household members.

Taken together, these findings have potential implications for health care providers and nutrition-based policies. Although CMM differences by child FS status do not reflect disparities in clinical disease, this pattern may contribute to a disproportionate burden of cardiometabolic complications among the most food-insecure Hispanic/Latino youth as they transition to adulthood. Consequently, health care providers should consider early screening for FI using the child FS measure to identify youth who may benefit from additional resources. Relatedly, policies targeting Hispanic/Latino families that facilitate uptake into food assistance programs are needed. In our study, FI was adversely associated with CMMs particularly among youth from families that did not receive any food assistance. Improving access and expanding eligibility to such programs may help curtail the potential negative health consequences of FI in this population.

This study has some strengths and limitations. The diverse sample of US Hispanic/Latino youth in our study increases the generalizability of our findings to heritage groups beyond Hispanics/Latinos of Mexican origin, because most previous studies that included Hispanics/Latinos primarily focused on this population. Additionally, the large sample size allowed us to test effect modification to identify groups within this population that may be facing greater health implications from FI. Given the cross-sectional nature of our data, however, we could not infer causality, substantiating the need for longitudinal studies and better causal approaches to directly evaluate the health implications of low FS. Our findings may have also obscured important differences by country of origin among youth with foreign-born parents. Our power was limited to evaluate these differences, but future research should consider the role that these social and cultural factors may play in terms of the associations we reported. Lastly, we did not adjust for multiple comparisons, which could have inflated the likelihood of observing false positives (type I error). Most multiple comparison adjustment methods, however, assume independence among dependent variables.[52] In our study, the dependent variables were biologically related. Employing an adjustment method that ignores these correlations may lead to overconservative adjustments, increasing the probability of false negative findings.[52] Nevertheless, because findings were more consistent for the child-versus-household FS measure, the statistically significant estimate for household FS and HDL-C should be interpreted with caution.

CONCLUSIONS

Our results suggest that Hispanic/Latino youth with severe FI (low/very low FS) have worse cardiometabolic profiles compared with their food-secure counterparts. These findings argue for exploring interventions to address FI among Hispanic/Latino youth, a fast-growing segment of the US population at high risk of cardiometabolic complications. Given the increase in FI that resulted from the coronavirus disease 2019 pandemic, especially for Hispanic/Latino immigrant families,[53] these findings may also foreshadow concerning trends for the health and well-being of Hispanic/Latino youth.

ABBREVIATIONS

CI: confidence interval
CMMs: cardiometabolic markers
DBP: diastolic blood pressure
FG: fasting plasma glucose
FI: food insecurity
FS: food security
HCHS/SOL: Hispanic Community Health Survey/Study of Latinos
HDL-C: high-density lipoprotein cholesterol
IR: insulin resistance
MetS: metabolic syndrome
SBP: systolic blood pressure
SNAP: supplemental nutrition assistance program
SOL Youth: Hispanic Community Children's Health Study/Study of Latino Youth
TGs: triglycerides
WC: waist circumference
WIC: Women, Infants, and Children

PEDIATRICS (ISSN Numbers: Print, 0031-4005; Online, 1098-4275).

Address correspondence to Sandra S. Albrecht, PhD, Department of Epidemiology, Columbia University Mailman School of Public Health, 722 West 168th St, New York, NY 10032. E-mail: ssa2018@cumc.columbia.edu

PEDIATRICS (ISSN Numbers: Print, 0031-4005; Online, 1098-4275).

FUNDING: Funding for the Hispanic Community Children's Health Study/Study of Latino Youth was supported by Grant R01HL102130 from the National Heart, Lung, and Blood Institute (NHLBI). The children and adolescents in the Study of Latino Youth are drawn from the study of adults, The Hispanic Community Children's Health Study/Study of Latinos, which was supported by contracts from the NHLBI to the University of North Carolina (N01-HC65233), University of Miami (N01-HC65234), Albert Einstein College of Medicine (N01-HC65235), Northwestern University (N01-HC65236), and San Diego State University (N01-HC65237). The following Institutes/Centers/Offices contributed to the HCHS/SOL through a transfer of funds to NHLBI: National Center on Minority Health and Health Disparities, the National Institute of Deafness and Other Communications Disorders, the National Institute of Dental and Craniofacial Research, the National Institute of Diabetes and Digestive and Kidney Diseases, the National Institute of Neurologic Disorders and Stroke, and the Office of Dietary Supplements. Additional support was provided by the Life Course Methodology Core at Albert Einstein College of Medicine and the New York Regional Center for Diabetes Translation Research (DK111022- 8786 and DK111022) through funds from the National Institute of Diabetes and Digestive and Kidney Diseases. Support for this study was provided by the NHLBI Institute Global Cardiometabolic Disease Training Grant (1T32HL129969-01A1), the National Institute of Diabetes and Digestive and Kidney Diseases (K01DK107791), and from the Population Research Infrastructure Program (R24 HD050924) awarded to the Carolina Population Center at the University of North Carolina at Chapel Hill by the Eunice Kennedy Shriver National Institute of Child Health and Human Development. Funded by the National Institutes of Health (NIH).

CONFLICT OF INTEREST DISCLOSURES: The authors have indicated they have no potential conflicts of interest relevant to this article to disclose.

REFERENCES

1. Rodríguez LA, Mundo-Rosas V, Méndez-Gómez-Humarán I, Pérez-Escamilla R, Shamah-Levy T. Dietary quality and household food insecurity among Mexican children and adolescents. *Matern Child Nutr.* 2017;13(4):e12372

2. Bickel G, Nord M, Price C, Hamilton W, Cook J. *Guide to Measuring Household Food Security, Revised 2000.* Alexandria, VA: US Department of Agriculture, Food and Nutrition Service; 2000

3. Kaur J, Lamb MM, Ogden CL. The association between food insecurity and obesity in children-the national health and

nutrition examination survey. *J Acad Nutr Diet.* 2015;115(5):751–758

4. Laraia BA. Food insecurity and chronic disease. *Adv Nutr.* 2013;4(2):203–212

5. Gundersen C, Lohman BJ, Garasky S, Stewart S, Eisenmann J. Food security, maternal stressors, and overweight among low-income US children: results from the National Health and Nutrition Examination Survey (1999-2002). *Pediatrics.* 2008;122(3):e529–e540

6. Thomas MMC, Miller DP, Morrissey TW. Food insecurity and child health. *Pediatrics.* 2019;144(4):e20190397

7. Coleman-Jensen A, Rabbit MP, Gregory CA, Singh A.; United States Department of Agriculture, Economic Research Service. Household food security in the United States in 2019. *Econ Res Serv.* 2020;ERR-275:1–39

8. Coleman-Jensen A, Rabbit MP, Gregory CA, Singh A.; United States Department of Agriculture, Economic Research Service. Household food security in the United States in 2017. *Econ Res Serv.* 2017;ERR-256:1–36

9. Nord M, Andrews M, Carlson S.; United States Department of Agriculture, Economic Research Service. Household food security in the United States, 2008. *Econ Res Serv.* 2009;ERR-83:1–58

10. Potochnick S, Perreira KM, Bravin JI, et al. Food insecurity among Hispanic/Latino youth: who is at risk and what are the health correlates? *J Adolesc Health.* 2019;64(5):631–639

11. Holben DH, Pheley AM. Diabetes risk and obesity in food-insecure households in rural Appalachian Ohio. *Prev Chronic Dis.* 2006;3(3):A82

12. Fitzgerald N, Hromi-Fiedler A, Segura-Pérez S, Pérez-Escamilla R. Food insecurity is related to increased risk of type 2 diabetes among Latinas. *Ethn Dis.* 2011;21(3):328–334

13. Gucciardi E, Vogt JA, DeMelo M, Stewart DE. Exploration of the relationship between household food insecurity and diabetes in Canada. *Diabetes Care.* 2009;32(12):2218–2224

14. Seligman HK, Laraia BA, Kushel MB. Food insecurity is associated with chronic disease among low-income NHANES participants. *J Nutr.* 2010;140(2):304–310

15. Seligman HK, Bindman AB, Vittinghoff E, Kanaya AM, Kushel MB. Food insecurity is associated with diabetes mellitus: results from the National Health Examination and Nutrition Examination Survey (NHANES) 1999-2002. *J Gen Intern Med.* 2007;22(7):1018–1023

16. Parker ED, Widome R, Nettleton JA, Pereira MA. Food security and metabolic syndrome in U.S. adults and adolescents: findings from the National Health and Nutrition Examination Survey, 1999-2006. *Ann Epidemiol.* 2010;20(5):364–370

17. Weigel MM, Armijos RX. Food insecurity, cardiometabolic health, and health care in U.S.-Mexico border immigrant adults: an exploratory study. *J Immigr Minor Health.* 2019;21(5):1085–1094

18. Pan L, Sherry B, Njai R, Blanck HM. Food insecurity is associated with obesity among US adults in 12 states. *J Acad Nutr Diet.* 2012;112(9):1403–1409

19. Nagata JM, Palar K, Gooding HC, Garber AK, Bibbins-Domingo K, Weiser SD. Food insecurity and chronic disease in US young adults: findings from the National Longitudinal Study of Adolescent to Adult Health. *J Gen Intern Med.* 2019;34(12):2756–2762

20. Hernandez DC, Reesor LM, Murillo R. Food insecurity and adult overweight/obesity: gender and race/ethnic disparities. *Appetite.* 2017;117:373–378

21. Golovaty I, Tien PC, Price JC, Sheira L, Seligman H, Weiser SD. Food insecurity may be an independent risk factor associated with nonalcoholic fatty liver disease among low-income adults in the United States. *J Nutr.* 2020;150(1):91–98

22. Kaiser LL, Melgar-Quiñonez HR, Lamp CL, Johns MC, Sutherlin JM, Harwood JO. Food security and nutritional outcomes of preschool-age Mexican-American children. *J Am Diet Assoc.* 2002;102(7):924–929

23. Papas MA, Trabulsi JC, Dahl A, Dominick G. Food insecurity increases the odds of obesity among young Hispanic children. *J Immigr Minor Health.* 2016;18(5):1046–1052

24. Jiménez-Cruz A, Bacardí Gascón M. Prevalence of overweight and hunger among Mexican children from migrant parents. *Nutr Hosp.* 2007;22(1):85–88

25. Holben DH, Taylor CA. Food insecurity and its association with central obesity and other markers of metabolic syndrome among persons aged 12 to 18 years in the United States. *J Am Osteopath Assoc.* 2015;115(9):536–543

26. Aschbacher K, O'Donovan A, Wolkowitz OM, Dhabhar FS, Su Y, Epel E. Good stress, bad stress and oxidative stress: insights from anticipatory cortisol reactivity. *Psychoneuroendocrinology.* 2013;38(9):1698–1708

27. Evans JL, Maddux BA, Goldfine ID. The molecular basis for oxidative stress-induced insulin resistance. *Antioxid Redox Signal.* 2005;7(7-8):1040–1052

28. Reina SA, Llabre MM, Vidot DC, et al. Metabolic syndrome in Hispanic youth: results from the Hispanic Community Children's Health Study/Study of Latino Youth. *Metab Syndr Relat Disord.* 2017;15(8):400–406

29. Walker SE, Gurka MJ, Oliver MN, Johns DW, DeBoer MD. Racial/ethnic discrepancies in the metabolic syndrome begin in childhood and persist after adjustment for environmental factors. *Nutr Metab Cardiovasc Dis.* 2012;22(2):141–148

30. Perreira KM, Ornelas IJ. The physical and psychological well-being of immigrant children. *Future Child.* 2011;21(1):195–218

31. Huang Y, Potochnick S, Heflin CM. Household food insecurity and early childhood health and cognitive development among children of immigrants. *J Fam Issues.* 2017;39(6):1465–1497

32. Nguyen BT, Shuval K, Bertmann F, Yaroch AL. The Supplemental Nutrition Assistance Program, food insecurity, dietary quality, and obesity among U.S. adults. *Am J Public Health.* 2015;105(7):1453–1459

33. Isasi CR, Carnethon MR, Ayala GX, et al. The Hispanic community children's health study/study of Latino youth (SOL youth): design, objectives, and procedures. *Ann Epidemiol.* 2014;24(1):29–35

34. Ayala GX, Carnethon M, Arredondo E, et al. Theoretical foundations of the Study of Latino (SOL) Youth: implications for obesity and cardiometabolic risk. *Ann Epidemiol.* 2014;24(1):36–43

35. Sorlie PD, Avilés-Santa LM, Wassertheil-Smoller S, et al. Design and

implementation of the Hispanic community health study/study of Latinos. *Ann Epidemiol.* 2010;20(8):629–641

36. Lavange LM, Kalsbeek WD, Sorlie PD, et al. Sample design and cohort selection in the Hispanic Community Health Study/Study of Latinos. *Ann Epidemiol.* 2010;20(8):642–649

37. Casey PH, Simpson PM, Gossett JM, et al. The association of child and household food insecurity with childhood overweight status. *Pediatrics.* 2006;118(5):e1406–e1413

38. Esposito K, Kastorini C-M, Panagiotakos DB, Giugliano D. Prevention of type 2 diabetes by dietary patterns: a systematic review of prospective studies and meta-analysis. *Metab Syndr Relat Disord.* 2010;8(6):471–476

39. Hoffmann K, Schulze MB, Schienkiewitz A, Nöthlings U, Boeing H. Application of a new statistical method to derive dietary patterns in nutritional epidemiology. *Am J Epidemiol.* 2004;159(10): 935–944

40. Grundy SM, Brewer HB Jr, Cleeman JI, Smith SC Jr, Lenfant C; American Heart Association; National Heart, Lung, and Blood Institute. Definition of metabolic syndrome: report of the National Heart, Lung, and Blood Institute/American Heart Association conference on scientific issues related to definition. *Circulation.* 2004;109(3):433–438

41. Magge SN, Goodman E, Armstrong SC; Committee on Nutrition; Section on Endocrinology; Section on Obesity. The metabolic syndrome in children and adolescents: shifting the focus to cardiometabolic risk factor clustering. *Pediatrics.* 2017;140(2):e20171603

42. Eisenmann JC. On the use of a continuous metabolic syndrome score in pediatric research. *Cardiovasc Diabetol.* 2008;7(1):17

43. Zimmet P, Alberti KG, Kaufman F, et al; IDF Consensus Group. The metabolic syndrome in children and adolescents - an IDF consensus report. *Pediatr Diabetes.* 2007;8(5):299–306

44. Fryar CD, Gu Q, Ogden CL; US Department of Health and Human Services, Centers for Disease Control and Prevention. Anthropometric reference data for children and adults: United States, 2011-2014. *Vital Health Stat.* 2016;3(39): 1–38

45. Cook S, Weitzman M, Auinger P, Nguyen M, Dietz WH. Prevalence of a metabolic syndrome phenotype in adolescents: findings from the third National Health and Nutrition Examination Survey, 1988-1994. *Arch Pediatr Adolesc Med.* 2003; 157(8):821–827

46. Dave JM, Evans AE, Saunders RP, Watkins KW, Pfeiffer KA. Associations among food insecurity, acculturation, demographic factors, and fruit and vegetable intake at home in Hispanic children. *J Am Diet Assoc.* 2009;109(4): 697–701

47. US Department of Health and Human Services. 2013 poverty guidelines. Available at: https://aspe.hhs.gov/ 2013-poverty-guidelines. Accessed August 21, 2013

48. US Department of Health and Human Services, Centers for Disease Control and Prevention. National health and nutrition examination survey: 2015-2016 data documentation, codebook, and frequencies. Available at: https://wwwn. cdc.gov/Nchs/Nhanes/2015-2016/ DEMO_I.htm. Accessed May 2, 2020

49. Uberti LJ. Stata tip 128: marginal effects in log-transformed models: a trade application. *Stata J.* 2017;17(3): 774–778

50. Chilton M, Black MM, Berkowitz C, et al. Food insecurity and risk of poor health among US-born children of immigrants. *Am J Public Health.* 2009;99(3):556–562

51. Van Hook J, Balistreri KS. Ineligible parents, eligible children: food stamps receipt, allotments, and food insecurity among children of immigrants. *Soc Sci Res.* 2006;35(1):228–251

52. Pocock SJ, Geller NL, Tsiatis AA. The analysis of multiple endpoints in clinical trials. *Biometrics.* 1987;43(3): 487–498

53. Waxman E, Gupta P, Karpman M; Urban Institute. More than one in six adults were food insecure two months into the COVID-19 recession: findings from the May 14-27 coronavirus tracking survey. Available at: https://www.urban.org/ sites/default/files/publication/102579/ more-than-one-in-six-adults-were-food-insecure-two-months-into-the-covid-19-recession.pdf. Accessed October 13, 2020.

Pediatric Formulas: An Update

Aamer Imdad, MPH,* Rida Sherwani, MBBS,† Kellie Wall, RD‡

*Division of Gastroenterology, Hepatology, Pancreatology, and Nutrition, Department of Pediatrics, Stead Family Children's Hospital, University of Iowa, Iowa City, IA

†Department of Pediatrics, State University of New York Upstate Medical University, Syracuse, NY

‡Division of Pediatric Gastroenterology, Hepatology, and Nutrition, Department of Pediatrics, State University of New York Upstate Medical University, Syracuse, NY

PRACTICE GAP

With the infant formula recall in 2022 and the resulting infant formula shortage, a new demand has evolved for alternative formulas, including infant formulas imported from Europe. There are recent developments in young child formula, including commercially made, food-based blenderized formulas and an increased interest in using plant-based milk during childhood. Pediatricians need to keep up to date with these changes to educate parents on infant and young child feeding.

OBJECTIVES *After completing this article, readers should be able to:*

1. Discuss the recent shortage of infant formulas in the United States and the availability of European formulas.

2. Discuss the older infant–young child formulas and pediatric formulas.

3. Discuss nonformula, plant-based (milk) drinks.

ABSTRACT

The recent shortage of pediatric formulas in the United States, caused by supply chain issues and contamination of formula products in 1 of the major manufacturing plants, led many families to seek an alternate formula for their children. The Food and Drug Administration (FDA) allowed import of infant formulas from selected European and non-European countries. The European infant formulas differ from those produced in the United States regarding the primary source of the formula, age category, mixing instructions, labeling requirements, and formula composition in terms of macronutrients and micronutrients. Although most European infant formulas are nutritionally adequate, pediatricians and families need to be aware of the differences between the European and FDA-regulated formulas for their correct use and preparation for infants and young children. Supplementation with cow milk is recommended for children beyond infancy, and older infant formulas are not recommended for otherwise healthy growing children. However, pediatric formulas have been used to support the nutrition needs of

AUTHOR DISCLOSURE: Drs Imdad, Sherwani, and Wall have disclosed no financial relationships relevant to this article. Even though the authors discuss formula feeding in infants and young children, we fully endorse the position of the American Academy of Pediatrics and the World Health Organization on breastfeeding and agree that human milk is the most optimal nutrition for infants. The names of some of the commercial products have been used in one of the tables. We do not endorse any specific formula for any infant or young child; the names used are for education.

ABBREVIATIONS

AAP	American Academy of Pediatrics
CDC	Centers for Disease Control and Prevention
EFSA	European Food Safety Authority
FDA	Food and Drug Administration
NASPGHAN	North American Society for Gastroenterology, Hepatology and Nutrition
OIYCF	older infant and young child formula

children with feeding difficulties, especially those dependent on tube feeding and with certain medical conditions. The FDA does not regulate the production of pediatric formulas beyond infant formula, and significant variations exist in their composition. The pediatric formulas are available as polymeric (intact), hydrolyzed, elemental, or food-based blenderized formulas. The plant-based nonformula (milk) drinks are being used increasingly for children. These products might not be nutritionally complete and should be avoided in infants and children dependent on liquid nutrition.

INTRODUCTION

The American Academy of Pediatrics (AAP) recommends that infants be breastfed exclusively for approximately the first 6 months of life and that, subsequently, breastfeeding should be supplemented with complementary foods, and continued as long as mutually desired, for at least 2 years and beyond. (1) The 2022 Centers for Disease Control and Prevention (CDC) breastfeeding report showed that for infants born in 2019, approximately 83% were fed initially by breastfeeding, and at 6 months, only approximately 56% were breastfeeding, with approximately 25% breastfeeding exclusively. (2) Globally, approximately 37% of children aged 6 to 24 months do not receive human milk. However, the percentage of children not receiving human milk is approximately 18% in lower-income countries, 34% in lower middle-income countries, and 55% in upper middle-income countries. (3) The Dietary Guidelines for Americans state that nonbreastfed infants should be offered iron-fortified infant formula during the first year of life. (4) In 2017-2019, approximately 216 million kg of powdered infant formula was purchased from major stores in the United States. Approximately 94% of these formula purchases were cow milk–based, and the remaining were soy-based. Of the cow milk–based formulas, approximately 68% had intact protein, and the rest had protein content either partially hydrolyzed (27%) or extensively or completely hydrolyzed (5%). (5) The diversity of breastfeeding practices and formulas used globally and in the United States underscores the importance of understanding the composition of pediatric formulas and the associated safety and health implications. In 2021-2022, the United States experienced a major infant formula shortage due to supply chain issues exacerbated by a large-scale product recall because of possible bacterial contamination of some powdered formula by *Cronobacter sakazakii*.(6)(7) This review discusses the recent formula shortages in the United States and the use of alternate formulas from Europe. We also discuss the young child formulas and the plant-based, nonformula (milk) drinks. The composition of infant formulas has been discussed in another *Pediatrics in Review* article and is not discussed in detail herein. (8) Table 1 gives the definitions of the most frequently used terms concerning formula feeding.

INFANT FORMULA SHORTAGE

The Food and Drug Administration (FDA) and the CDC investigated 4 cases of *C sakazakii*–related illness reported by consumer complaints from September 20, 2021, to February 24, 2022. Four infants were admitted to the hospital, resulting in 2 deaths due to infection with *C sakazakii*.

C sakazakii is a rod-shaped, gram-negative bacteria that can exist in the environment and survive in very dry conditions. (17) *C sakazakii* can cause sepsis/meningitis in very young infants, and infection may present as fever, poor feeding, fussiness, lethargy, and seizures. The diagnosis is confirmed on blood or cerebrospinal fluid culture (no special media is required for growth). The treatment is with broad-spectrum intravenous antibiotics that can be tailored based on sensitivities from the bacterial culture. (17)(18)

All 4 cases of *C sakazakii*–related illness were traced back to formula produced in a manufacturing plant from Abbott Nutrition's Sturgis, Michigan, facility, resulting in a national recall of the products produced in that plant. (6) This recall accounted for approximately 20% of US formula production. Apart from the large-scale recall, other factors that contributed to the infant formula shortage had to do with supply chain issues, including the strict regulation of imports and labor shortages during the COVID-19 pandemic. It is also important to note the significance of the market concentration of the manufacturing capacity for infant formulas: just 4 companies manufacture 99% of the formula in the United States. A multipronged approach might be required to prevent future infant formula shortages with a combined effort from governments and nutrition-related organizations and input from families and providers. (19)(20)

The risk of contamination with *C sakazakii* is only with powdered formula and not with premade, liquid, or concentrate formula. To minimize the risk of contamination, the FDA enforces quality control for the infant formula produced in the United States through regulatory and engineering protocols to minimize the risk of contamination at the production site. However, contamination of powdered formula with *C sakazakii* may occur not only during

Table 1. Terms and Definitions

TERM	DEFINITION (COMMENTS)
Infant formula	"A food which purports to be or is represented for special dietary use solely as a food for infants by reason of its simulation of human milk or its suitability as a complete or partial substitute for human milk." (9)
Older infant–young child formulas	Milk-based drinks or plant protein–based formulas intended to partially satisfy the requirements of children aged 1–3 y. The terms *follow on* or *follow up* or *weaning formulas* or *toddler milk, growing-up milk, or formula for young children toddler's milk, growing up milk, or formula for young children* are synonyms to older infant and young child formula. (10)(11)
Medical food	Medical foods are specially formulated and processed products that provide partial or sole-source nutrition, may be consumed orally or via feeding tube, and provide nutrition for an individual who, due to a chronic medical condition, has impairments in ability to "ingest, digest, absorb, or metabolize ordinary foodstuffs or certain nutrients, or who has other special medically determined nutrient requirements, the dietary management of which cannot be achieved by the modification of the normal diet alone." (12)
Specialty formula	"Specialty formulas are intended for use by an infant with an inborn error of metabolism, low birth weight, or who otherwise has an unusual medical or dietary problem." The formulas meant for inborn errors of metabolism, renal failure, and cow milk allergy are considered specialized formulas. (9)(13)
Hydrolyzed formula	Hydrolyzed formulas contain hydrolyzed proteins, which may include a mixture of amino acids, peptides, polypeptides, and denatured proteins obtained by chemical, enzymatic, and thermal hydrolysis of proteins.
Partial, extensive, and completely hydrolyzed	Partially hydrolyzed formulas contain ~30% of total protein that is hydrolyzed, extensively hydrolyzed have 90%, and completely hydrolyzed have 100% of the proteins hydrolyzed. The completely hydrolyzed formulas are also called amino acid–based formulas. (13)(14)
Hypoallergenic formula	Extensively hydrolyzed and completely hydrolyzed infant formulas are considered hypoallergenic formulas. (13)(15)
Enteral nutrition	Provision of nutrients to the gastrointestinal tract, bypassing the oral cavity, via a tube, catheter, or stoma. (14)(16)
Blenderized formula	Commercially produced or homemade formulas, administered via feeding tube, composed of foods and liquids blended to a thin consistency. (14)
Dietary reference intakes	Set of nutrient-based reference values used to assess nutrient intake of healthy people. (14)

formula production but also once the formula containers are opened and exposed. Hence, health-care workers must support and educate caregivers about contamination risks with *C sakazakii* and other microorganisms during formula preparation. (21)(22) Table 2 summarizes recommendations from the FDA about the safe preparation of powdered formula.

The European Formulas

European formulas were in use in the United States before the infant formula shortage; however, most of these were imported by families via purchase on the Internet. (15)(23)(24) After the formula shortage, the FDA adopted an enforcement discretion to increase infant formula supplies in the United States. (7) Enforcement discretion by the FDA is issued in selective situations in which the FDA can use its discretion to enforce certain regulations and may choose not to enforce certain regulations if it believes that the risk to public health is low or if it believes that the benefits of the product outweigh the risks. In the case of formula shortages in the United States, exercise of this discretion meant that certain foreign-produced infant formulas could be exempted from particular statutory and regulatory requirements set by the FDA for infant formula production. (25) The FDA regulations for infant formula produced in the United States include multiple requirements to ensure safety

Table 2. Summary of Recommendations from the Food and Drug Administration (FDA) about the Safe Preparation of Pediatric Formula (9)

- Provider should wash hands before preparing the bottles or feeding the baby. The workspace should be cleaned and sanitized.
- Bottles should be cleaned and sanitized.
- If warming the bottle, provider should not use a microwave. Microwaves heat unevenly and risk burning the baby's mouth and throat. To warm the bottle, the bottle should be placed under running warm water.
- If using powdered infant formula, water should be from a safe source.
- Prepared infant formula should not be left at room temperature for more than 2 h.

and suitability of infant formula. The FDA requires that a formula company must present evidence that an infant formula provides adequate nutrition for health and adequate growth for infants. An infant formula regulated by the FDA must meet set, minimum amounts for 30 nutrients (including macronutrients and micronutrients). The FDA oversees the manufacturing practices of infant formula with controls to prevent adulteration and requires an annual audit of the production site. The labeling requirement by the FDA stipulates that the label must include directions for preparation and use, a pictogram showing the major steps for preparing infant formula, and a "use by" date. As part of the enforcement discretion, the FDA sought information from interested foreign companies on the listing of and amount of all nutrients and other ingredients, a copy of the product label and description of packaging, current or anticipated inventory of the formula, microbiological testing results, and facility inspection history. The FDA used this information to consider on a case-by-case basis whether to exercise enforcement discretion and approve formula imports from companies in Europe, Australia, New Zealand, and Mexico. (9)(26)

Although non-European companies were allowed to export formula to the United States, because most infant formulas were from Europe we now discuss the difference between regulations by the FDA for infant formulas and regulations by the European Food Safety Authority (EFSA) for European infant formulas. (9)(27) Table 3 summarizes the main differences between EFSA- and FDA-regulated infant formulas. The key differences include the primary source of the formula, age category, mixing instructions, labeling requirements, description of iron-fortified formula, and composition of formula in terms of macronutrients and micronutrients. (9)(27) European formulas include a goat milk–based formula option not available in the United States; age category, with the choice of different formula for the first 6 months called infant formula and a follow-on formula for 6 to 12 months available in Europe but not in the United States. Most European formulas are prepared with a 1:1 ratio (with 1 scoop of formula in 1 oz of water), and most FDA-regulated formulas are prepared with a 1:2 ratio (with 1 scoop of formula in 2 oz of water). This oversight of ratio differences could result in making a diluted or concentrated formula, leading to electrolyte imbalances, seizures, and potential death with long-term use. The FDA sets the degree of iron fortification at 1 mg of iron per 100 cal, and some European formulas may not be fortified to this level. (15) The amounts of macronutrients, vitamins, and minerals are fairly similar, with some differences, such as the mandatory addition of docosahexaenoic acid in European formulas but not in the United States, although many US formulas contain docosahexaenoic acid. (8)(27)(28) Most of the European formulas are safe in terms of risk of infections; however, cases of transmitted infection, including that of *Salmonella,* have been reported. (29) Overall, the European formulas cleared by the FDA can be safely used in the United States with necessary counseling to the families on the issues noted herein.

Approach to Formula Replacement in Case of Shortage

The shortage of infant formula in the United States left multiple families without formula, thereby requiring families to seek substitutes. In the event of a formula shortage, a pediatrician should be prepared to recommend an alternate formula to an affected family should the need arise. We suggest following the steps in the Fig to determine the best alternative for a given formula. The standard cow milk–based formula can be replaced with any other available brand from the United States or from Europe cleared by the FDA. (7) In the case of a specialized formula, additional considerations might be required. The definition of specialized formulas is available in Table 1, and a further description is available in a previous *Pediatrics in Review* article. (8) When using a specialized formula for treating cow milk allergy, an extensively hydrolyzed formula can be replaced with a similar alternative or with a completely hydrolyzed formula or amino acid–based formula. In the case of completely hydrolyzed formula, a similar alternative might be required unless the infant is approximately 1 year of age, when a significant proportion of infants outgrow cow milk allergy. If a soy-based formula is used to treat cow milk allergy, it could be replaced with an alternate soy-based formula or with an extensively hydrolyzed or completely hydrolyzed formula. A formula meant to treat an inborn error of metabolism should be replaced with a similar formula from another brand. The North American Society for Gastroenterology, Hepatology and Nutrition (NASPGHAN) maintains a complete list of alternate formulas that is available online, (30) and the FDA lists the companies that have been allowed to import formulas to the United States. (26)

The FDA and the CDC discourage using homemade formula or diluting existing formula in case of formula shortage, as cases of severe malnutrition (31) and illness have been reported using homemade formula. (31) For infants 6 to 12 months of age who are on a regular cow

Table 3. Differences between Formulas Regulated by the EFSA versus the FDA

DOMAIN	FDA-REGULATED FORMULAS (9)	EFSA-REGULATED FORMULAS (27)
Type of formula	Cow milk, soy-based, partially, and extensively hydrolyzed, amino acid–based formulas.	Cow milk–based, soy-based, partially hydrolyzed, extensively hydrolyzed formulas. Option for goat milk formula.
Age category	The same formula is used for all infants aged 0–12 mo.	Different formula for 0–6 mo, called infant formula, and 6–12 mo, called follow-on formula.
Mixing instructions	Most formulas have mixing instructions in a 1:2 ratio of formula concentrate (scoops) to water, and mixing instructions are given as formula per ounce.[a]	Most formulas have mixing instructions in a 1:1 ratio and mixing instructions are given as formula per milliliter.
Labeling requirements	Instructions must be in English and should include directions for preparation, a pictogram showing the major steps for formula preparation, an expiration date, and whether water should be added to prepare the formula.	Instructions may be in a language other than English as well.
Iron fortification	Iron content minimum 0.15 mg/100 kcal, maximum 3.0 mg/100 kcal. To be labeled as iron-fortified, the formula should have ≥1 mg/100 kcal of formula.	Iron content varies based on formula type, with 0.3 mg/100 cal for infant formula (0–6 mo) and 0.6–1.7 mg/100 kcal for follow-on formula (6–12 mo).
Macronutrient requirement: protein	Minimum 1.8 g/100 kcal, maximum 4.5 g/100 kcal[b]	Cow milk–based: minimum 1.8 g/100 kcal, maximum 2.5 g/100 kcal. Soy-based: minimum 2.25 g/100 kcal, maximum 2.8 g/100 kcal.[c]
Macronutrient requirement: fat	Minimum 3.3 kcal/100 kcal, maximum 6.0 kcal/100 kcal Linoleic acid is required.	Minimum 4.4 kcal/100 kcal, maximum 6.0 kcal/100 kcal Linoleic acid, α-linolenic acid, and docosahexaenoic acid are required.
Macronutrient requirement: carbohydrate	No limit	Minimum: 9 g/100 kcal, maximum 14 g/100 kcal.
Micronutrient requirement: vitamins	FDA regulates minimum levels of vitamins A, C, D, E, and K; thiamine (B$_1$); riboflavin (B$_2$); vitamin B$_6$; vitamin B$_{12}$; niacin; folic acid; pantothenic acid; and biotin[b]; and maximum values of vitamins A and D.	EFSA regulates minimum and maximum values of vitamins A, C, D, E, and K; thiamine (B$_1$); riboflavin (B$_2$); vitamin B$_6$; vitamin B$_{12}$; niacin; folate; pantothenic acid; and biotin.
Micronutrient requirement: minerals	FDA regulates minimum values of calcium, phosphorus, magnesium, iron, zinc, manganese, copper, iodine, selenium, sodium, potassium, and chloride and maximum values of iron, iodine, selenium, sodium, potassium, and chloride.	EFSA regulates minimum and maximum values of calcium, phosphorus, magnesium, iron, zinc, manganese, copper, iodine, selenium, sodium, potassium, and chloride and only maximum values of molybdenum and fluoride.

EFSA=European Food Safety Authority, FDA=Food and Drug Administration.

[a]1 oz=30 mL.

[b]Certain other amino acids, such as choline and inositol, might be required for nonmilk US-based recipes; also, if the biological quality of the protein is less than that of casein, the minimum amount of protein shall be increased proportionately to compensate for its lower biological quality. For example, an infant formula containing protein with a biological quality of 75% of casein shall contain at least 2.4 g of protein (1.8/0.75), as is the case for soy-based formulas produced in the United States.

[c]Additional amino acids might be required for specific formulas, such as goat-based formulas; also, the amount of protein might differ for hydrolyzed formula. Each of the indispensable and conditionally indispensable amino acids must be available in amounts at least equal to that contained in the dietary reference.

milk–based formula, if the family is unable to obtain an alternate formula as an urgent replacement, regular whole cow milk can be used on a short-term basis (1 week). (32)(33) However, the long-term use of cow milk during infancy should be avoided because the use of cow milk in infancy is associated with a risk of gastrointestinal blood loss and iron deficiency anemia. (34) In case of formula shortage for infants with cow milk allergy who are on a hypoallergenic formula, we suggest using an electrolyte rehydration solution for emergency situations when an alternate hypoallergenic formula is unavailable, but for no more than 24 to 48 hours with the aim of finding another alternate for the hypoallergenic formula.

OLDER INFANT AND YOUNG CHILD FORMULAS

At 1 year of age, human milk and infant formulas are no longer complete sources of nutrition for children, (1)(4) and the AAP and Dietary Guidelines for Americans recommends

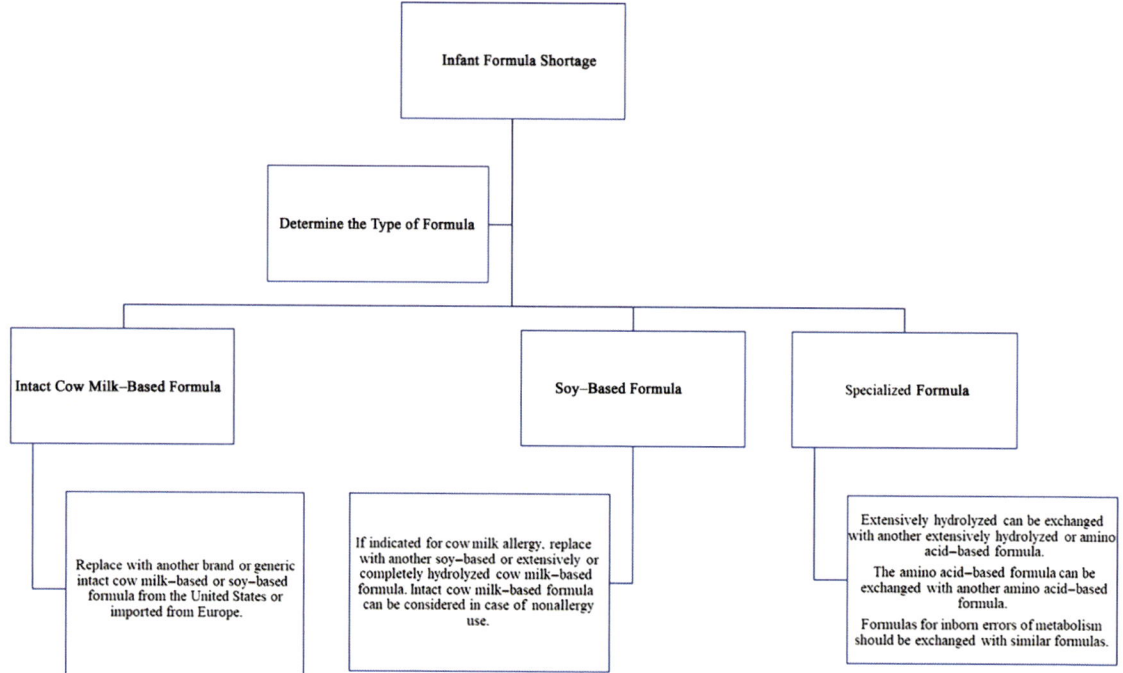

Figure. Approach to alternate infant formula in case of shortage. This guidance is based on expert opinion and is meant for infant formula. Specialized formulas herein are formulas with extensively hydrolyzed proteins or amino acid formulas or those used for treating inborn errors of metabolism.

that infants should be transitioned to pasteurized whole milk at 1 year of age in addition to appropriate solid foods for this age. (1)(4)(10) Whole milk is an essential staple in a toddler's nutrition as it provides a consistent protein source, hydration, calcium, and vitamin D for bone growth, and fat for growth and brain development. (35) The term *older infant and young child formula (OIYCF)* is used interchangeably with *follow on* or *follow up* or *weaning formulas* or *toddler milk, growing-up milk,* or *formula for young children.* (10)(14) The use of OIYCFs is discouraged in otherwise healthy infants or children younger than 3 years. (10)(11) The regulation of young child formulas is less strict compared with FDA regulation for infant formulas because the FDA considers noninfant, young child formulas as medical foods (definitions in Table 1). Because of the lack of uniform regulations of OIYCFs, there is significant variation in the composition of these formulas from both the United States and Europe. (11)(14)(36) It is, therefore, important for health-care professionals to interpret with caution the package labeling and claims made by formula manufacturers of OIYCFs because nutritional deficiencies have been described in children on enteral nutrition. (14)(11)(37)(38) A clinical report from the Committee on Nutrition of the AAP discourages the marketing of OIYCFs with names similar to infant formulas and recommends OIYCFs be clearly distinguishable from infant

formulas in terms of promotional material, logos, product names, and packaging and should not be kept on store shelves next to infant formulas. The labeling should not be similar to that of infant formulas, and the name of the product should be something such as *follow on drink* or *follow on beverage* rather than *follow on formula* or *toddler formula.* (10)

PEDIATRIC FORMULAS

Although formula feeding is not recommended beyond 1 year of age, certain groups of older children might require support from formula feeding, such as those with feeding difficulties, especially those dependent on tube feeding; children with certain medical conditions such as eosinophilic gastrointestinal disorders, inflammatory bowel disease, short-bowel syndrome, and oropharyngeal dysphagia; and those with multiple severe food allergies. (4)(13)(14) The medical or therapeutic use of enteral formula in these circumstances is justified; however, these formulas should be differentiated from OIYCFs, which are mainly used for transition from infancy to early childhood (Table 4). The formulas used for a medical indication are nutritionally complete and could be used as the sole source of nutrition for children. (14) We will use the term *pediatric formulas* for these formulas. The nomenclature around the pediatric formulas varies. Due to the multiple products available in the

Table 4. Differences among Infant Formula, OIYCFs, and Pediatric Formulas

NAME	INFANT FORMULA (8)	OIYCFs (10)	PEDIATRIC FORMULAS (14)
Regulation	The FDA regulates infant formula production in the United States and the EFSA in Europe.	This category is treated as a medical food by the FDA, and regulation is applied just like any other food item considered medical food.	It is treated as a medical food by the FDA
Age	Infant formulas are used for infants aged <12 mo.	Most used as a transitional milk for children aged 9–36 mo.	Most used for children aged 1–13 y.
Indication	Infant formula is recommended when a baby is not receiving human milk in the first year after birth	There is no medical indication for use of OIYCF for an otherwise healthy infant and young child.	There is no medical indication for a pediatric formula for an otherwise healthy child; however, it can be used for a medical or therapeutic indication.
Composition	Infant formulas could be cow milk–based or soy-based. The macronutrient content varies for different types of infant formulas, with options available with reduced lactulose, high MCT content, or hydrolyzed protein. Infant formula could be used as a sole source of nutrition in the first 6 mo of age, could be continued along with introduction of solid food.	The composition varies significantly, with no standard set by the FDA or the EFSA. Most of these formulas are not nutritionally complete and cannot be used as the sole source of nutrition for a medical indication.	Pediatric formulas could be cow milk–based, soy-based, and commercially produced plant-based blenderized formulas. Most pediatric formulas are nutritionally complete and could be used as the sole source of nutrition. The composition varies based on type of formula, as given in Table 5.

EFSA=European Food and Safety Authority, FDA=Food and Drug Administration, MCT=medium-chain triglyceride, OIYCF=older infant and young child formula.

market and the fact they are constantly changing, it is not feasible to cover each formula product. We, however, provide a general nomenclature described by the American Society for Parenteral and Enteral Nutrition. (39) The pediatric formulas can be classified into intact or polymeric, extensively hydrolyzed or peptide, completely hydrolyzed or elemental, and blenderized food-based (Table 5). It is important to note that these categories are not inclusive of all the products available and that some of the formulas could include more than 1 category, for example, some of the blenderized formulas could be extensively or completely hydrolyzed.

The most widely used and least expensive pediatric formula is the standard polymeric (intact) formula, primarily available in sterile, ready-to-use form. (14)(40) The polymeric formulas are available in standard (1 kcal/mL), low (~0.6 kcal/mL), or high (1.2–1.5 kcal/mL) calorie density formulations. Most of the polymeric formulas could be used as sole sources of nutrition and meet the dietary reference intakes for essential vitamins and minerals if adequate volumes are administered, typically between 750 and 1,500 mL, depending on the specific formula and the age of the child. (14) The polymeric formulas could be delivered via tube feeds. Polymeric formulas can be an attractive option for oral supplementation as multiple options with different flavors, including vanilla, chocolate, strawberry, and banana, are available. (16)(41) The carbohydrate content typically provides 44% to 53% of the required daily total

calories. Although the carbohydrate source may vary, the polymeric formulas typically include carbohydrates from a combination of corn maltodextrin, rice syrup solids, sugar, and cornstarch. (14)(16)(41) Most of the polymeric formulas are considered lactose-free and could be used in children with lactose intolerance; however, these formulas are not suitable for patients with galactosemia because a small amount of lactose (<4 g/L) is present in the cow milk–based pediatric formulas. (14) The protein source in polymeric formulas could include cow milk, soy, and pea, and the proteins typically contribute approximately 12% to 15% of the required daily total calories. Some of the cow milk–based formulas could have soy in them, so parents of formula-fed children should check the labels for sources of protein if their child needs to avoid soy. (14) The polymeric formulas are not appropriate for patients with a cow milk, soy, or corn allergy. Most of the polymeric and pediatric formulas are gluten-free. Polymeric formulas contain fat derived from plant oils, contributing 35% to 45% of the required daily total calories in a standardized polymeric formula. (14)(16)(41) Some of the pediatric formulas contain only protein and carbohydrates and some micronutrients but no fat (also called clear formulas), and these formulas are not a complete source of nutrition. They should be avoided in patients who are completely dependent on formula feeding. (14)

The hydrolyzed protein formulas contain proteins hydrolyzed by adding enzymes that break down peptide bonds. The hydrolyzed formulas may contain hydrolyzed

Table 5. Description of Commonly Used Pediatric Formulas

CHARACTERISTIC	POLYMERIC/ STANDARD/INTACT PROTEIN FORMULAS	HYDROLYZED	ELEMENTAL	BLENDERIZED
Caloric density, kcal/mL; kcal/oz	0.6–1.5; 18–45	1–1.5; 30–45	0.8–1; 24–30	1–1.3; 30–39
Carbohydrate, % kcal	44–55	48–54	40–63	32–43
Sources of carbohydrate	Corn maltodextrin, rice syrup solids, sugar, cornstarch	Corn maltodextrin, sugar, cornstarch	Solid corn syrup, tapioca starch, potato starch	Fruits, vegetables, rice
Protein, % kcal	12–20	12–14	12–15	11–20
Sources of protein	Milk, soy, pea (Pea protein formulas lack dairy, soy, and corn)	Milk, pea	Amino acids	Milk, peas, beef, poultry, quinoa, fish, brown rice, hemp, oats, molasses, etc
Fat, % kcal	25–45	35–60	25–45	34–57
Sources of fat	LCTs (canola oil, soybean oil, safflower oil, sunflower oil, flaxseed oil, coconut oil) MCTs	LCTs (canola oil, soybean oil, safflower oil, sunflower oil, flaxseed oil, coconut oil, fish oil) MCTs	LCTs (safflower oil, soybean oil, coconut oil, palm kernel oil, sunflower oil) MCTs	LCTs (canola oil, olive oil, flaxseed oil, fish oil, almond butter, grapeseed oil, beef, poultry, sesame seeds, sunflower seeds, fish, egg, hemp powder, etc) MCTs
Volume to meet DRIs, mL				
Ages 2–8 y	750–1,300	750–1,000	1,000–1,500	900–1,000
Ages 9–13 y	1,500–1,680	1,500	1,500–1,900	1,200–1,500
Osmolality, mOsm/kg (mmol/kg)	300–600 (300–600)	250–450 (250–450)	390–675 (390–675)	500–780 (500–780)
Potential indications	Children with normally functioning gastrointestinal tracts who cannot meet their nutritional needs with an age-typical diet.	Children with intolerance to polymeric formulas or with altered gastrointestinal tract function.	Children with allergies.	Might be better tolerated in patients with gastrointestinal symptoms. Fulfills any caregiver preference for plant-based food.
Market examples	Boost® Kid Essentials™, PediaSure®, Kate Farms®, Compleat® Pediatric	Peptamen Junior®, PediaSure® Peptide, Kate Farms® Pediatric Peptide	EleCare®, Alfamino®, Neocate®	Compleat® Pediatric Organic Blends, Nourish, PediaSure® Harvest, Real Food Blends®
Retail price, $				
Per ounce	0.26–0.48	0.78–0.86	0.67–0.72	0.57–0.82
Per 1,000 kcal	7.80–13.60	25.87–28.70	22.45–24.00	15.80–18.00
Special considerations	Lactose-free but contains <4 g of lactose per liter, so contraindicated in galactosemia	Poor palatability	Poor palatability	Poor palatability, if undiluted, requires 12 or 14 Fr or large-diameter enteral access device

DRI=dietary reference intake, Fr=French gauge, LCT=long-chain triglyceride, MCT=medium-chain triglyceride.
Modified with permission from Klepper et al. (14)

protein consisting of a short chain of amino acids and free amino acids, and the elemental formulas contain completely hydrolyzed proteins in the form of free amino acids. (14)(42) Some formulas may use porcine enzymes to hydrolyze the proteins, and, therefore, these formulas are not considered halal or kosher. (43) Information on the mode and extent of hydrolysis might be available on the label of the product, and if so, could be used to help families who prefer to use a formula that is halal or kosher. The calorie density for hydrolyzed formulas ranges from standard 1 kcal/mL to high

1.5 kcal/mL. Elemental formulas could be available in either low 0.8 kcal/mL or standard 1 kcal/mL calorie form. The carbohydrate content makes 48% to 54% of the hydrolyzed formula and approximately 40% to 60% of the elemental formulas. (14) The carbohydrate sources are similar to polymeric formulas except that some hydrolyzed formulas may contain tapioca starch and potato starch. The protein source in hydrolyzed formula is from milk and peas. The hydrolyzed and elemental formulas have a higher proportion of medium-chain triglycerides and a small proportion of long-

Table 6. Nutritional Comparison of Cow Milk and Plant-Based Nonformula Milk (Drinks)

PER 1 CUP (240 mL)	COW MILK	ALMOND	CASHEW	COCONUT	FLAXSEED	HEMP	OAT	PEA	RICE	SOY
Calories	150	30–100	25–80	45–90	55	70–170	130	115	110	90
Protein, g	8	1–5	0–1	0–1	0	2–4	4	8	1	6
Fat, g	8	3	2–3.5	5	2.5	5–6	2.5	5	2.5	3.5
Carbohydrates, g	13	9–22	1–20	8–13	9	1–35	24	11	20	15
Sugar, g	12	7–20	0–18	0–9	9	0–23	19	10	13	9
Calcium, mg	300	300	100–450	100–450	300	400	350	450	300	400
Vitamin D, IU	120	110	125	125	100	150	120	150	120	120

Reprinted with permission from Merritt et al. (56)

chain fatty acids. This is important to know because fat absorption can be facilitated via medium-chain triglycerides in cases of malabsorption such as seen with severe cholestasis and pancreatic insufficiency (patient may still need enzyme replacement therapy for pancreatic insufficiency). (14)(42) Elemental formulas are considered anallergenic because they do not contain intact proteins. Consequently, such formulas could be used with patients who are allergic to cow milk. Elemental formulas could also be used with patients who have certain eosinophilic gastrointestinal disorders, for example, as exclusive enteral nutrition in individuals with eosinophilic esophagitis. (14) The hydrolyzed formula can also be used in children with intolerance to standard intact formulas. Both the hydrolyzed and elemental formulas are available in powder form but are less palatable for oral use compared with polymeric formulas, although flavored versions of the hydrolyzed and elemental types have become available recently. The osmolality of elemental formulas is high (390–675 mOsm/kg [390–675 mmol/kg]) and can lead to loose stools. The cost of hydrolyzed or elemental formulas is higher than intact formulas, and the insurance coverage varies based on the amount needed, route administered, and type of insurance. (16)(42)(44)

Although administration of home-based blenderized foods is a common practice that was accepted by the medical community, commercially produced blenderized feeds have recently become available. (45)(46) Blenderized feeds are made of whole foods, and the contents may include vegetables, fruits, meat, legumes, whole grains, and dairy/dairy alternatives that have been blended or liquified for enteral feeding. (14)(47) The commercially blenderized formulas are also available in hydrolyzed form and in combination with intact cow milk–based formulas, called *hybrid formulas.* The available evidence on the use of blenderized feeds suggests better tolerability, lower need for medications, improvement in chronic respiratory symptoms, decreased emergency department visits, and adequate growth. (42)(48)(49) However, generally speaking, randomized controlled trials comparing different formula types are lacking, although we did identify a few ongoing trials comparing thickened formulas/feeds to improve outcomes in children with aerodigestive problems. (50)(51)(52) The plant-based formulas also give families the option of whole food–based formulas. However, plant-based blenderized formulas have limited palatability, and due to their increased viscosity, there might be challenges to administering the formula, especially with smaller-diameter tubes. (14)(41) Families interested in making blenderized feeds at home should consult a dietitian to help with recipes to ensure the adequacy of nutrients in the blenderized feeds while still under the supervision of a medical provider. (53)(54)

PLANT-BASED NONFORMULA MILK (DRINKS)

Plant-based, nonformula milk is increasingly used by parents and caregivers of infants and young children as an alternative to cow milk. (55) The term *milk* is technically reserved for the fluid secreted from the mammary glands of mammals, (28)(56) and the term *plant-based drink* might be more appropriate for plant-based fluids meant for nutritional support. (57) The FDA considers the plant-based, nonformula drinks to be medical food, and the macronutrient and micronutrient components of these products vary significantly compared with infant formula regulated by the FDA. (56)(57) Families might be interested in using plant-based drinks in the setting of cow milk allergy during infancy, concerns for lactose intolerance, and concerns related to the presence of unsaturated fat in cow milk or because of a preference for plant-based products as part of a lacto-ovo-vegetarian diet or the social preference(s) in certain cultures. (57)

Table 6 gives an overview of available plant-based drinks and their comparison with cow milk. The number of calories per 240 mL (1 cup) varies among the plant-based products; most do not have equivalent calories as the same volume of cow milk. The amount of protein also varies, with some products having very little protein, such as flaxseed- and rice-based drinks, and other products, such as soy-based drinks, might have an equivalent amount of protein compared with cow milk. In addition to the variation in the available protein in a given volume, the protein quality in terms of the protein efficiency ratio also varies among different plant-based beverages. (58) For example, compared with the most abundant protein in cow milk, casein, the protein efficiency ratio value is 80% for soy, 72% for oat, 66% for coconut, 60% for rice, 57% for pea, and only 16% for almond protein. (56) This means that the bioavailability of the protein from plant-based drinks could be lower compared with the same amount of protein from cow milk. The amount of fat and carbohydrates also varies, and different products might have sugar as a flavor additive. Finally, the level and diversity of fortification also varies. Although these products may have adequate amounts of calcium and vitamin D, other micronutrients might not meet the dietary reference intake. (57) Although adding some of the plant-based drinks such as soy (nonformula), pea, and oat-based drinks to a child's diverse and nutritionally adequate diet might be reasonable, the plant-based beverages are not nutritionally complete. Plant-based beverages should be avoided during infancy and for children on enteral nutrition who are dependent on liquid food. Plant-based, nonformula drinks should also be avoided as a replacement for cow milk for toddlers and young children, and if there is a need for replacement of cow milk, a pediatric formula might be a more appropriate replacement. Future studies must assess whether plant-based drinks are adequate to promote growth and bone mineralization in young children. (56)(57)

CONCLUSIONS

Significant advances have been made in the available formula products for infants and children, with a substantial increase in demand and supply leading to a multibillion-dollar industry. Although there are clear guidelines for infant formula production from the FDA and the EFSA, there is a lack of universal regulation for formula products beyond infancy. The lack of universal regulations for producing OIYCFs and pediatric formula has led to significant variation in these products with concerns for excess and deficiency of certain micronutrients. (11)(38) With an increasing number of products available in the market, it is highly challenging for pediatricians to have complete knowledge of each product. There is a need for a registry that should encompass basic information for each product

that should be publicly available to medical providers and families. There is a need for universal regulation of pediatric formula with clear guidance on the indications for their use, composition, labeling requirements, and safety. Finally, the terminology around OIYCFs and plant-based drinks should be regulated, and the terms *formula* and *milk* should be prohibited for these products to avoid confusion with FDA-approved infant formula and mammalian-source milk, respectively.

Summary

- The European pediatric formulas imported under Food and Drug Administration (FDA) guidance differ from those produced in the United States in certain aspects (15); however, they are comparable with formulas produced in the United States in their nutritional value. (9)(27) (Based on some research evidence)

- Older infant and young child formulas or pediatric formulas are not recommended for otherwise healthy children. (10)(14) (Based on some research evidence as well as consensus among experts)

- Thickened plant-based blenderized pediatric formulas may help with aerodigestive problems in children dependent on tube feeding. (42)(48)(49) (Based on some research evidence)

- The plant-based nonformula (milk) drinks are not nutritionally complete and should be avoided in infants and children dependent on liquid nutrition. (56) (Based on some research evidence and consensus among experts)

Acknowledgment

We thank Dr Michael Rebagliati for his help with review of the manuscript.